THE H⬤T
DETOX PLAN

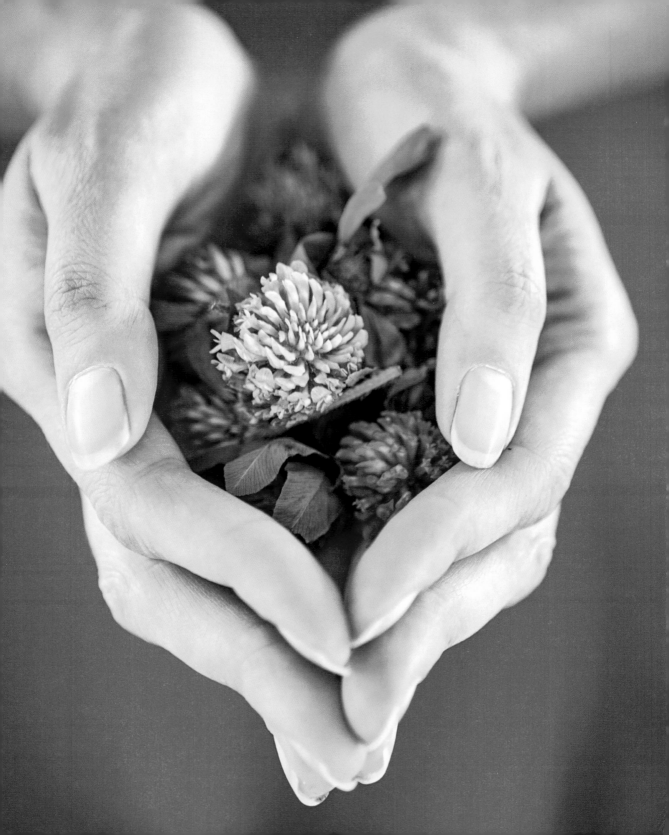

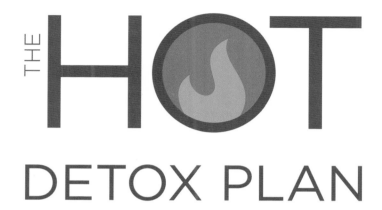

THE HOT

DETOX PLAN

Cleanse Your Body and Heal Your Gut with Warming, Anti-inflammatory Foods

Julie Daniluk

HAY HOUSE, INC.
Carlsbad, California • New York City
London • Sydney • Johannesburg
Vancouver • New Delhi

Copyright © 2017 by Julie Daniluk

Published and distributed in the United States by: Hay House, Inc.: www.hayhouse.com® • *Published and distributed in Australia by:* Hay House Australia Pty. Ltd.: www.hayhouse.com.au • *Published and distributed in the United Kingdom by:* Hay House UK, Ltd.: www.hayhouse.co.uk • *Published and distributed in the Republic of South Africa by:* Hay House SA (Pty), Ltd.: www.hayhouse.co.za • *Distributed in Canada by:* Raincoast Books: www.raincoast.com • *Published in India by:* Hay House Publishers India: www.hayhouse.co.in

Indexer: Ruth Pincoe
Cover design: Tricia Breidenthal • *Interior design:* LINDdesign • *Interior illustrations:* Julie Daniluk and Leanne Chan

All photographs © Shannon J. Ross, with the exception of the following: pages ii, viii, 5, 50, 82, 115, 262, 342 © Christine Bujis; page 209 © iStock; page 275 © Julie Daniluk and Alan Smith. All rights reserved.

Cataloging-in-Publication Data is on file at the Library of Congress.

Tradepaper ISBN: 978-1-4019-5195-5

10 9 8 7 6 5 4 3 2 1
1st Hay House edition, January 2017

Printed in the United States of America

SUSTAINABLE FORESTRY INITIATIVE
Certified Chain of Custody
Promoting Sustainable Forestry
www.sfiprogram.org
SFI-01268
SFI label applies to the text stock

Dedication

dedicate this book to you. Trust that your higher power, in concert with nature, will transform any obstacle into a clearing of tremendous blessing. Our health struggles make us more compassionate, more sensitive and more grateful when the breakthroughs arrive.

I also dedicate this book to my family. First and foremost, my husband, Alan Smith, who wore every hat in the creation of the Hot Detox! He helped manage the recipe testing and edited every word to ensure it reached maximum clarity. He is the salt of the earth, providing nourishment, grounding and most of all great taste to this culinary joyride. You are my Alpha and Omega, and I love you forever!

My sister, Lynn Daniluk, is my great protector and without her, I could not bring my message to the world with such grace. Her consistent insight into detoxification and recipe contributions was fantastic. Here

is to becoming supercentenarian wonder twins!

My mom, Elaine Daniluk, taught me so much about intuitive cooking. Thanks for all your recipe testing, love, healing and cheerleading.

My father, Neil Daniluk, shows up on an emotional level and restores my confidence in humanity. Thanks for our precious Sunday morning sessions of wise advice and sharing.

My brother and yoga instructor, Yogi Shambu (Steven Daniluk), provided a wonderful hot detox yoga flow to accompany the Hot Detox. He is my lighthouse keeper and I owe him my lucidity.

My nephews, Christian, Kaydn, Taevan, Eli, Aiden, Finn and Coltan, and nieces, Jade, Audrey, Ashlynn and Amelie, remind me that the future is so bright. Our mission to protect the environment from toxins stems from the need to provide them a safe world.

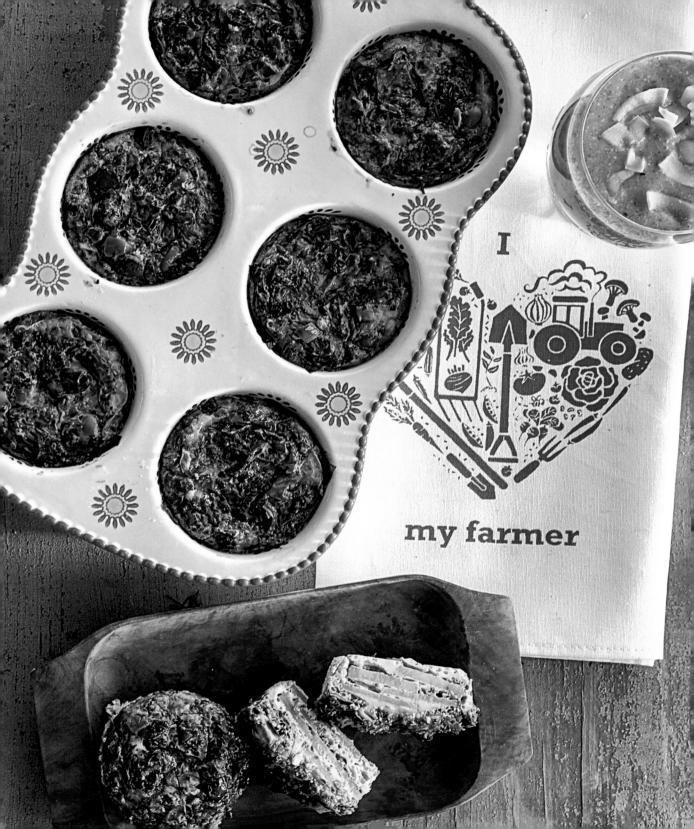

Contents

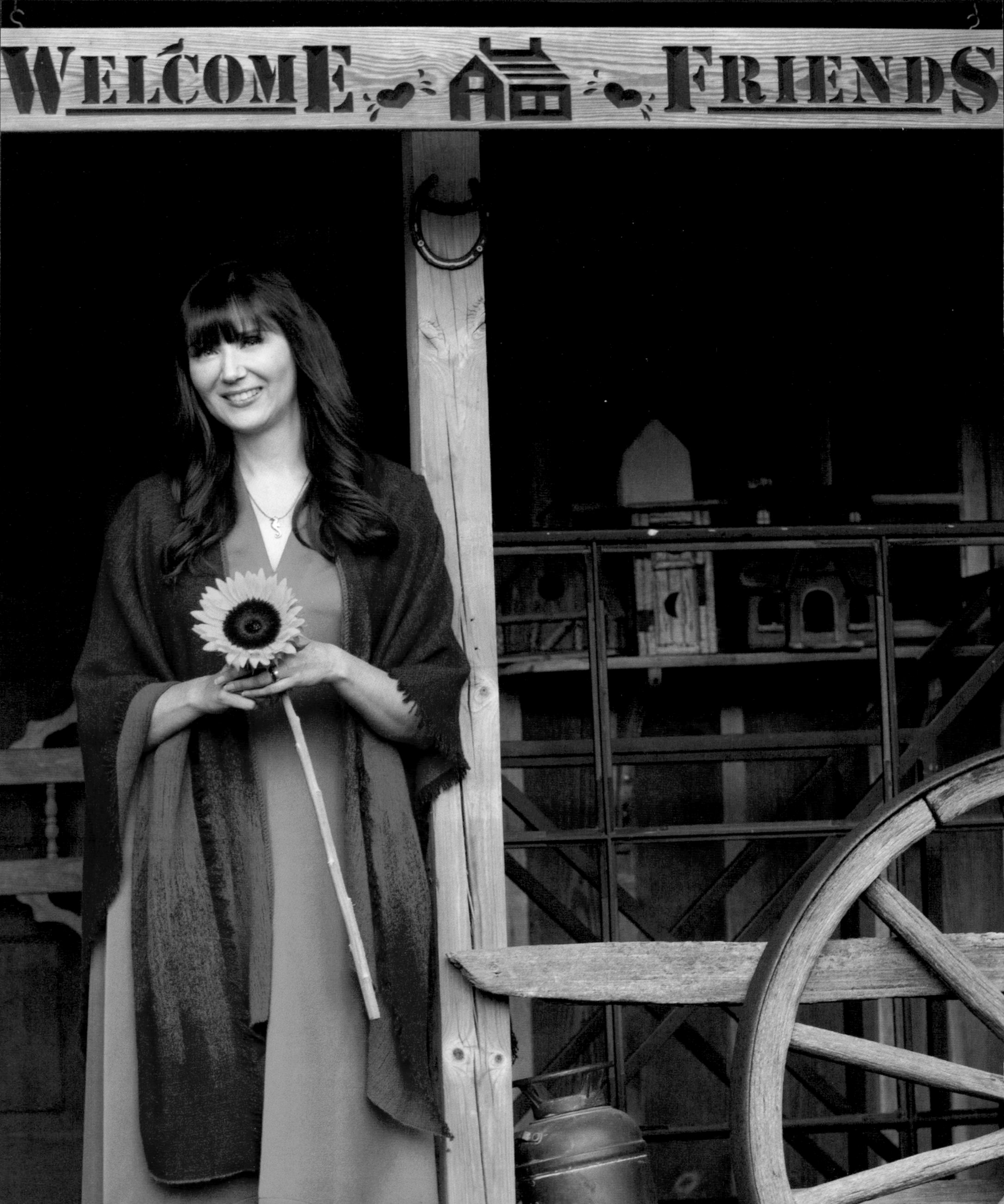

Introduction

Are you ready to eat hot, comforting foods, feel a warm happy glow and look hotter than you have in years?

Let me introduce you to the Hot Detox, an incredible tool that has the potential to truly transform your life. I have seen so many people benefit from it, whether they had allergies, belly bloating, hormonal imbalance, skin disorders or irritable bowel syndrome (IBS). The Hot Detox works by taking stress off your digestive system until it is restored, through incorporating foods that heal and avoiding foods that can potentially be harmful.

The Hot Detox is a deep cleansing program that serves up a delicious warming menu with anti-inflammatory remedies that spark digestive vitality. Results are not obtained through deprivation, special supplements or depleting your body of its essential nutrients. You can have delicious, healing food with a balanced approach over 3, 10 or 21 days instead of a crash diet or fast that will leave you jonesing for sugary or fried junk food. Plus, following the Hot Detox offers you the opportunity to lose weight, improve your skin and boost your mood, ensuring you look smoking hot!

The Hot Detox embraces the ancient wisdom of India and China, applying the time-tested practice of warming up the body's core. Many detox programs are created in California or other consistently warm climates where consuming cold smoothies, juices and raw salads is desirable and healthy. But when it is cold outside, a standard "cold" detox program does not support you. It may cause you to feel rundown, slow your metabolism or aggravate a digestive condition.

Whether you live in a warm or a cool climate, utilizing the heat of a warming diet is the key to alleviating many common concerns such as IBS, low immunity, hormone imbalance and chronic pain. And for those who live in a warm climate, have a hot constitution or suffer from a fiery inflammatory condition such as dermatitis, the cooling superfoods recommended in this book will balance the menu to ensure great results.

My Detox Story

I come by detoxification very naturally. When I was young, I spent every summer with my grandmother and was intrigued by her commitment to cleanse. She was a follower of Dr. Paul Bragg, a health advocate who began his work in the 1950s. For 50 years, until she was well into her 80s, my grandmother detoxified a few days a week. This allowed her insulin receptors to become fully primed so that when she went back to regular food it was metabolized very easily. At 94, her blood sugar was incredibly balanced, with the insulin sensitivity of a person half her age. Her skin was silky smooth and her hair stayed dark and strong.

Since those summers with Grandma, I have explored the most popular methods of detoxification. I have done water fasting, the lemonade "master cleanse" fast, the macrobiotic brown rice cleanse, the cold juice fast, the kichadi cleanse, the candida diet, the gallbladder flush, parasite programs, herbal cleanses and even an extreme Ayurvedic cleanse with a saltwater purge. Sadly, the more extreme cleanses left me depleted, which primed my gut for inflammation. Water fasting doesn't provide any protection from the free radicals that are produced through the process of metabolism. The lemonade "master cleanse" sent my blood sugar flying only to crash an hour later, and after a week on the fast, my mouth was full of canker sores and my moods erratic. The brown rice cleanse was too high in carbohydrates and was so incredibly boring that I binged at the end. Cold juice fasting taxed my digestive fire and left me with indigestion.

The lack of nutrition in these popular detox plans can prevent you from detoxifying safely. This is why I developed the Hot Detox: to ensure that the nutrition the body requires is always present to effectively run the detox pathways of the elimination organs. It is time to focus on the nutrition your body needs to repair, rebuild and revitalize.

I created the Hot Detox because I truly believe that this method of detoxification will take your health to the next level. I want you to have an Olympic life even if you never set foot in a gym. The focus of the Hot Detox is longevity and performance enhancement. The type of performance I am talking about is always being able to find the right words to say because your mind is razor sharp, taking that hike on your bucket list because you can breathe easily and climb effortlessly, and having so much energy that you create that dream project that is deep inside you. Now that I have felt the difference between being riddled with inflammation and being pain-free and filled with authentic energy, I want to share this feeling with you!

Let's hear from Arlene B., who had incredible results:

Julie's 3-Day Detox and the 21-Day Detox is such a preparation for the rest of one's life. It is a guide for anyone in search of health, energy and emotional well-being. Before the program, I felt like I was sipping daily on a huge inflammatory cocktail that sent pain bubbling through my veins and tissues, creating fibromyalgia, osteoarthritis, osteoporosis, macular degeneration, depression, anxiety and deep, deep fatigue.

I am 73 now and I thank God a precious wave came along and pushed my misguided craft towards Julie and her life-saving program waiting on the Island of Wellness. Her island full of delicious food is one of No Return. This is how I visualize it ... never, never, never going back to the delusional and deceptive shores of inflammatory foods.

I was fortunate to experience weight loss, an increase in energy and a decrease in my pain level. The most surprising and remarkable benefit of the Hot Detox was the elimination of brain fog. Now I can really zero in and concentrate on living a happy life.

What do you want to create in your life? A more vibrant career? A more joyous relationship? More energy to take on your life mission? Absolutely anything you want to create has to come through the gateway of vitality. Without your health, manifesting your vision into reality is nearly impossible.

Need more evidence? Wayne A. literally got his life back by doing the Hot Detox:

I was diagnosed with rheumatoid arthritis 10 years ago. Last year, I started seeing a naturopath who recommended your program. I can honestly and happily say to you that this is the best that I have felt since being diagnosed. I am now pain-free! My wife and I really enjoy your recipes. Your enthusiasm and zest for life is contagious.

Thank you for your dedication and for helping so many people with similar stories to mine. I have not needed a Rituxan infusion and I have been off methotrexate for 6 months. My last visit to my rheumatologist was my most successful ever. He said it was the best that he has ever seen me. Thank you for your tireless efforts. You are appreciated oodles. Gut healed and RA symptoms banished!

Rest assured, I sing your praises daily to any and all who will listen — family, friends and strangers. I tell them it truly does matter what goes in your mouth.

I have tackled this new chapter in my life and I am determined to stay off my liver- and kidney-killing meds. I am excited and encouraged about recapturing my health.

Thank you, Julie. May you continue to flourish.

Going Back to Move Forward

I created the Hot Detox as a radical revisit of the two ancient healing systems that brought me back to life. When I had post-infectious colitis and chronic joint pain, I found raw food went straight through me undigested. Salad would leave me with a terrible bellyache. Dr. Sun, my traditional Chinese medicine doctor, taught me that my digestion, or what she called my "spleen meridian," had been impaired by a microbial infection and that I should cook my food with warming spices to heal it. I started to incorporate more recipes from my yoga practice and found the two Eastern traditions very complementary. After months of eating warming, soothing cooked food, my digestive system started to get stronger

Why Hot Detox?

Here is a summary of the typical symptom relief and transformational results that clients have reported by following my program:

- Greater commitment to long-term health

- Balanced blood sugar levels/reduction in type 2 diabetes

- Greater flexibility/reduction of stiffness

- Improved athletic performance

- Improved digestion, including reduction of irritable bowel syndrome and inflammatory bowel disease symptoms

- Improved grip strength

- Increased interest in vegetables

- Improved kidney, liver and gallbladder function

- Improved libido

- Improved memory, sharper focus and greater attention span

- Better moods, including reduced anxiety and depression

- Improved skin texture and color, including reduction in acne and eczema

- Improved thyroid function/balanced hormones

- Pain relief, including migraine and headache relief

- Reduced bloating and swelling

- Reduced food sensitivities and seasonal allergies

- Reduced asthma

- Less muscle and joint inflammation

- Lower blood pressure and blood cholesterol

- Stronger hair and nails

- Stress relief

- Weight loss

and I could incorporate more cold and raw foods. I am now in complete remission and pain-free!

In this book, I want to share with you how to strengthen your body by cleansing your organs with both Ayurvedic remedies from India and traditional Chinese medicine techniques from Asia. These anti-inflammatory solutions spark digestive vitality. By following the Hot Detox program you will detox and strengthen your spleen, lungs, liver, kidneys, skin and bowel without the common symptoms of other deep cleanses. This is a food cleanse, not a radical, purging fast. The Hot Detox is a soul-satisfying detox that uses metabolism-boosting spices to reduce bloating, heal digestion and reset your vitality.

As Grandma used to say, "*Ya tebe lyublyu. Davayte yisty zdorovu yizhu!*" which means, "I love you. Let's eat healthy food!" Go say that to yourself in the mirror, and let's get started.

Happy cleansing!

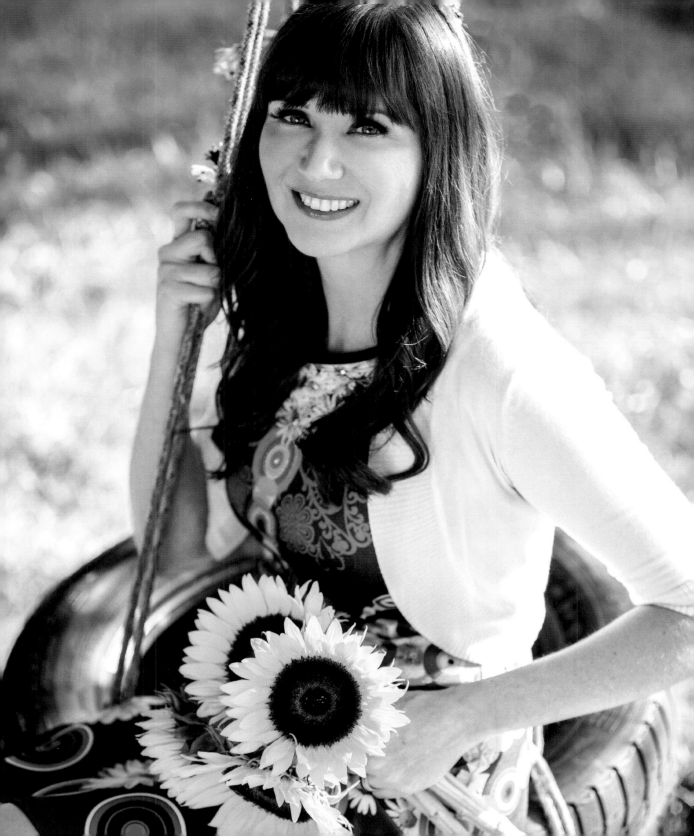

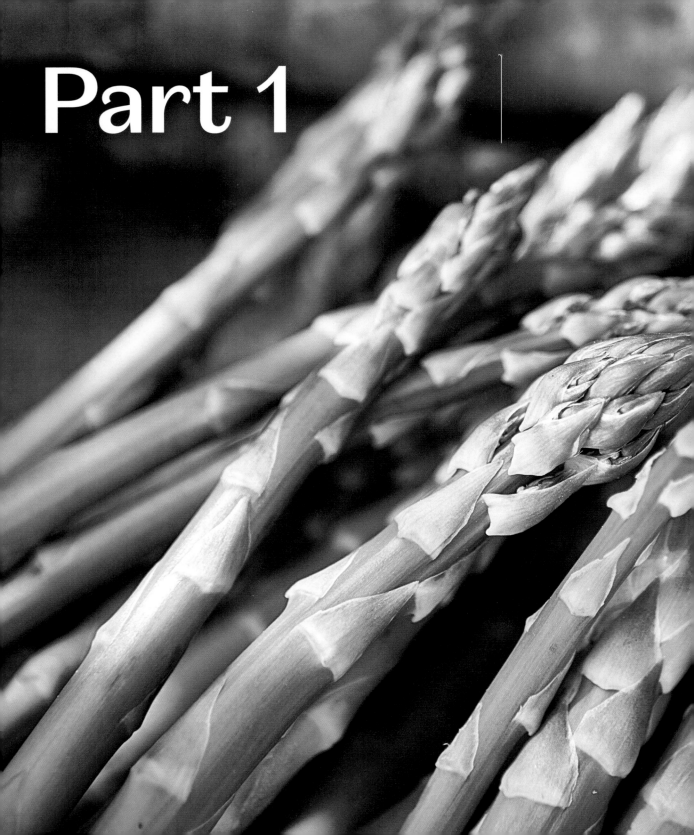

Part 1

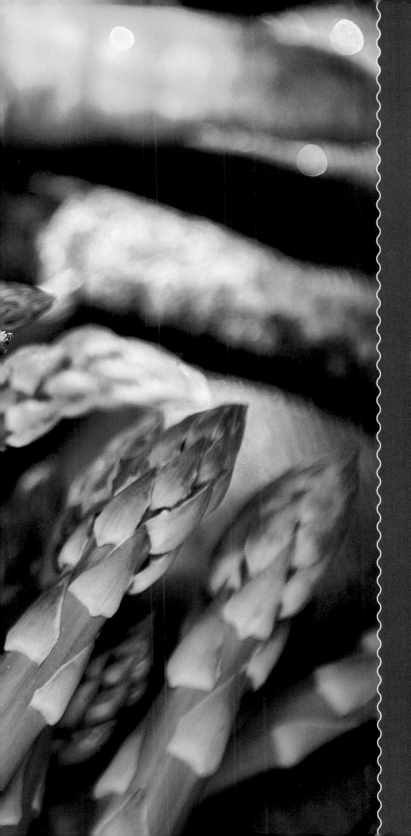

The Science of Detox

"I started to adjust my diet based on Julie's guidance, and I noticed a remarkable change in my level of pain! I was astounded — I never would have thought that food could be affecting me that way! While I will always walk with a limp due to severe osteoarthritis, [afterwards] the pain was nominal. I could walk, I could climb stairs, I could do things that before drained me. I was ecstatic — I found a way to help ease my pain without medication!"

—Debbie S.

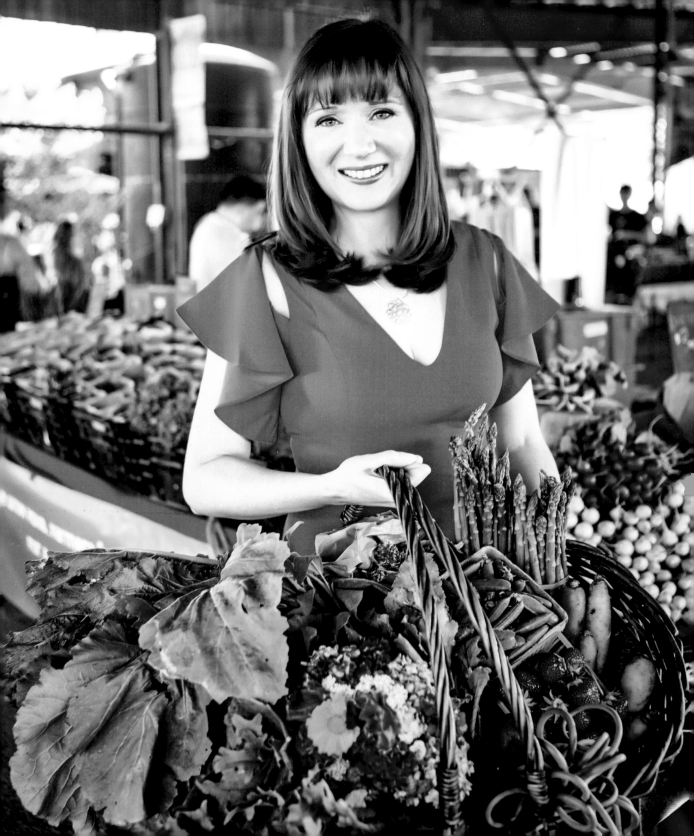

Creating Fire: The Benefits of the Hot Detox Program

Set your life on fire.
Seek those who fan your flames.
—Rumi

Our digestive fire (called *agni* in Ayurveda) is the power of our digestive organs to process and absorb what we eat while burning off waste products. If we have a strong digestive fire, we are able to easily digest food and absorb its nutrients. If we have a weak digestive fire, our body won't digest well, creating an inflammatory environment. In turn, inflammatory foods can dampen the digestive fire by promoting negative microbes that disrupt the healthy microbiome of our gut ecology. In fact, an inflammatory digestive environment can cause such a dramatic disturbance that we have a terrible time digesting and absorbing the foods we eat. We rely on our gut microbes, and if they are disrupted by poor eating habits, they can't assist us with digestion. Essentially, we are what we absorb.

Traditionally, detoxification was done in the spring and fall when temperatures were moderate and fresh greens were plentiful. However, the popularity of New Year's resolutions in January pushes many people to want to cleanse in the heart of winter. But this desire to diet goes against common sense. In the winter, we need to keep the fires burning within us to cope with a cool climate. Have you ever started your day with a frozen banana smoothie and ended up feeling bloated and tired by noon?

Eating cold foods can also damage our digestive fire. To understand how, let's look at physiology for just a minute. Digestion can be split into two main categories: mechanical and chemical. Mechanical digestion involves a process called peristalsis (synchronized muscle contractions) that moves food along the intestinal tract. The contractions of peristalsis are initiated by motor action potentials (electrical impulses that produce a contraction in a muscle). And the temperature of your meal affects the frequency of these motor action potentials. A cold meal reduces the frequency of motor action potentials in the gut, whereas a warm meal increases them. We may have evolved over 200,000 years, but we haven't eaten frozen or cold foods until the last 200 years. And we wonder why we have so many digestive issues!

When you start to chew, the chemical process of digestion starts with enzymes called amylase and lipase in the saliva. After you swallow your food, the stomach produces an essential chemical compound called hydrochloric acid. Exposure to hydrochloric acid inside the stomach activates the enzyme pepsin. Hydrochloric acid mixes with water and the digestive enzymes pepsinogen and gastric lipase to break down our food from large chunks into a slippery mixture called *chyme*. Therefore when people take antacids, they dramatically reduce their body's ability to break down food and absorb nutrition. Medications, cold food and refined foods such as sugar and flour can also shut off this chemical digestive process and impair the ability to absorb the nutrition our body needs to heal. An optimal digestive system is able to break down all food—cold and warm. Unfortunately, by constantly eating inflammatory and cold foods, we dampen our digestive fire.

Many inflammatory foods also affect our digestion because they are so acidic that they lower our pH levels. For example, raw cane juice might be full of minerals, but once you suck those minerals out and turn it into a white crystalline powder (i.e., white sugar), it becomes highly acidic when consumed, which makes it difficult to balance our pH. We require a balanced pH in order to maintain a healthy gut microbiome. The healthy range for the body's pH is 7.35–7.45 (slightly alkaline), and if it is lower than that, meaning the body is acidic, there is greater vulnerability to some disease.

Your pH Balancing Act

An optimal pH cannot be discussed without talking about the acid–alkaline balance, which is important to digestive health. In the acid camp, we have foods like sugar, flour, polished rice, pasta and bread. Refined foods are more acidic due to their lack of minerals. Even worse, these acidic foods rob your body of the nutrients it needs to maintain health. For example, acid can affect bone resorption (the process by which something is reabsorbed), leading to bone loss disorders such as osteoporosis.

You can create an alkaline state in your body by including high-mineral foods in your diet—the minerals are what make them alkaline. Our alkaline friends include all leafy greens, full-mineral sea salt, all fruit and all root vegetables. But you need

The pH Scale

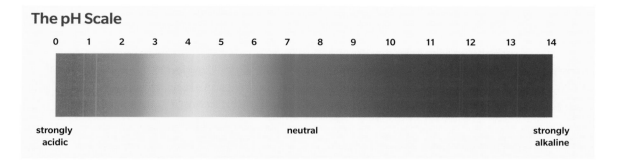

| | | | | | | | | | | | | | | |
|0|1|2|3|4|5|6|7|8|9|10|11|12|13|14|

strongly acidic   neutral   strongly alkaline

the digestive fire to absorb all the alkaline minerals and nutrients from these foods. For example, kale is the highest food on the ANDI (Aggregate Nutrient Density Index) scale, a scoring system that rates foods from 1 to 1,000 based on their concentration of nutrients such as vitamins and minerals. If your digestive system is working properly, a raw kale salad would do you wonders. The person who is digestively compromised, however, can't effectively absorb the nutrients and benefit from the pH-balancing effects of raw kale. This is why the Hot Detox program focuses on heating foods up through steaming, stewing and broiling.

Preparing foods in this way assists digestion and thereby absorption.

On the Hot Detox plan, we're going to be avoiding anything processed or white (i.e., sugar, bread, alcohol)—the acidic, energetically cold foods. Instead, we're going to be choosing beautiful bright-colored produce to keep us alkaline, and we're going to warm them up to aid with digestion.

Fueling the Digestive Fire

We're also going to add certain foods to further enhance digestion, such as bitter herbs and sour foods. Sour foods help

Acid-Forming Foods	Alkaline-Forming Foods
Alcohol	Most fruits
Animal products (meat, fish,* poultry,* dairy)	Most vegetables
Coffee	Leafy greens
Grains (wheat, rice, corn, flour, bread)	Some nuts and seeds
Legumes (beans, lentils)*	Herbs and spices
Refined sugars and carbohydrates	Non-dairy milk (hemp, almond, coconut)
Processed foods	Spring water
Soda	

* Although fish, poultry and legumes are acid-forming, they are included in the Hot Detox plan to provide essential amino acids for detoxification. As long as 80 percent of a meal is alkaline, the body can accommodate these acid-forming foods.

trigger bicarbonate (the alkaline compound in your small intestine) to aid digestion. The bicarbonate works like an antacid, immediately buffering the acid that comes out of the stomach. After the stomach enzymes have done their work, the pancreatic bicarbonate in the small intestine breaks down the food further into tiny particles. These particles contain the nutrients that our body needs from food. If they have been broken down properly and if our digestive system is healthy, the nutrients can move easily across the bowel lining into the blood, where we absorb them.

Leaky Gut and Inflammation

When someone has a digestive issue such as leaky gut (also known as intestinal hyperpermeability), ulceration in the bowel, Crohn's disease or colitis, they may not absorb only the nutrients from the food—food particles themselves may pass into the bloodstream. This may seem like a non-issue, but nutrients and food particles are not one and the same. Food should never cross into the bloodstream—only nutrients. Our body forms an autoimmune reaction to food particles in the bloodstream, triggering inflammatory cytokines and histamine responses, which results in pain. We feel a food reaction in all areas of our body. These "harmless" food particles are thus connected to the pain of arthritis, bursitis, fibromyalgia, chronic fatigue and similar disorders.

This is why we really need to be careful to make sure our digestion is working properly. If it's not working, inflammation increases across our whole body. If it is working, inflammation is essentially non-existent.

I am excited to introduce you to the Hot Detox because not only does it aid with digestion, it also lowers inflammation. Through cooking foods, adding spices, bitters and sour foods, and with proper mastication (using kitchen appliances and/or our teeth to soften and break down our food), we can unburden our digestive system. The Hot Detox allows a respite from refined and raw food until our digestive system renews itself. Once restored, it will be able digest foods that may have been troublesome to digest before.

The Hot Detox is quite different from the raw diets made popular in California in the last decade. Many raw food advocates believe that food is best eaten in its raw state. While I am all for eating raw foods, we must have the digestive power to benefit from them. Raw foods can be cold in nature and if eaten straight out of the fridge or freezer may weaken our digestive fire. This cleanse will strengthen your digestion and allow you to enjoy more of the healthy foods you love.

Stoking the Fire: How the Hot Detox Promotes Long-Term Health

When you are young, your digestive juices are in their prime and work powerfully. As you age, changes occur in your digestive tract. These changes lead to a decrease in digestive acid and enzymes, making it difficult to efficiently digest your food. It is typically at this stage in life when we begin to experience a host of health problems, allergies, food sensitivities or food intolerances. The Hot Detox provides a solution by fixing indigestion with food, instead of

Is Leaky Gut Getting You Down?

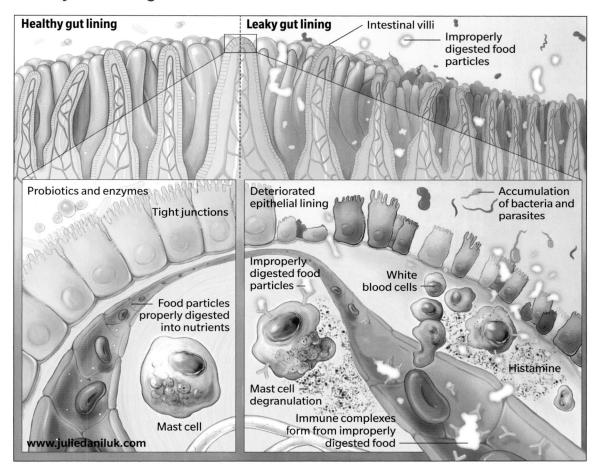

antacids or protein pump inhibitors that don't increase digestive juices at all. Utilizing these products allows all kinds of food particles into the bloodstream, continuously sabotaging the health you are trying to recover. It's a vicious cycle, but it doesn't have to be that way.

A good example of how healing food can be is with respect to stomach ulcers. Most stomach ulcers are caused by an infection—up to 90 percent by *H. pylori* bacteria.

An *H. pylori* overgrowth can be killed off by antibiotics, but also by certain foods such as berries, cranberries and unrefined extra virgin olive oil. We want to avoid relying heavily on antibiotics because they destroy our microbiome further, causing low acidophilus stores. And what happens then? We're not able to absorb our food effectively, leading to food particles in the bloodstream that cause inflammation.

Where East Meets East: Ayurvedic and Chinese Healing

Chinese and Indian cultures have a great deal of healing knowledge regarding warming foods. They each have a 5,000-year-old healing tradition with a similar belief system around the concept of digestive fire. One of these beliefs is that if you have a digestive disorder (which they often consider a cold, damp condition), you should eat warming foods to counteract poor digestive fire. This is in tune with my findings in *Meals That Heal Inflammation* and *Slimming Meals That Heal*: warming foods such as ginger and cinnamon are anti-inflammatory and help to heal the gut.

To understand the wisdom of these cultures, let's begin with the Ayurvedic healing system of India. According to Ayurveda, a person is a combination of three energetic elemental types, called *doshas*, that make up one's constitution: *vata*, *pitta* and *kapha*. A *vata* dosha is ruled by wind and space. When *vata* becomes out of balance, a person can suffer from digestive conditions including bloating, gas, indigestion and irritable bowel syndrome. A person who is ruled by *vata* is often attracted to dry and crispy foods filled with air, like popcorn, cold cereal and kale chips. I see so many of my fellow yogis attracted to dry crispy foods and the raw food diet. A person with *vata* imbalance needs to pacify the *vata* by avoiding cold foods, as they are difficult to digest and will only exacerbate digestive symptoms.

Personally, as someone who has dealt with *vata* imbalance, I found tremendous benefit from following a warming diet. When I struggled through my own healing crisis I experienced terrible digestive distress, and I eventually chose to avoid cold, raw food and dry crispy foods like popcorn in order to heal my gut. I followed an anti-inflammatory diet, and also stopped eating *vata*-increasing foods like raw salad, which is strange for a nutritionist to do. But my stomach simply couldn't tolerate the cold, raw food, especially the lettuce leaves, and I found that salad led to loose stools. I can certainly eat a raw salad now, because I've healed my gut, but back then I had to give my digestive system a rest and puree my foods to take the stress off my stomach. By heating my meals, I transformed them into something digestible, something that was easy on my body.

The *pitta dosha* is ruled by fire, tempered with water. A person who has this fiery constitution may be more tempted by hot foods like chili peppers and fried foods. Unfortunately, eating hot foods can cause an imbalance that may lead to inflammatory conditions in the body such as eczema, psoriasis, painful heartburn and bloodshot eyes. People who enjoy superspicy foods may be surprised that the Hot Detox does not use any hot peppers or black pepper. This is because we want to warm the body, but not overheat it. The Hot Detox menu also incorporates some optional cooling foods listed as boosters in the recipes that can assist in balancing *pitta*.

The *kapha dosha* is ruled by water and earth. A person with this "go with the flow" constitution typically holds onto excess weight and water, and is often tempted to overeat sweet and dairy-laden foods. People with an imbalance of *kapha* frequently suffer from excess mucus and sluggish bowel movements. The bitter greens, warming spices (ginger and turmeric) and broth-based soups in the Hot Detox menu are perfect for balancing *kapha* as they can increase elimination and reduce excess mucus. Many people report finally losing stubborn weight they have struggled against for years. This is why the Hot Detox works for most people. It is nice and balanced!

From a food science perspective, heating something (or breaking it down in the blender) opens the cellular structure of food, making the nutrients more accessible—easier to digest and assimilate. For example, the beta-carotene in a carrot is far more absorbable when you cook the carrot and pour oil on it than if you just eat the carrot raw. By cooking the carrot, you break open the cellulose and make the beta-carotene accessible. Then the oil helps transport the beautiful beta-carotene into your system. It changes the way the food is digested in your body.

Another good example is broccoli, a great source of sulforaphane. This compound has a unique ability to stimulate Phase 2 liver detox, a very important phase for the removal of harmful compounds and excess estrogens from the body (see Chapter 3). Sulforaphane also activates cell suicide, playing a big role in preventing replication of cancer cells. You don't activate the sulforaphane in broccoli until you masticate it. If you don't chew or puree the broccoli well, you miss the opportunity to activate an enzyme called myrosinase, which converts glucoraphanin into sulforaphane. By putting some lovely oil on broccoli and chewing it to mush or pureeing it into a soup, you help your body absorb it. In this way, the cold, hard food is transformed into warm, highly beneficial food. This is the power of the Ayurvedic tradition: cooking food or making a soup or stew makes it easier to digest.

The Ayurvedic and Chinese traditions show a lot of crossover when it comes to foods to avoid or foods to enjoy. Both support the belief that raw vegetables are hard to digest. They also recommend staying away from refined cereal, pasta and rice cakes. Ice cream, as another example, is considered "triple yin death" in traditional Chinese medicine. This is because it contains sugar and dairy, and it's frozen, all three of which are very hard on your gut. Ice cream is two tough-to-tolerate substances wrapped in a frozen delivery system—and then we wonder why we get a bellyache when we eat it! Similarly, Ayurvedic tradition suggests leaving treats like ice cream to the hottest days of the year because in the bright sun, you have more digestive fire. You might be able to handle a frozen coconut treat when the summer sun is at high noon, but otherwise, ice cream could wreak havoc. Thus these two ancient traditional systems complement each other.

Hot Foods versus Cold Foods

Much of the theory behind the Hot Detox is rooted in the Ayurvedic and Chinese wisdom about why warming foods are so beneficial to the body. Two particularly inspiring books on this topic are *Between Heaven and Earth: A Guide to Chinese Medicine* by Harriet Beinfield and *Ayurvedic Cooking for Self-Healing* by Usha Lad and Dr. Vasant Lad.

Is It a Hot Pot or Not?

	Warming foods	Neutral foods	Cooling foods
Proteins	**Meat and poultry:** beef, chicken, lamb, organ meat, turkey, venison **Fish and seafood:** anchovy, mussel, shrimp, trout **Vegan proteins:** chestnut, flaxseed, lentil, most nuts and seeds, pine nut, sesame seed, sunflower seed, walnut	**Meat and poultry:** chicken egg, duck, goose, pork, quail, veal **Fish and seafood:** Arctic char, carp, halibut, herring, lobster, mackerel, oyster, salmon, sardine, shark, tuna, whitefish **Vegan proteins:** almond, most beans (adzuki, black, fava, kidney, pinto), Brazil nut, cashew, chia seed, chickpea, hazelnut, hemp, macadamia nut, peas, pistachio, pumpkin seed	**Meat and poultry:** rabbit **Fish and seafood:** clam, cod, crab, octopus, scallop **Vegan proteins:** lima bean, mung bean, navy bean, soybean and soy products (e.g., miso, tempeh, tofu)
Fruits and vegetables *Note: Many raw fruits and veggies are cooling in nature but can be warmed with heat and spice*	**Fruits:** avocado, cherry, date, dried fruits, guava, hawthorn fruit, kumquat, longan, lychee, nectarine, peach, raspberry **Vegetables:** chive, kale, leek, onion (including green onion, shallot and scallion), most root vegetables (beet, Jerusalem artichoke, jicama, kudzu root, parsnip, rutabaga, yacon root, yam) pumpkin, winter squash	**Fruits:** apricot, cranberry, fig, goji berry, grape, loquat, olive, papaya, pineapple, plum **Vegetables:** artichoke, cabbage, carrot, cauliflower, celeriac root, celery, kohlrabi, mushrooms, okra, potato, string bean, sweet potato, taro root, turnip	**Fruits:** apple, banana, bilberry, blackberry, blueberry, cantaloupe, citrus fruits, currant, elderberry, gooseberry, kiwi, mango, monk fruit, mulberry, passion fruit, pear, persimmon, plantain, rhubarb, strawberry, watermelon **Vegetables:** asparagus, bamboo shoot, bell pepper, broccoli, cucumber, eggplant, most leafy greens (arugula, bok choy, collard, dandelion, lettuce, rapini, sorrel, spinach, Swiss chard, watercress, wild greens), radish, sea vegetables (including seaweed and kelp), snow pea, spirulina, sprouts, tomato, zucchini

Is It a Hot Pot or Not? (*continued*)

	Warming foods	Neutral foods	Cooling foods
Herbs, spices and condiments	Angelica, basil, bay leaf, black pepper, caraway, cardamom, cayenne, chili, Chinese ginseng, cinnamon, clove, cumin, curry, dill, fennel, garlic, ginger, horseradish, milk thistle, mustard, nutmeg, oregano, paprika, perilla, rosemary, safflower, sage, spearmint, star anise, thyme, turmeric	Alfalfa, carob, chamomile, coconut oil, coriander (seed), honey, licorice, maple syrup, marjoram, olive oil, parsley, rose hip, saffron, vanilla	Cilantro, dandelion, horsetail, lavender, lemon balm, nettle, peppermint, salt, sesame oil, soy sauce, tarragon, yellow gentian
Grains	Quinoa	Amaranth, corn, millet, oat, rice (brown, white and rice bran), rye, spelt	Barley, buckwheat, kamut, wheat and wheat bran
Others	Butter, capers, chocolate, cocoa, coconut meat and milk, coffee, ghee, goat cheese and milk, sorghum, unrefined sweeteners, vinegar, wine	Cow's milk cheese, stevia	Agar-agar, beer, black and green tea, fruit juice, ice cream, cow's milk and soy milk, sauerkraut, sugar (white) and sugar cane, yogurt

The Energetics of Food: A Theory from the Far East

The chart opposite and above shows a summary of energetics of food from a traditional Chinese medicine perspective. The warming foods are the focus of this book. Cooling foods will be cooked or placed alongside warming spices to heat them up and make them easier to digest. For example, dandelion is sautéed with garlic to warm it up.

Interestingly, if we look at the cooling foods in the chart, we can see they include foods that many people have allergies or intolerances to, such as dairy, wheat, sugar and soy. In fact, many of these cooling foods also cause inflammation in the body, as

I explain in my books *Meals That Heal Inflammation* and *Slimming Meals That Heal*, whereas warming foods tend to be anti-inflammatory. Refined cooling foods often cause inflammation because, according to traditional Chinese medicine, they dampen the spleen energy, which governs the digestive system. Many of us live in a stressed spleen energy state because we center our meals on refined cooling foods. It is important to understand that natural cooling foods, such as greens and fruit, are healing and are important to eat daily. Unfortunately, the damage caused by refined cooling foods means most people with digestive problems need to pair natural cooling and warming foods in the same meal to bring their systems from a cold and damp state to a more balanced one.

Heat It Up! How Cooking Food Supports the Body

The way food is prepared and cooked is also important. Cooling foods are often eaten raw, cold or frozen. Warming foods, on the other hand, are most beneficial when prepared by steaming, blanching, sautéing, broiling, stewing, roasting or baking. We can actually change the way we absorb food by how we process it. We can take a healthy food that might be considered cool, like a raw apple, and transform it into a beneficial warming food by cooking and pureeing it. Applesauce is easy to digest and soothing to the gastrointestinal tract. You can also achieve this change by adding beautiful spices and oils for a comforting snack.

We want to avoid grilling and frying as both can cause inflammation. Cooking meat at the high temperatures used for grilling and frying creates heterocyclic amines (HCAs) and polycyclic aromatic hydrocarbons (PAHs), compounds that have been linked to some cancers. When you grill that steak on the barbecue, you are creating very high concentrations of both HCAs and PAHs. The hotter the grill, the higher the content of HCAs and PAHs in the meat. HCAs can also form when you fry food at a high temperature over a long period of time. That is why we will be sticking to healthy cooking methods and avoiding fatty meat during the Hot Detox.

The Yin and Yang of Food

Contractive foods (foods that grow in small spaces) are often warming and hold heat in the body. Warming foods typically take longer to grow (beets, sweet potatoes, parsnips) and are often red, orange or yellow. They are traditionally served warm and easy to chew. Root vegetables that grow in the earth are contractive and have a natural warming effect on the body. It's not surprising that we often crave root vegetable–based meals during the winter months. Expansive foods (foods that grow up towards the sky or down towards the earth) include shoots, fruits that hang from trees, melons, cucumbers and other vine-grown foods. These are cooling foods that dispel heat from the body. Cool produce grows quickly (lettuce, cucumber) and contains cooler tones of blue, green and beige. These are usually the foods we serve raw and crave during the warm summer months.

Does the inflammatory nature of refined cooling foods mean you should eat only hot foods 100 percent of the time? Of course not. I recommend the 80–20 principle: during winter (or cool months) you enjoy 80 percent warming foods and 20 percent cooling foods. During summer, it might be the opposite. It's important to enjoy a bit of both worlds at all times of the year, because there are incredibly beneficial foods on both lists. For our purposes in the Hot Detox, however, I recommend eating mostly warming foods. You will still enjoy some detoxifying cooling foods during this process, but they are always cooked or served with warming spices. Once you are finished with the cleanse, you can start to reintroduce some cold foods and see how your body tolerates them.

No one can accurately predict how another person will feel or react when eating certain foods — everything is individual. Self-observation is important in this program, and I encourage you to journal

How Toxins Enter and Exit the Body

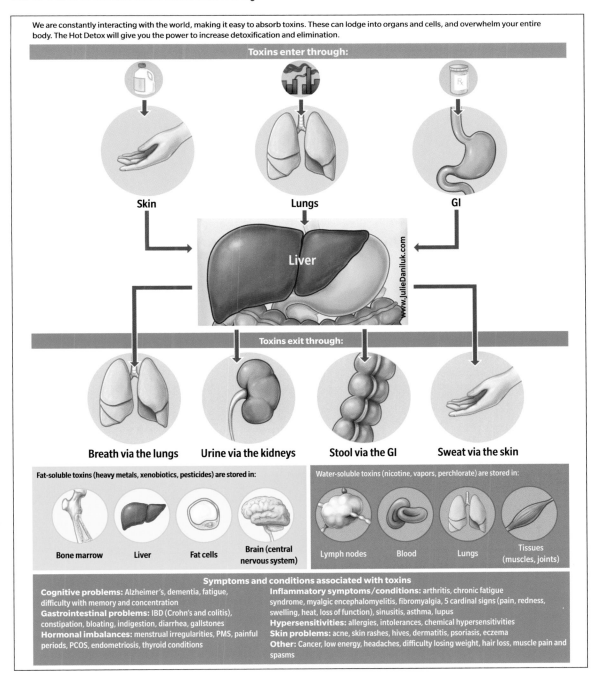

We are constantly interacting with the world, making it easy to absorb toxins. These can lodge into organs and cells, and overwhelm your entire body. The Hot Detox will give you the power to increase detoxification and elimination.

Toxins enter through:

Skin   Lungs   GI

Liver

www.JulieDaniluk.com

Toxins exit through:

Breath via the lungs   Urine via the kidneys   Stool via the GI   Sweat via the skin

Fat-soluble toxins (heavy metals, xenobiotics, pesticides) are stored in:

Bone marrow   Liver   Fat cells   Brain (central nervous system)

Water-soluble toxins (nicotine, vapors, perchlorate) are stored in:

Lymph nodes   Blood   Lungs   Tissues (muscles, joints)

Symptoms and conditions associated with toxins

Cognitive problems: Alzheimer's, dementia, fatigue, difficulty with memory and concentration
Gastrointestinal problems: IBD (Crohn's and colitis), constipation, bloating, indigestion, diarrhea, gallstones
Hormonal imbalances: menstrual irregularities, PMS, painful periods, PCOS, endometriosis, thyroid conditions

Inflammatory symptoms/conditions: arthritis, chronic fatigue syndrome, myalgic encephalomyelitis, fibromyalgia, 5 cardinal signs (pain, redness, swelling, heat, loss of function), sinusitis, asthma, lupus
Hypersensitivities: allergies, intolerances, chemical hypersensitivities
Skin problems: acne, skin rashes, hives, dermatitis, psoriasis, eczema
Other: Cancer, low energy, headaches, difficulty losing weight, hair loss, muscle pain and spasms

How Toxins Wreak Havoc in the Body

Toxin	Harm
Xenoestrogens such as insecticides, solvents, herbicides, pesticides, dyes, pigments, food flavorings, perfumes, plastics and resins. There are over 70,000 synthesized chemical compounds, most of which have hormonal effects in addition to toxic effects.	Exposure to too many xenoestrogens can ultimately lead to hormonal imbalances, neurological and reproductive problems, cancers, cardiovascular diseases, chronic inflammation and obesity.
Metals such as lead, cadmium, aluminum, mercury and arsenic	Cadmium increases inflammation in the liver and kidneys, and mercury exposure causes the immune system to attack its own immune cells. Countries like Taiwan, Bangladesh and Mexico that have high levels of arsenic in their water supply also have a high prevalence of diabetes. High levels of arsenic reduce the uptake of glucose by cells, leading to hyperglycemia (high blood sugar) and a corresponding high insulin secretion.
Titanium dioxide (found in paint, artificial food coloring, and sunscreen) and **tetrachlorodibenzo-p-dioxin** (the active compound in herbicides)	These compounds contribute to chronic inflammation and pain by promoting the release of pro-inflammatory cytokines such as IL-1ß, IL-6, and TNF-α. Several of our internal organs such as the liver, kidneys and lungs respond to this toxicity by sounding the alarm bells of inflammation.
Benzene, present in gasoline, and **toluene**, a component of many adhesives and solvents	These toxins are stored in our fat cells and are difficult to eliminate, which can lead to systemic infections and a state of chronic inflammation. In fact, studies have shown that when overweight and obese people lose weight, many of those entrapped toxins are liberated into their bloodstream.
Atrazine, a compound found in many herbicides	Atrazine has been linked to obesity, type 2 diabetes and belly fat. By affecting major hormones involved in weight control (i.e., leptin, testosterone, insulin and the thyroid hormones), many toxins can contribute to weight gain. The link between toxins and obesity is so strong that it was called "chemobesity" by researchers in 2010.

how you feel after eating your meals. The Hot Detox online program provides additional support for this, but essentially I want you to enjoy the ratio of warming to cooling foods that works for you. It's not about restriction, but about exploring to find the right menu for your body. After all, variety is how we prevent nutritional deficiency, and is vital to a healthy lifestyle.

Why Should You Cleanse?

Every day we are bombarded by infomercials, websites and magazine articles about the urgent need to get rid of our entrapped toxins, but what evidence is there to motivate you to give the Hot Detox a try?

Once I watched a medical doctor on television claim detox programs were a complete waste of money and time. He said there was no science to support their benefit and that the body can detoxify itself. I wanted to yell at the TV, "Sure, maybe back before the industrial revolution our body knew how to detoxify, but you are doing a disservice to your viewers if you don't look at the hard science to see the benefit of helping the body detoxify in our present world." His opinion made me realize that despite the good science that supports the benefits of a detoxification program, many people don't know it or perhaps don't trust it.

Whatever the reason, my goal is to shed light and understanding so that doing a detox can be as regular an activity as using an app on your smartphone. To quote my favorite Vulcan, Spock, "Logic is the beginning of wisdom, not the end." So let's dig into the logical science of detoxification and see what wisdom we might find.

A Scientific Perspective

Clinical studies in humans have found that well-designed detoxification programs are incredibly helpful in mitigating pain and reducing disease symptoms. For instance, in a study published in *Alternative Therapies in Health and Medicine*, researchers put a group of chronically ill patients on a detox program that focused on gastrointestinal healing and liver detoxification. Another group of patients received a low-calorie and hypoallergenic diet. Compared to the second group, the patients on the detox plan had fewer symptoms of their disease at the end of the 10-week study period. Other studies have shown that detox diets improve liver function and general well-being.

Firefighters who had been exposed to intense toxins by an explosion were evaluated for exposure to polychlorinated biphenyls (PCBs). During the study at the University of Southern California, 14 firefighters followed an experimental detoxification program consisting of a supervised diet, exercise and sauna. After completing the detoxification program, the firemen had improved neurobehavioral and memory test scores compared to the group that did not participate in the program.

Other studies show benefit from detox diets for those suffering from fibromyalgia, a chronic inflammatory condition characterized by muscular and joint pain and fatigue. For example, in one U.S. study, 8 women between the ages of 48 and 74 consumed a diet that promotes detoxification for 4 weeks. This "elimination diet" has many elements of the program outlined in the Hot Detox, including phytonutrient-rich foods such as fruits and vegetables. At the end of the study, the women reported less pain, less muscle stiffness and better pain tolerance than at the beginning of the program. Furthermore, throughout the study the women had eliminated entrapped mercury and arsenic via the urine.

It is logical to assert that eliminating toxins from the body is a good thing to do. Since you are reading this book, I imagine you are pleased to know that your body will be reaping some serious benefits. Get ready for more energy, brighter moods and increased vitality!

> In 1992, after a motor vehicle accident, I felt like I had lost everything: my health, my job and my love of life. I was diagnosed with fibromyalgia and lived with chronic pain, debilitating headaches, aching muscles and joints, severe fatigue, feelings of depression and being overwhelmed. I called it the two-step dance — one step forward and two back. I felt like I had no choice except to live like this. I just hurt in body, mind and soul.
>
> After years of suffering, I found Julie.
>
> Within just a year, I no longer needed the 650 milligrams of acetaminophen I used to take 10 times daily for pain, my CPAP (continuous positive airway pressure) for my sleep disorder is down from a 14 to a 7, and I have lost 80 pounds.
>
> I have a better quality of life that also enriches my life with my husband. We love to travel and are planning a trip to Costa Rica, where I will no longer be an observer but an active participant, climbing the mountain and hiking trails through the jungle with him. This is how I continue to see my future.
>
> Julie, I don't know how to thank you for all you have done for me.
>
> — Heather M.

This is why the Hot Detox program is so important — it ensures that when you liberate these toxins, you have the elimination pathways open to excrete them.

What You Have in Store

This book will explore the process of detoxification through many different applications of heat — both external (heat therapy) and with food. While the detox menu plan itself is 21 days, the total time you spend on this detox program can be as short as 3 days or up to 1 month. Before starting the program, a lead-up "sets the table" and prepares you.

In the first days after you successfully complete the Hot Detox, there will be an assisted reintegration of the foods you avoided during the cleanse. During this "exit" phase, you can test out inflammatory foods and other foods you avoided to see how your body handles them and what causes you digestive distress. This testing will help you come up with your own list of "safe" and "harmful" foods based on how your own body reacts.

The next few chapters discuss how detoxification works in each major system of the body. In the next chapter you are going to learn a great deal about how food interacts with your gut lining. It is fascinating, and I hope you really soak in the information so you have more tools to heal with. Knowing how your body reacts to and absorbs food is fundamental in creating what I call juicy vitality.

2

Start with the Gut

An empty stomach is not a good political adviser.
—Albert Einstein

One of the biggest ways we interface with the outside world is through our gastrointestinal tract, whose entire surface area is approximately equal to that of a football field. It plays a huge part in the immune system as the place where the outside world (microorganisms, plants, animals and water) has passage into the inside world (our body). Recent research has found that up to 70 percent of our immune system is located in our gut. When we use healing food choices to soothe the inflammation of the digestive lining and balance the immune system, it translates into reduced inflammation throughout the whole body.

All the cells of your body, as well as your organs (including the major organ of detoxification, the liver), rely upon a well-functioning bowel. Bowel cleansing is the first and most important thing to focus on, as it opens the highway of detoxification. If you do not have a properly functioning bowel, you will have a multiple-car pileup on the freeway out of your body. The Hot Detox will get your bowels working and moving properly by clearing this traffic congestion.

Your Food's Big Adventure

Before I discuss how the Hot Detox can fight inflammation in the gut, I am going to tell a tale of acid rains, turbulent seas and Sahara desert conditions. It's a voyage where nothing that enters ever comes out the same way again—it's the story of digestion.

Everything we eat must be broken down into smaller molecules of nutrients in order to be absorbed by the body. Your digestive system processes foods and drinks into their smallest parts in order to use their components to build and repair cells and to manufacture energy. This unique system consists of a series of hollow organs joined and coiled inside your abdominal cavity in a long, twisted tube. The gastrointestinal tract runs from your mouth to your anus, via your esophagus, stomach, and small and large intestines. Your liver, gallbladder and pancreas are also involved in digestion, by producing juices and enzymes that help break down food.

Down the Hatch

Let's start by traveling along the gastrointestinal tract. Picture yourself as if you were riding atop a popular lunch item: a roast beef sandwich. First, teeth sink into the sandwich, cutting off a bite and grinding it into smaller pieces. Salivary glands spit out enzymes like a waterfall, unleashed by all the wonderful smells and flavors coming from the sandwich. These enzymes work like scissors to cut up the starchy bread into simple sugars. The sandwich is chewed for about five seconds, though many digestive complaints would be relieved if this time increased to 30 seconds. Taking the time to thoroughly chew your food allows salivary enzymes to access more of its surface area and saturate it. The more physical contact between enzymes and food, the better food is digested. As the food softens, the tongue pushes the ball of food to the back of the throat and into the esophagus. A trapdoor closes off the trachea (windpipe) to make sure that you and the sandwich go down the right chute.

Though swallowing is a voluntary action, the movement of food through the esophagus is involuntary and proceeds under the control of autonomic nerves. Just like squeezing a tube of toothpaste, the wet mass of food (called a bolus) goes down the esophagus in a series of contractions called peristalsis. Like an ocean wave traveling through the muscle layer of the esophagus, the muscle layer contracts, narrowing the tube and propelling you down the esophagus. The valve to the stomach (known as the cardiac sphincter muscle) opens, and the gooey sandwich finally lands in the stomach. If this valve gets inflamed, acid from the stomach can escape up the esophagus, producing heartburn or acid reflux.

Acid Bath

Now imagine being inside a small muscular sack (the stomach), sloshing back and forth in an ocean of half-digested pulp, and getting mixed in with digestive juices. Doesn't it remind you of a wave pool at a water park? Just when you think you've got your balance back, the walls of the stomach contract and fold in again. Over and over for up to 4 hours, you get crushed under waves that mix food with digestive juices and dissolve it into teeny tiny bits. Hydrochloric

How Toxins Are Removed by the GI System

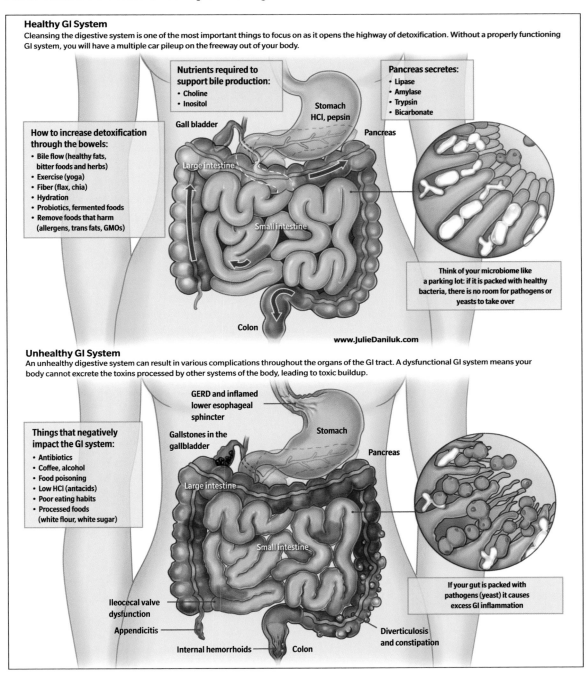

Healthy GI System
Cleansing the digestive system is one of the most important things to focus on as it opens the highway of detoxification. Without a properly functioning GI system, you will have a multiple car pileup on the freeway out of your body.

Nutrients required to support bile production:
- Choline
- Inositol

Pancreas secretes:
- Lipase
- Amylase
- Trypsin
- Bicarbonate

Stomach
HCl, pepsin

Gall bladder

Pancreas

How to increase detoxification through the bowels:
- Bile flow (healthy fats, bitter foods and herbs)
- Exercise (yoga)
- Fiber (flax, chia)
- Hydration
- Probiotics, fermented foods
- Remove foods that harm (allergens, trans fats, GMOs)

Large intestine

Small intestine

Think of your microbiome like a parking lot: if it is packed with healthy bacteria, there is no room for pathogens or yeasts to take over

Colon

www.JulieDaniluk.com

Unhealthy GI System
An unhealthy digestive system can result in various complications throughout the organs of the GI tract. A dysfunctional GI system means your body cannot excrete the toxins processed by other systems of the body, leading to toxic buildup.

GERD and inflamed lower esophageal sphincter

Gallstones in the gallbladder

Stomach

Pancreas

Things that negatively impact the GI system:
- Antibiotics
- Coffee, alcohol
- Food poisoning
- Low HCl (antacids)
- Poor eating habits
- Processed foods (white flour, white sugar)

Large intestine

Small intestine

If your gut is packed with pathogens (yeast) it causes excess GI inflammation

Ileocecal valve dysfunction

Appendicitis

Diverticulosis and constipation

Internal hemorrhoids

Colon

Do You Have Enough Lighter Fluid for the Fire?

When people complain of digestive troubles, a popular treatment is to suppress the digestive juices. What may surprise you is that the very thing that seems to be the culprit is actually the solution. Let's look at what happens when you have too little of the main ingredient in our digestive juices: hydrochloric acid.

- Your digestion is impaired. More strain is placed on the other digestive organs as they take on the task the stomach acid was supposed to do — preparing food for assimilation. Most notably, the pancreas is forced to synthesize and secrete a higher volume of enzymes to digest the food particles.

- You absorb fewer nutrients. Having undigested food entering the small intestine compromises the amount and quality of nutrients the body can ultimately absorb. In fact, low stomach acid has been associated with an increased risk of deficiencies in nutrients such as vitamin B12, vitamin C, calcium, iron and magnesium.

- You become vulnerable to pathogens unknowingly ingested with your food, which can occur from accidentally eating undercooked meat or rancid and moldy food. Potentially harmful parasites, worms, yeasts, molds or bacteria present in those contaminated foods can burrow into the tender walls of your stomach or the rest of your gastrointestinal tract. This type of damage may contribute to ulcer formation, leaky gut syndrome or irritable bowel syndrome. (This is what happened to me from terrible food poisoning in Thailand, where a virulent bacterium nearly killed me and instigated post-infectious colitis.) Healthy levels of hydrochloric acid in the stomach would normally sterilize your food and kill these intruders to prevent such an infection. Remember that immune cells are present all along your intestines, and if in good working condition, should be able to catch and protect you from most pathogens. However, parasites and other pathogens present in the gut will trigger inflammation and negatively affect your good intestinal bacteria.

acid rains down from the crimson walls of the stomach to help break down large food particles into smaller pieces, preparing the semi-solid bolus for more complete digestion. Don't worry — the stomach is protected by a coat of mucus to keep the acid from wearing it out. After a few hours in the hard-working stomach, the bolus is converted into chyme. Chyme is a strongly acidic liquid mixture of unrecognizable predigested food and stomach secretions (hydrochloric acid, enzymes and mucus).

Since the sandwich has now been crushed up like a tin can in a trash compactor, you will be suspended in a slippery liquid for the rest of the ride. Like Luke Skywalker, who escaped the Death Star garbage compactor just in the nick of time, you are now heading directly into the small intestine. Several factors affect the rate at which the stomach will empty. What was the emotional state when the ride started? How strong is the muscular action of the stomach? What were the ingredients in the sandwich you rode in on? A sandwich is a tricky food because carbohydrates spend the least amount of time in the stomach, whereas proteins and fats stay in the stomach longer. As the sandwich churns in the stomach, the rest of the digestive organs, as well as the brain (which helps to orchestrate the digestive symphony), are busy preparing the small intestine for completing the subsequent steps in the digestive process with the help of enzymes and juices produced by the pancreas, liver and small intestine. Hormones and neurotransmitters course through veins to signal the pancreas to produce and secrete enzymes, sodium bicarbonate, insulin and other hormones. In addition, specialized cells lining the small intestine begin to make enzymes to help break down carbohydrates and fats.

If you are lucky enough to be in a good, healthy stomach, then once the sandwich is liquefied into chyme, another muscular valve (called the pyloric sphincter) at the base of the stomach will open to allow the predigested acidic mash to enter the lumen, the inner region of the small intestine. In a happy, healthy digestive system, the muscles that make up the gastrointestinal wall dependably synchronize peristaltic movements to keep the food mixing and moving along smoothly.

Through the Intestines

Now that you and the sandwich chyme are in the small intestine, you can see the pancreas (the main digestive gland in our body) squirt out some sodium bicarbonate to neutralize the strong hydrochloric acid from the stomach. This incredible change from acid to alkaline could not come too soon. Now you are comfortable and ready for a gentle rain of pancreatic enzymes, including amylase to break down carbohydrates, steapsin to break down fats and trypsin to break down proteins. If the pancreas is stressed from overeating, consuming too much refined food or alcohol, or eating when stressed, it may have a difficult time making the enzymes that are essential for proper digestion.

As you continue down the digestive river, the ride is about to get more exciting: bright yellow bile swishes into the mixture. The liver produces bile continuously throughout the day, and it gets stored and concentrated in the gallbladder between meals. The gallbladder squeezes out bile through the bile ducts and into the intestine when it senses food. Bile helps with the digestion of fats, and also has the important function of lubricating the intestines and stimulating peristalsis. You are happy to see all the fats mix with the bile that aids the digestive journey. Bile emulsifies large globs of fat into tiny enzyme-accessible droplets, much as detergent dissolves grease from a frying pan, allowing other enzymes to break it down even further.

While it's at work, the small intestine is much like an exciting waterpark slide. From the inside, the small intestine looks like a thick carpet with long fibers sticking out. The inner walls are folded into small fingerlike projections called villi. In turn, the villi are also covered with projections, this time microscopic, called microvilli. Villi and microvilli increase intestinal surface area to maximize efficiency of nutrient absorption. Picture spilling wine on a thick plush carpet versus a vinyl floor. The carpet fibers will absorb a lot more wine than the smooth vinyl, making it much more difficult to deal with the stain. As long as the microvilli are in good working order, a tremendous amount of vitamins, minerals, proteins and carbohydrates will cross over the digestive lining into the bloodstream to nourish all the cells in the body.

The leftover part of your sandwich boat that is not able to be absorbed in the small intestine has one final significant door to go through: the ileocecal valve. This valve is located between the ileum, which is the last portion of your small intestine, and the cecum, which is the first portion of your large intestine. Normally, it is a one-way valve that allows digested food to pass into your large intestine while preventing waste from re-entering the small intestine once it has passed out.

However, when the ileocecal valve is stuck open (which can happen if this area of the intestines becomes inflamed), waste products can back up into the small intestine, disturbing digestion and causing toxins to accumulate. If the small intestine gets irritated by rough fiber, the ileocecal valve can also be stuck closed. This can be dangerous as it prevents waste from moving forward into the large intestine. A malfunctioning ileocecal valve can be the underlying reason for many digestive complaints including irritable bowel syndrome (IBS) and indigestion.

But wait, the journey isn't over yet. The next part is much wider and drier as you venture through the large intestine. The role of the large intestine is much like that of a dehydrator: water from the remaining mass of food is extracted and recycled back into the body. Leftover food, older cells and loads of bacteria are baked for 18 hours into a drier loaf, which ends up being between a third to a fourth of the size it was at the beginning of the journey. At the end of the

expedition—a trip that's more than 25 feet long from top to tail!—food leaves the body by way of a bowel movement.

The time it takes for food to complete this journey is known as the intestinal transit time. Transit times vary among people based on their intestinal health, diet, hydration and lifestyle, but can range from 12 to 48 hours. A transit time that is outside this range should be addressed by a health practitioner, especially if it continues for more than a few days. By increasing the amount of beneficial microbes (probiotics) and good fats you consume, you can assure a balanced transit time.

Making Friends with Your Doo-Doo

Even more important than transit time when it comes to bowel health is the condition of your stool. They might not be pleasant to think or talk about, but stools have many different shapes, forms and consistencies, and all of them tell a different digestive story. Observing your stool is one way of knowing how well your digestive system is functioning, your overall health, and what's happening inside your body. Most people think that as long as they are passing a stool once or twice a day, then they must be healthy—but this is not always the case.

For example, you might be going to the washroom regularly but only passing stringy, pencil-thin stools. This can be an indication of an allergic response to a food. Inflammation creates such a thin and restricted passageway in the colon that it can only handle eliminating tiny bits of feces at a time—which produces the pencil-thin stool. Another unhealthy sign is small, dry, pellet stools, which signal dehydration. On the other end of the spectrum, chronic diarrhea indicates that the food is being passed undigested, which can be dangerous if prolonged and unresolved.

Nicely formed, wide, sausage-like stools that move easily through the colon are your goal. The stool should be medium brown, uniform in texture, smooth and soft, formed into one long shape. Ideally it is one to two inches in diameter and up to 18 inches long. It is S-shaped because it holds the shape of your lower intestine. It should make a gentle dive into the water and sink slowly. It should have a natural smell that does not clear a room. If you really have great digestion, your s%&* doesn't stink! These kinds of perfect bowel movements can be achieved by following the Hot Detox because the program is soothing and comforting to the digestive system and can heal and restore digestive health.

Hot Detox Solutions

Now that you have experienced the digestive processes, let's look at solutions to some typical problems. In the Hot Detox, you are going to see a number of solutions for detoxification. Don't feel you have to do all of them. Just like a restaurant, I am giving you a menu to choose from. If you ordered one of everything, your meal out would stop being an enjoyable experience. If you are new to cleansing, simply layer in the suggestions as you feel ready for them. Always consult a health care provider before taking any herbs or supplements. Just following the very first solution is enough to produce good results!

Hot Detox Solution #1: Removing Foods That Harm

Gut permeability plays a big role in detoxification. Hyperpermeability (or leaky gut) allows increased absorption of xenobiotics (substances with a biological activity that are found as pollutants in the natural environment, such as petroleum and pesticides) and toxins, which then need to be processed by the liver. The Hot Detox improves gastrointestinal integrity through the increase of prebiotics (e.g., fiber) and probiotics that occur in fermented foods, which protect and soothe the digestive lining.

The most important thing with detoxification is to understand that certain foods cause an allergic response. This response can cause inflammatory swelling of the intestines and stops peristalsis from working correctly. You must learn which foods are causing distress and get rid of them. Before we add in cleansing remedies, we have to take out the foods that cause irritation to the bowel. That's why on the Hot Detox we are stripping away inflammatory foods (the complete list of foods to avoid can be found on page 48).

Hot Detox Solution #2: Hydration

After eliminating harmful and inflammatory foods, the next thing to consider is hydration. The food you eat floats down your digestive highway on a blanket of water, much like a water slide, as we just saw. Dehydration leads to constipation, and as your digestive system becomes distressed, detoxification is impaired.

To avoid dehydration, it is ideal to drink 6 to 10 cups of fluid daily (depending on your size). Some people may find this easy. To others, this may sound like torture. I don't like the taste of plain water, so I flavor it to make it enjoyable and effortless to drink my eight cups a day. I splash it with lemon, or add blueberries, an herbal teabag or an ounce of real fruit or veggie juice. Avoid sugar-laden fruit juices or "calorie-free" powdered, aspartame-heavy flavored drink mixes, as these harm the body. Instead, make your own delicious flavored water or my delicious Detox Lemonade from *Meals That Heal Inflammation.* Just add 2 tablespoons of lemon juice and 10 drops of stevia liquid to 2 cups of warm water. Hydration doesn't need to be boring. The Hot Detox contains many healing hydration options that help you attain the ideal liquid intake, from warming teas to super shakes and soups.

The final thing to remember when it comes to hydration is what you drink from. Avoid plastic water bottles at all costs. Drinking from plastic water bottles increases your intake of xenoestrogens, which cause toxicity and hormonal imbalance in your body. It is best to consume filtered water from a glass container. Mason jars (aka canning jars) are perfect, since most have measurements indicating how much liquid they hold. Some people drink from stainless steel, but personally I find it tastes like you're kissing a robot. There is also the potential that nickel and heavy metals in the stainless-steel bottle could leach into your drink. In summary: glass is the best way to go.

Hot Detox Solution #3: Fiber

We've all heard of fiber and some of the wonderful benefits of increasing fiber in our diet, but what exactly is it? Fiber is a carbohydrate that humans can't digest because we lack the enzymes to break it down. This is why it fills us up and helps to control hunger. Fiber is important in detoxification because it binds to the bile acids that carry toxins out of the body and helps to eliminate them in the stool. This allows for faster transit times and less reabsorption and damage to the intestinal lining. Not enough fiber in the diet can lead to mild constipation and toxin reabsorption.

You may not be aware that there are different types of fibers, which do not work the same for every person. When people think of fiber, they typically think of wheat or oat bran. But these fibers may not be the healthiest choice for most. Wheat bran is very harsh and can feel like razor blades to the colon for some people. Both wheat and oat bran are high-allergen foods because they contain gluten (oat bran is often contaminated with wheat gluten in processing), making them troublesome to the bowel.

Fiber Twin Powers, Activate!

Fiber comes in two forms: soluble and insoluble. Soluble fiber forms a gel when mixed with liquid, while insoluble fiber passes through our intestines largely intact. Both kinds of fiber are beneficial. Soluble fiber binds with fatty acids. It prolongs stomach-emptying time so that sugar is released and absorbed more slowly, which helps regulate blood sugar for people with diabetes. It also lowers total cholesterol and

What Is the Best Fiber?

The year 1890 could be called the year the human diet started to go downhill. It was the year a new milling technique swept North America that removed fiber from whole grains to produce refined flour. Although celebrated as progress, the new milling technique displaced beneficial nutrients and created a modern diet in which large amounts of refined carbohydrates are consumed, contributing to an increased risk of many inflammatory diseases. From diabetes to heart disease to inflammatory bowel disease (IBD), we can often trace the root cause back to deficiency of nutrients and an excess of empty carbohydrates.

You may need to test out different fibers to find the one that works best for you. For example, if you find that fiber constipates you, you may need a much gentler fiber. Pectin fibers from fruit or ground flax or chia (where the insoluble fiber is ground fine and soluble fiber dissolves) can be easier on the system. If you cannot tolerate fiber at all, I recommend partially hydrolyzed guar gum. It is ideal for even the most sensitive people, including those with IBS, IBD, diarrhea and leaky gut. If you are currently using bran, which is not recommended on this cleanse, you can substitute psyllium. Gentle fibers should be included in our diets on a regular basis. No matter what your state of health or condition, there is a fiber that will work wonders for you!

LDL cholesterol (low-density lipoprotein, the "bad" cholesterol), thus reducing the risk of heart disease. Finally, it promotes friendly bacteria, which feed on soluble fiber. Insoluble fiber moves bulk through the intestines. By promoting regular bowel movement and preventing constipation, it moves toxic waste through the colon in less time. It also controls and balances the pH (acidity) in the intestines, which helps prevent colon cancer by preventing microbes from producing cancerous substances.

During the Hot Detox program, we're going to steer clear of both wheat and oat bran, and rely more on ground seed fibers, which are low-allergy, high-nutrient solutions. Flax and chia seeds are some of my favorite fibers because they are the perfect balance between the soluble and insoluble. These mucilaginous fibers sweep the bowels clean in a very gentle way—picture a soft bristle broom sweeping out the toxins and waste from the digestive tract.

Legumes, seeds and vegetables are the richest sources of fiber. We require 0.88 to 1.23 ounces (25–35 grams) of fiber a day for optimal health! However, if you have diverticulitis or IBD (inflammatory bowel disease), consult your health care practitioner to establish the safe amount of fiber for your condition.

Good Health from Good Friends

Although we cannot digest fiber, our microscopic friends can. Our gut microbiota digest the fiber we eat into short-chain fatty acids. SCFAs can activate detoxifying and antioxidative enzymes, including glutathione S-transferases and sulfur-transferase, that help eliminate carcinogens.

Keep that in mind that you must consume lots of fruit and vegetables, as these contain fiber that becomes prebiotic, meaning it feeds the probiotics (beneficial bacteria) in our gut. Some of the best sources of fiber in produce comes from artichoke, asparagus, jicama and burdock.

Fiber food	Grams of fiber	Soluble	Insoluble
Acorn squash	0.2 oz (6 g)/cup	○	○
Apple	0.16 oz (4.4 g) ea.	○	○
Artichoke	0.4 oz (10 g) ea.		○
Asparagus (chopped)	0.14 oz (4 g)/cup		○
Brown rice	0.14 oz (4 g)/cup		○
Burdock root	0.19 oz (5.5 g)/cup	○	○
Butternut squash	0.25 oz (7 g)/cup	○	○
Chia seeds	0.39 oz (11 g)/oz	○	○
Chickpeas	0.99 oz (28 g)/cup	○	○
Cinnamon	0.14 oz (4 g)/Tbsp		○
Coconut meat	0.25 oz (7 g)/cup		○
Cooked kale	0.10 oz (3 g)/cup		○
Cooked spinach	0.14 oz (4 g)/cup		○
Eggplant	0.10 oz (3 g)/cup	○	○
Flaxseed	0.10 oz (3 g)/Tbsp	○	○
Grapefruit	0.10 oz (3 g) each	○	○
Jicama root	0.21 (6 g)/cup	○	○
Lentils	1.23 oz (36 g)/cup	○	○
Mung beans	1.20 oz (34 g)/cup	○	○
Navy beans	0.67 oz (19 g)/cup	○	○
Pineapple	0.08 oz (2.3 g)/cup	○	○
Psyllium husk	0.14 oz (4 g)/Tbsp	○	○
Raspberries	0.29 oz (8 g)/cup		○
Sweet pepper	0.10 oz (3 g) each		○
Zucchini	0.10 oz (3 g)	○	○

If your beneficial bowel microorganisms do not have enough produce to munch on, they can actually start to eat away the mucus lining in your gut. We need lots of brightly colored produce in our diet to ensure that our gut functions well. People who eat a high-meat, low-produce diet encourage growth of the wrong types of microbes. People who eat a high flour and sugar diet create a very large candida population. This is why the Hot Detox program recommends 7 to 10 vegetables each day, even past the 21 active days. The Hot Detox recipes use psyllium, flax, chia, pineapple and fermented and cooked vegetables to provide the pre- and probiotics needed for balancing the microbiome, minimizing toxin production from pathogenic bacteria.

Hot Detox Solution #4: Probiotics

The human gastrointestinal tract contains approximately a thousand different species of bacteria. Probiotics make up to 60 percent of your stool, making them absolutely necessary to the detoxification process. The probiotics you eat and nourish inside your gut are essential for digestive balance. The modern world makes it tough to maintain a high amount of probiotics in the body because we encounter so many things that kill off these beneficial bacteria. Antibiotics, antibacterial hand gels, meat with antibiotic residues, tap water or swimming pools that are heavily chlorinated, and ingesting inflammatory foods such as yeast, white flour, white sugar and high-fructose corn syrup common in processed foods will all tip the scales in favor of the negative microbes. This can cause beneficial bacteria to die and harmful bacteria to thrive.

Where to Find Probiotics

Base ingredient(s)	Fermented foods	Health benefits
Beans	Miso (soy, red bean) Natto (soy)	• Increases the absorption of vitamins and minerals through the intestinal lining • Acts as the first line of defense for the immune system • Reduces certain types of cancers • Improves intestinal tract health
Fish	Rakfisk (Arctic char, trout)	
Fruits	Nata de coco (coconut) Sicilian green olives	
Grains	Amazake (rice) Injera (teff) Miso (brown rice) Ogi (millet, sorghum) Pao cai (rice congee) Sourdough	
Honey	Jun (fermented with green tea)	
Milk (dairy or non-dairy)	Buttermilk Cheese Kefir Quark Yogurt	
Seeds	Ogiri (egusi seed, sesame seed)	
Vegetables	Fermented juices (beet, cabbage, carrot, celeriac) Kimchi (cabbage, radish/daikon, scallion, cucumber) Kvass (beet) Unpasteurized pickles (vinegar-free vegetable blend) Poi (taro root) Sauerkraut (cabbage)	

"Preserving" Your Health

Want to know the secret to preserving your health? It turns out that the traditional methods of preserving food are teeming with health benefits. People enjoyed fermented foods for their tangy flavors well before refrigeration kept food from spoiling. Being Ukrainian, I was raised watching my grandma make sauerkraut from scratch. Indians enjoy a predinner yogurt drink called *lassi*. All of Asia enjoys pickled fermentations of cabbage, turnips, cucumbers, onions, squash and carrots. Northern Europeans are known for their high consumption of yogurt and kefir and its effects on their longevity.

Indeed, natural pickling may mean that you get more out of your food, because fermented foods have a higher bioavailability and activity of nutrients. The digestibility of nutrients is improved by the bacteria found in fermented foods. The fermentation of fiber-rich components produces active compounds that are anti-inflammatory and have a positive impact on your immune system and blood sugar levels. A study has found that, compared to unfermented juices, fermented vegetable juices contain a higher mineral content (iron, zinc, manganese, copper), 16 percent more soluble iron, and a decrease in phytates (which inhibit the absorption of iron). Among other nutrients critical for well-being found in fermented foods are vitamin B12, most of the B vitamins, folate and vitamin C.

Fermented foods can help ease anxiety and other mental health concerns. Yes, the bacteria in your gut can explain your mood, due to the gut-microbiota-brain connection. Studies have shown that when you eat fermented food products regularly, you have a lower risk of anxiety and depression. In addition, fermented foods significantly increase the available GABA content (gamma-aminobutyric acid is a messenger in the brain that helps to reduce anxiety).

Fermented foods can also help reduce the risk of certain cancers. This occurs through increasing beneficial bacteria (which in turn detoxify carcinogens), producing compounds that play a role in programmed cell death (apoptosis, which is important in killing cells that are abnormal or cancerous), and enhancing the immune system. *Lactobacillus acidophilus* is an important probiotic that can decrease polyps (which can be a precursor to cancers), adenomas and colon cancers.

Since the digestive tract is an important component of the immune system (it contains the MALT, mucosa-associated lymphoid tissue, which is the largest part of the immune system), these two systems go hand in hand. The introduction of beneficial bacteria from fermented foods will benefit both digestion and immune function. Fermented foods can in fact reduce the incidence and duration of respiratory tract infections.

Fermented foods also have an anti-inflammatory effect and can help decrease allergies. These foods have been shown to promote anti-inflammatory messengers called cytokines (e.g., interleukine-10). A study using probiotic cereal has shown to prevent early allergies by balancing T-cell response. T helper cells, white blood cells made by the thymus, come in two types. Th1 and Th2 cells each create and release different messengers that are either inflammatory or anti-inflammatory. A healthy immune system will have a balanced T-cell response, switching from Th1 to Th2 or vice versa as needed. The problem is when our immune system gets "stuck" in one of these responses, leading to a production of only certain specific messengers, which can lead to conditions such as asthma, eczema, allergies and autoimmune diseases. Through consuming fermented foods and an anti-inflammatory diet that supports the lymphatic system, we can get unstuck and rebalance the Th1 and Th2 cells. Fermented foods can also help alleviate symptoms of a milk protein allergy by assisting in the breakdown of lactose.

Where Do We Get Good Bacteria?

There are multiple ways to help restore reserves of good bacteria. Taking a supplement is one way, but we shouldn't rely on supplementation alone, as we want to get many different species of good bacteria back into the colon. Hot Detox recipes such as Coconut Cashew Yogurt (page 158), Pretty Purple Sauerkraut (page 208), Beet Kvass

Be a Detox Detective

My mother, Elaine Daniluk, is a potter, painter and costume designer who has always been the life of the party. You can imagine my frustration when she was struck down with colitis. After consulting with health expert Bryce Wylde, she discovered she suffered from an overload of cadmium, a metal used in pottery glaze and paint that prevents probiotics from establishing in the gut.

He suggested following the Hot Detox plan (omnivore without grains or legumes) and taking billions of probiotic bacteria a day. He also suggested she include partially hydrolyzed guar gum as a soluble fiber to feed the probiotics because it is gentle enough for colitis patients. She went from horrific diarrhea up to 14 times a day to having normal stool in less than 2 weeks.

This taught me a good lesson. Never give up looking for the underlying cause of a condition. Consult with the best practitioners and invest in diagnostic tools like metal testing and stool analysis that help you be your very own Sherlock Holmes!

(page 206) and Ginger Kimchi (page 206) are all amazing food sources of good bacteria—and they are delicious! Fermented soy tempeh and miso are other good sources of healthy microbes, though we don't use them in the Hot Detox as many people have problems digesting soy. If you want to experiment with fermented soy foods, you can do so after the cleanse.

Why Have Lots of Different Types of Probiotics?

The trick in this detox program is to keep your sources of probiotics varied so that you rebalance your microbiome as quickly as possible. For example, *Lactobacillus acidophilus* lives in the small intestine and inhibits the growth of many pathogens (salmonella, *E. coli*, listeria and staphylococci). *Bifidobacterium longum* lives in the colon and increases glutathione S-transferase activity, helping you detoxify. *Bifidobacterium bifidum* lives in the stomach and intestines, and offers antibacterial activity against *H. pylori*, the bacteria that cause ulcers. It also alleviates IBS symptoms and improves quality of life.

It is important to learn about the different kinds of bacteria, both good and bad, and what they do for our microbiome. For example, it's a common belief that yeast is the enemy, but not all yeast is bad. *Saccharomyces boulardii*, a type of yeast, has been known to have great benefit in the treatment and prevention of gastro-intestinal disorders, including travelers' diarrhea, acute and chronic diarrhea, and antibiotic-associated diarrhea. We need to stop believing that all yeast is bad and all bacteria are to be fought. We coexist with trillions and trillions of bacteria and yeasts every day. Our microbiome is an ecosystem that we need to love and nourish in order to recover from allergies, heal our gut lining, and open up our digestive pathways for elimination and detoxification. For a detailed chart of the different benefits of probiotic strains, consult the Hot Detox online program at www.JulieDaniluk.com.

Getting Down and Dirty

Another place we pick up good bacteria is through soil-based organisms. Don't be afraid to eat snap peas, raspberries or herbs directly from the garden (providing you have access to an organic harvest). You might think this is strange, since we've been taught that soil is "dirty" and to wash our hands after being outside, but it's been shown that allergenicity is directly tied to how sterile our world is. Let us relinquish our fear of dirt to restore balance in the gut. That said, you must thoroughly wash produce from a store. If other people have handled your produce with a food-borne pathogen, you could get sick.

Hot Detox Solution #5: Lubrication

Now that we have eliminated harmful foods, added delicious beverages, introduced fiber into our diet, and are starting to build up our good bacteria with probiotics, the next big thing to do is lubricate the bowels. Beyond hydration, consuming good-quality oils helps the stool to easily slip out of the body. Many people do not have enough good-quality oil in their diet to accomplish this. This is where fish oil is highly beneficial; I tend to avoid flax oil as it goes rancid quickly. To avoid oxidation, keep all omega-3 oils in the freezer (they will get cloudy but won't freeze solid). Keep them cold, consume them regularly and they will serve you, and your bowel, well.

Another wonderful fatty substance that I want to touch on is lecithin. Lecithin contains two critical nutrients: choline and inositol. I've recommended lecithin to many of my clients who needed to increase their production of bile (choline is a critical constituent of bile). Both choline and inositol also dramatically increase stool size. Note, however, that because lecithin promotes bile flow it is best avoided if you suffer from an active gallstone.

The incredible flavor of the Hot Detox recipes comes from the large amount of coconut. You will have the chance to try lots of recipes that incorporate not just the tasty flakes but also coconut butter, oil, milk, beverage, cheese and yogurt. According to traditional Chinese medicine, coconut is warming in nature, so coconut is an ideal pairing with cool green produce to bring a dish into balance. It also is rich in medium chain triglycerides (MCTs) that convert to beta-hydroxybutyrate. BHB is an alternative fuel source to carbohydrates that your body uses to make energy. More important, BHB forms ketones, which protect the brain, reduce inflammation and directly increase liver detoxification. For more information on how a ketosis menu may benefit you, be sure to check out the Hot Detox online program at www.JulieDaniluk.com.

Boosting Your Hot Detox: On to the Liver

Making the recipes in the Hot Detox will cover all five solutions, but if you need extra help getting your bowels moving then it might be time to move some liver *qi* (your circulating life force, pronounced "chee"). If your liver is sluggish and needing a little extra encouragement, the next chapter will explain how to wake it up.

Give Back to Your Liver

Life loves the liver of it.
—Maya Angelou

The liver is the main organ responsible for processing all the toxins that both occur naturally and enter the body (through ingestion, inhalation or absorption). Did you know that the liver performs over 400 functions a day? Can you imagine having to multitask that much? One of the amazing things that it does is convert fat-soluble toxins (such as benzene, a carcinogen in the fumes from your car exhaust) into water-soluble compounds that can then be eliminated from the body via your kidneys or bowels. We are quite lucky that the liver can deal with such a wide range of toxic chemicals, drugs, solvents, food additives and pesticides. Even more remarkable, it's one of the only organs in our body that can regenerate itself. It continues to function even when 80 percent of liver cells are damaged or removed.

It's time to give your liver some love. Liver cleansing is one of the most incredible things you can do for yourself, no matter where you stand in terms of overall health. If you have robust health, it's a good idea to do at least two liver cleanses a year to keep your liver working optimally and to prevent diseases further down the road. If you're suffering from any kind of health challenge such as hepatitis, chronic fatigue or an inflammatory condition that prevents the uptake of nutrients, then you should be very gentle with yourself when going through the process of liver detoxification. Otherwise, cleansing toxins too quickly can cause a healing crisis. This occurs when the cells release toxins into circulation but the elimination organs (liver, kidneys and bowels) are not able to eliminate them fast enough. The toxins remain in circulation, leading to fatigue, fever, headaches, nausea and poor coordination. Because the Hot Detox is a gentle, food-based program, it is much less likely to cause a healing crisis, but you should still move at your own pace.

Phase 1 and Phase 2 of Liver Detoxification

Liver detoxification works through two phases: Phase 1 is oxidation and Phase 2 is conjugation, or joining together. The enzymatic reactions of Phase 1 convert incoming toxins into substances that Phase 2 can process out of the body. Ideally, both phases work in sync, creating a flow that efficiently removes toxins from the body. However, Phase 1 speeds up in response to drugs, alcohol and coffee because your body wants to get rid of these substances as fast as possible. The problem is that Phase 2 may not have sped up at the same rate as Phase 1, potentially creating a huge pileup of toxins in the liver.

To understand the process, try to imagine your liver as a conveyor belt in a factory. At the beginning of the conveyor belt, you have Phase 1. This phase processes a toxin (a pesticide, for example) and sends it on to Phase 2 to pick up the rest of the work. This handoff of toxins from Phase 1 to Phase 2 is called the intermediate phase. Phase 2 does

most of the heavy lifting, with six different pathways that require specific nutrients to function optimally and to successfully process the toxin out of the body. If you are deficient in nutrients or proteins or have a genetic variation that makes that detox pathway weak, your Phase 2 does not have the materials that it requires to work and the conveyor belt hits a standstill. You end up with a buildup of toxins. Let's get Phase 2 working efficiently with the nutritious meals found in the Hot Detox!

A Deeper Look at Detox Pathways

We are about to geek out on some cool science in this section. I want to arm you with the facts because you may hear people say that cleanses are not scientifically validated. The fact is, your detox pathways are complex mechanisms that don't always operate at peak efficiency. It is just incredible how many nutrients you really need to run your detox pathways, and the Hot Detox program will provide them all! I encourage you to read this in-depth investigation, but if you are short on time and trust that I have your back with all this research, you can jump to the next section.

Phase 1: Oxidation

The Phase 1 pathway uses enzymes as part of the cytochrome P450 system to oxidize toxins, making them more soluble in water (most toxins are fat soluble and cannot be eliminated without this process). Phase 1 can also convert toxins via hydrolytic and reductive reactions, but for the sake of simplicity we will focus on oxidation. There are a

How the Liver Processes Toxins

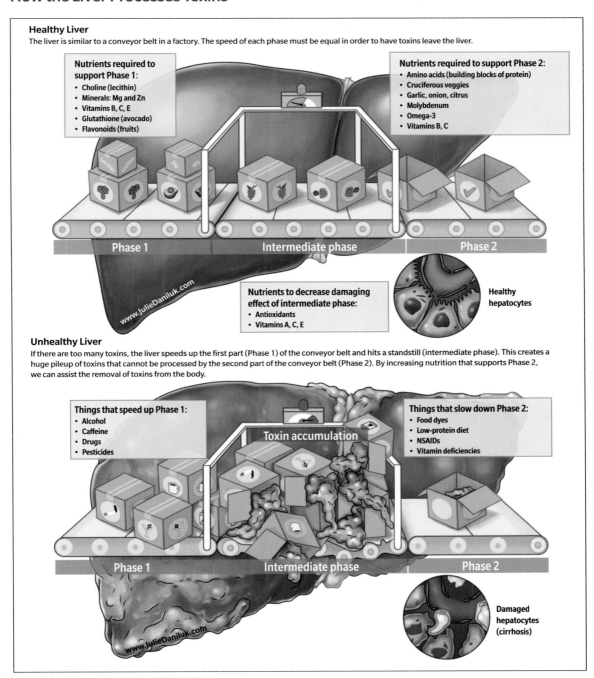

Healthy Liver

The liver is similar to a conveyor belt in a factory. The speed of each phase must be equal in order to have toxins leave the liver.

Nutrients required to support Phase 1:
- Choline (lecithin)
- Minerals: Mg and Zn
- Vitamins B, C, E
- Glutathione (avocado)
- Flavonoids (fruits)

Nutrients required to support Phase 2:
- Amino acids (building blocks of protein)
- Cruciferous veggies
- Garlic, onion, citrus
- Molybdenum
- Omega-3
- Vitamins B, C

Phase 1   Intermediate phase   Phase 2

www.JulieDaniluk.com

Nutrients to decrease damaging effect of intermediate phase:
- Antioxidants
- Vitamins A, C, E

Healthy hepatocytes

Unhealthy Liver

If there are too many toxins, the liver speeds up the first part (Phase 1) of the conveyor belt and hits a standstill (intermediate phase). This creates a huge pileup of toxins that cannot be processed by the second part of the conveyor belt (Phase 2). By increasing nutrition that supports Phase 2, we can assist the removal of toxins from the body.

Things that speed up Phase 1:
- Alcohol
- Caffeine
- Drugs
- Pesticides

Toxin accumulation

Things that slow down Phase 2:
- Food dyes
- Low-protein diet
- NSAIDs
- Vitamin deficiencies

Phase 1   Intermediate phase   Phase 2

www.JulieDaniluk.com

Damaged hepatocytes (cirrhosis)

The Nutrition We Need to Run Our Lives — Phase 1

Pathway	What it detoxifies	Nutrients required	Inducers	Inhibitors
Phase 1 (Cytochrome P450 enzymes) **Reactions:** • Oxidation • Reduction • Hydrolysis • Hydration • De-halogenation	**Drugs** • Codeine • Warfarin • Amitriptyline • Atorvastatin • Steroids • Ibuprofen • Acetaminophen **Food** • Caffeine • Vanillin **Nutrients** • Fatty acids • Arachidonic acid **Environment** • Alcohol • Benzopyrenes • Insecticides	• Vitamin C • Magnesium • Protein • Riboflavin • Niacin • Pyridoxine • Folic acid • Vitamin B12 • Glutathione • Flavonoids • Phospholipids	**Drugs** • Alcohol • Nicotine • Steroids • Acetylsalicylates • Caffeine **Food** • Cabbage • Brussels sprouts • Broccoli • High-protein diet • Oranges **Nutrients** • Vitamin C • Niacin **Herbs** • St. John's wort **Environment** • Paint fumes • Pesticides • Exhaust fumes	**Drugs** • Montelukast • Antihistamines • Stomach acid secretion–blocking drugs **Food** • Grapefruit juice • Curcumin • Onions (quercetin) • Red chili peppers (capsaicin) • Dill, celery, caraway and parsley **Other** • Aging • Intestinal bacteria toxins • Charcoal-broiled meats

number of different P450 enzymes, and each one acts on a different set of compounds (such as drugs, insecticides, pollutants, etc.).

The cytochrome family of enzymes plays an important role not only in the detoxification of drugs, but also in drug interactions. Interestingly, although Phase 1 is a necessary step in the elimination process, it can actually increase free radicals and create products that are even more dangerous than those being detoxified if Phase 2 cannot keep up and finish the job. The good news is the Hot Detox helps take the burden off the Phase 1 pathway by avoiding alcohol and excessive caffeine.

Intermediate Phase

As the toxins are processed in Phase 1, they become metabolites that are highly reactive. The toxins produce more free radicals once they have been oxidized. In a perfect world, the metabolites from Phase 1 pass into Phase 2 pathways and are excreted. But it is dangerous if this brief transfer becomes a "holding tank." If the metabolites are not able to move along to Phase 2, a toxic pileup can occur on the only road out of town. Let's hit that home again: if you are missing the necessary nutrition to run the Phase 2 pathway efficiently, free radicals can damage your liver cells. This is why a diet high in antioxidants (such as vitamins A, C and E) is important for liver protection at this stage. Fortunately, there are many foods and supplements that balance out these two pathways, clearing out toxin traffic jams. The Hot Detox program is rich in these important nutrients.

Phase 2: Conjugation

During Phase 2, the now oxidized toxic compounds are combined with another substance (such as sulfur or cysteine) to render them less harmful and able to be eliminated via urine or stool. Phase 2 reactions include glutathione conjugation, glucuronidation, amino acid conjugation, acetylation, methylation, sulfation and sulfoxidation. These pathways are outlined in the table and explained below. Phase 2 requires both energy and specific nutrients for proper functioning.

Glute a Thigh On

Glutathione is an antioxidant compound created from the amino acids glutamate, cysteine and glycine. It is mainly involved in the detoxification of heavy metals, carcinogens and xenoestrogens (foreign chemicals that can mimic hormones) through a process called glutathione conjugation. This is the act of joining together the toxic chemicals with glutathione via an enzyme called glutathione S-transferase.

Numerous substances have been shown to support glutathione levels, including N-acetylcysteine (NAC), beta-hydroxybutyrate (BHB), S-adenosyl-methionine (SAMe), milk thistle and vitamin C. Glutathione levels can be depleted if a highly active Phase 1

(due to a high intake of caffeine, alcohol or drugs) creates increased levels of free radicals. Acetaminophen is also well known for depleting glutathione levels.

Run That Nation

Glucuronidation is a critical detoxification step in which glucuronic acid (an oxidized substance with a chemical structure that is similar to glucose) is joined with hormones, drugs, pollutants or bile acids. The enzyme UDP-glucuronosyltransferase increases this detoxification pathway, while the enzyme beta-glucuronidase minimizes it. Research has shown that calcium D-glucarate and glucaric acid inhibit beta-glucuronidase, which supports detoxification. These compounds are found in apples, citrus, milk thistle and cruciferous vegetables like broccoli, rapini, collards, cauliflower, bok choy, kale and cabbage. Elevated beta-glucuronidase activity is associated with an increased risk of hormone-dependent cancers (breast, prostate) and colon cancer, possibly due to a decrease in this detox pathway.

Congrats Amigo

Amino acid conjugation describes how numerous amino acids, such as arginine, glutamine, glycine, ornithine and taurine, combine with toxins to neutralize them. Glycine is one of the most important amino acids for Phase 2 detoxification, but taurine, glutamine, arginine and magnesium are also important nutrients.

ACE-lebration

Acetylation is a process that removes drugs and carcinogens from the body by joining acetyl coenzyme A with toxins via

The Nutrition We Need to Run Our Lives — Phase 2

Pathway	What it detoxifies	Nutrients required	Inducers	Inhibitors
Glutathione	**Drugs** • Acetaminophen • Nicotine **Environment** • Insecticides • Epoxides (derived from polycyclic aromatic hydrocarbons) • Heavy metals • Carcinogens • Xenoestrogens	• Glutathione • Vitamins B2 and B6 • Vitamin C • N-acetylcysteine • Glycine • Cysteine • Glutamine • Methionine • Zinc • Copper • Manganese • Selenium	**Food** • Brassicas • Limonene **Herbs** • Citrus, dill, caraway • Gingko	**Nutrients** • Deficiency of vitamin B2, glutathione, selenium or zinc
Glucuronidation	**Drugs** • Acetaminophen • Morphine • Muscle relaxants • Coumarins	• Glucuronic acid • Glucaric acid • Calcium D-glucarate • Glutamine • Magnesium • Vitamins B3 and B6	**Drugs** • Birth control pills **Food** • Fish oils • Limonene **Environment** • Cigarettes • Phenobarbital	**Drug** • Aspirin
Amino acid	**Drug** • Aspirin **Environment** • Benzoate (food preservative)	• Glycine • Taurine • Glutamine • Arginine • Ornithine • Magnesium	**Nutrient** • Glycine	**Food** • Low-protein diet
Acetylation	**Environment** • Sulfonamides • Mescaline	• Acetyl coenzyme A • Vitamins B1, B2, B5 and C		**Nutrients** • Deficiency of vitamins B2, B5 or C
Methylation	**Drugs** • Dopamine • Epinephrine • Histamine • Cancer drugs	• Folic acid • Choline • Vitamins B12 and B6 • S-adenosyl-methionine	**Nutrients** • Choline • Methionine • Betaine • Folic acid • Vitamin B12	**Nutrients** • Deficiency of folic acid or vitamin B12

The Nutrition We Need to Run Our Lives — Phase 2 (*continued*)

Pathway	What it detoxifies	Nutrients required	Inducers	Inhibitors
Sulfation and sulfoxidation	**Drugs** • Estrogen • Acetaminophen • Serotonin • Steroids **Food** • Sulfites • Garlic compounds **Nutrients** • Vitamins C and D **Environment** • Aniline dyes	• Cysteine • Methionine • Molybdenum • Taurine • Zinc • Copper • Manganese • Selenium • Sulfur • B vitamins	**Nutrients** • Cysteine • Methionine • Taurine	**Food** • Tartrazine (yellow food dye) **Nutrient** • Molybdenum deficiency **Drug** • Non-steroidal anti-inflammatory drugs

the enzyme N-acetyltransferase. People with impaired acetylation often have drug reactions (for instance, to sulfa drugs) and can be helped with increased vitamin B1, vitamin B2, vitamin B5 and vitamin C.

Math Elation

Methylation is the addition of a methyl group (a single carbon and three hydrogens) to another molecule. SAMe is the primary methyl donor and requires adequate levels of methionine, vitamin B12 and folic acid for synthesis. Methylation is important for the metabolism of several pharmaceuticals as well as neurotransmitters. It also plays a role in excreting heavy metals and regulating gene expression (which is critical for longevity). People who carry gene variations as seen in MTHFR (methylenetetrahydrofolate reductase) gene mutations can have poor methylation. We must do our due diligence to assist this pathway through

healthy nutrition. Our mental well-being and long-term health depend on it.

Surf's Up

The mineral sulfur is essential for both the sulfation and sulfoxidation parts of this pathway. Sulfation is the pathway used to metabolize sulfur-containing molecules (drugs or foods) and to enzymatically eliminate and detoxify sulfite preservatives. Sulfation increases the capacity to dissolve bile acids and enhance excretion of toxins through the kidneys and bowels. The enzyme sulfur-transferase is in charge of eliminating hormones, neurotransmitters and drugs like acetaminophen. Sulfites (a preservative in processed foods, wine and drugs) are processed by sulfoxidation via the enzyme sulfite oxidase. The mineral molybdenum is an important cofactor for sulfite oxidase and ensures optimal detoxification.

Gold at the End of the Rainbow

After exploring all those pathways, I hope you have a better understanding of the importance of good nutrition in order to have all the required vitamins, minerals, amino acids and antioxidants for an effective detoxification. This is why juice cleanses and fasts are not as effective in detoxification, because they lack fiber, amino acids (from protein) and possibly other crucial nutrients. Adding supplements such as NAC and milk thistle, and eating cruciferous vegetables (for their sulfur and selenium content) can help improve the result of your detox by inducing the Phase 2 pathway and protecting against free radicals. However, all of the nutrients necessary for an effective detoxification are part of the Hot Detox, which is why it is so amazing and beneficial. Here are some more solutions to boost your liver.

Hot Detox Solution #1: Eat a Rainbow

Give your liver a good cleanse by focusing on real, whole foods. Focus on organic produce because it contains many phytonutrients that assist the liver in detoxification. This is why during the Hot Detox, we will be eating 7 to 10 servings of vegetables and 2 to 3 servings of fruits per day. You might be thinking, How on earth am I supposed to get that many servings of organic fruits and vegetables every day? It's actually quite easy when you incorporate juicing and blending into your daily routine. We will be relying heavily on blended shakes and soups. And the food in the Hot Detox is absolutely delicious—so much so that you'll want to continue to relish the recipes even after the cleanse!

Sour and bitter foods are especially important for liver detoxification because they encourage the flow of bile, which increases the elimination of toxins from the body. Certain herbs and teas, called cholagogues (substances that promote the discharge of bile, such as turmeric and dandelion) can be great in assisting with liver detoxification. But some of the cholagogues are bitter, and who wants to eat bitter foods? Actually, if you pair something bitter with something sweet, you'll fall head over heels in love with it! For example, chocolate is the most craved food in the universe, and the most consumed beverage on the planet is coffee. Both are highly bitter substances, but when we pair them with something sweet, we love them. Other great examples of delicious bitter foods include arugula, dandelion, rapini and burdock. The Hot Detox pairs bitter foods with sweetness so that you can fall in love with the recipes and help your detoxification pathway at the same time.

We will also concentrate on foods that are especially detoxifying to maximize the cleansing power: carrots, dark leafy greens of all kinds, beets and cruciferous vegetables. Cruciferous vegetables, in particular, contain sulforaphane and indole-3-carbinol, both of which assist specific pathways of detoxification. Cruciferous vegetables should be prepared by chopping and cooking them gently to maximize benefit.

Hot Detox Solution #2: Give Yourself an Oil Change

Liver detoxification is improved when we include good-quality fats in our diet. In today's world, most people eat poor-quality

or rancid fats, which cause terrible disso-
nance in the liver. On this cleanse, we're
going to give you an oil change by eliminating harmful, rancid fats and enjoying
healing omega-3s. Omega-3s make the
body's cell membranes less rigid and
more permeable, allowing toxins to be
effectively exchanged in and out of the
cell. Safe sources include algae, flax, chia,
walnut, camelina and sacha inchi seeds.
Due to their powerful anti-inflammatory
benefit, sustainable fish (such as ancho-
vies, black cod, herring, mackerel, salmon
and sardines) are included in the Hot
Detox menu during Phases 1 and 3. It is
also important to enjoy lots of coconut oil
because you can utilize it as a fuel source
without burdening the liver.

Hot Detox Solution #3: Bulk Up with Fiber

Soluble fiber is a key factor in both liver and
bowel detoxification. It dissolves in water
and can be found in flaxseeds, chia seeds
and foods high in pectin (apple, citrus), to
name a few. Soluble fiber can help the gallbladder and bowel flush excess bile, allowing
the liver to function more easily. Soluble fiber
mixes easily into shakes or warming soups.
How much is enough? Women need a minimum of 1 ounce (28 grams) of fiber and men
need 1.27 ounces (36 grams) of fiber daily.

Hot Detox Solution #4: Look for Nutrients

Certain antioxidants and nutrients really
help the liver perform its job correctly.
NAC is one of the more powerful nutrients
required for Phase 2 detoxification of the
liver, but there are many others, such as
alpha-lipoic acid, l-taurine, methionine,

Eat the Rainbow

Beyond being a feast for the
eyes, every color brings with
it a nutritional strength. By
eating a rainbow of foods,
you are sure to ingest nature's
finest multivitamins.

7–10 servings per day

RED	Red onion Red bell pepper Strawberries Tomato	**LYCOPENE/VITAMIN C** Reduces free radicals Prevents cancer Prevents heart disease
ORANGE	Carrots Mango Pumpkin Sweet potato	**BETA-CAROTENE** Neutralizes free radicals Heals gastrointestinal tract, skin and lungs
YELLOW ORANGE	Grapefruit Lemon Orange Peach	**VITAMIN C/FLAVONOIDS** Boosts immune system Promotes collagen production Has anti-cancer properties
GREEN	Collard greens Kale Spinach Swiss chard	**B-VITAMINS** Help prevent cancer Reduce homocystine Help repair DNA
PALE GREEN	Broccoli Brussels sprouts Cabbage Cauliflower	**INDOLES/LUTEIN** Help prevent cancer Reduce the risk of macular degeneration
BLUE	Blackberries Blueberries Blue algae Concord grapes	**ANTHOCYANINS** Are powerful antioxidants Have anti-cancer properties Promote heart health
RED PURPLE	Acai berries Purple grapes Plum Purple carrots	**RESVERATROL** Fights free radicals Helps control inflammation Lowers blood pressure
WHITE	Chives Garlic Leek Onion	**SULFUR COMPOUNDS** Help remove toxins Help improve circulation Suppress inflammation
BROWN	Amaranth Flax Kasha Quinoa	**FIBER** Helps control blood sugar Regulates bowel movements Helps remove toxins

selenium, zinc and choline, that also support Phase 2.

We need to also make sure we are getting adequate vitamins to assist with liver cleansing, including vitamins A, C and E. These vitamins are available through quality food sources. Sources of vitamin A include dark leafy green and orange vegetables, while we get vitamin C from our orange and red fruits, and vitamin E comes from delicious nuts and seeds. The Hot Detox menu plan will ensure that you will get loads of the vitamins and nutrients required for liver detoxification because it is based around whole foods.

Note: If you would like to take supplements while on the Hot Detox, look for natural vitamins that are free of genetically modified corn, fillers, binders and other added ingredients. Artificial, chemically derived vitamins can add an extra burden to your liver.

Hot Detox Solution #5: Enjoy Herbs and Spices

Certain herbs and spices can actually protect your liver, making them great choices to include during the Hot Detox program. Milk thistle, schisandra and turmeric are some of my favorites. Burdock and artichoke are also popular choices, as is dandelion. Many of the recipes in the Hot Detox menu include these herbs and spices, but they can also be taken as supplements. A complete list of powerful herbs and their specific detox benefits can be found in the Hot Detox online program at www.JulieDaniluk.com.

Hot Detox Solution #6: Drink More Fluids

Like bowel cleansing, liver cleansing requires good hydration. Water helps everything stay lubricated and assists the bowels with carrying away liver toxins. The good news is that the Hot Detox includes adequate amounts of fluid through healing teas, shakes and soups — which will benefit both your bowel and liver.

Your Gallbladder: The Unsung Hero

You can't talk about the heroic role of the liver without mentioning its trusty sidekick, the gallbladder. The gallbladder is a pear-shaped hollow structure located on the right side of the abdomen directly under the liver. Its primary function is to act as a reservoir to store and concentrate bile (the digestive liquid produced by the liver) that is not immediately used for digestion. When food enters the small intestine, a hormone called cholecystokinin is released, which signals the gallbladder to contract and secrete bile into the small intestine through the common bile duct. As we saw in Chapter 2, bile helps the digestive process by emulsifying fats and neutralizing acids in partially digested food.

An excess of cholesterol, bilirubin or bile salts can cause the stored bile to crystallize and form gallstones. Gallstones are small, hard deposits inside the gallbladder. A person with gallstones will rarely feel any symptoms until the gallstones reach a certain size, or unless the gallstones obstruct the bile duct. If this occurs the gallbladder can become inflamed and infected (a condition known as cholecystitis).

Risk Factors for Gallstones

Did you know that 20 percent of women will have a gallstone by the time they are 60? In fact, before menopause women are twice as likely to develop them than men. Why? Women experience different periods of hormonal flux in a lifetime, and gallstones are more likely to form during pregnancy, use of birth control pills and hormone replacement therapy. There is also an increased risk with age, obesity, diabetes and rapid weight loss. Genetics plays a large role in the prevalence of gallstones, and people with African or Native heritage should take extra care.

It might come as a surprise to you, but hidden food allergies can negatively affect your gallbladder. For instance, people who have celiac disease have reduced cholecystokinin release, meaning that their gallbladder doesn't receive the signal to release bile for digestion. Their bile sits in the gallbladder much longer than normal, and therefore has a higher chance of causing gallbladder issues. Unfortunately, people are not always aware of what foods they are sensitive to, so it is important to discover what those might be. This can be done through paying attention to how you react to certain foods after coming off the Hot Detox. Blood tests for food intolerances (IgG) and food allergies (IgE) are available through your naturopathic doctor.

Attack of the Stones

The pain of a gallbladder attack may be dull or sharp and excruciating, and can be so intense that it can take your breath away. The pain may be experienced on the right

How Do You Know?

Certain symptoms may indicate that your gallbladder is starting to form stones:

- An excess amount of gas, bloating, and abdominal distention
- Pale stools that are fatty and float to the surface
- Stools with a more rancid smell than usual
- Increase in belching
- Indigestion or vomiting
- Abdominal pain, particularly on the right side under the ribcage
- Loss of appetite, or sudden nausea after meals

Headaches, severe fatigue and anxiety are also quite common during a gallbladder attack. If you have more than three of these symptoms in conjunction, or if any of these symptoms are very severe, it's a good idea to get an ultrasound scan of your gallbladder to make sure you don't have gallstones.

side near the liver or in the center of the abdomen, but it may also radiate to the back right shoulder blade or between the shoulder blades. It is common for gallbladder attacks to start late in the evening and go through until morning. Interestingly, this correlates with the time (11 p.m. to 1 a.m.) that traditional Chinese medicine says vital energy flows through and cleanses the gallbladder. If you are consistently waking up between 12 a.m. and 3 a.m., your body might be telling you your gallbladder or liver needs attention.

As soon as you start to experience symptoms, you should avoid eating or drinking.

Natural Gallstone Prevention and Relief

The suggestions below are for people who may be at high risk of developing gallstones and those who have small gallstones that do not need medical treatment.

Foods to avoid:

- High-fat foods (especially unhealthy fats such as trans fats, hydrogenated fats, denatured-pasteurized and processed vegetable fats, excessive amounts of saturated animal fats and fried foods). Note: If you are presently experiencing gallstones, you may need to reduce healthy fats until your symptoms are under control.

- Dairy (especially high-fat cheeses, milk, ice cream)

- Sugar (refined cane, beet and corn sweeteners)

- Gluten-containing grains (wheat, spelt, kamut, barley and rye)

- Certain enzyme supplements that can inflame gallbladder symptoms (check with your naturopathic doctor)

- Eggs

- Bananas

Foods to increase:

- Pure water. Before a meal, drink warm water with lemon juice or apple cider vinegar. This aids in tonifying the digestive system, encourages motility and helps the small intestine absorb nutrients better.

- Green and yellow vegetables, squash, beets, dandelion greens and root, fruit, fresh lemon juice, roasted or stewed lean meats, poultry and fish. You may need to lightly steam or cook your vegetables before eating them because raw vegetables can be harder on your gallbladder. Be sure to chew your food very well to assist in the digestive process.

- Bitter herbs and vegetables such as globe artichokes, dandelion, gentian, turmeric, cardamom, burdock and ginger, which help flush bile from the body.

- One tablespoon of lecithin once a day before a meal, which helps you produce more bile. Sunflower lecithin is best because it is not genetically modified.

- Slippery elm bark, which helps to heal the lining of the digestive system. Add slippery elm powder to applesauce or make into a tea.

Even drinking water can inflame your gallbladder and aggravate your symptoms. Herbal remedies and supplements can force the gallbladder to work harder, so they should also be avoided until you are symptom-free. One of the most helpful things to do if you think you are having a gallbladder attack is to lie face down with your stomach on a heating pad. The heat and weight will help soothe the spasms in the gallbladder and bile ducts, and mitigate the pain. If this method relieves your symptoms, then you are most likely dealing with a gallbladder issue as opposed to a digestive complaint.

During an attack, you want to reduce the inflammation and spasms to decrease the chance that a stone is pushed out into the bile ducts. I recommend a tissue salt protocol of natrum sulph, calcarea phos, natrum phos, and magnesia phos. These can be taken individually or combined in a formula. Take four small tablets of each remedy every 10 to 15 minutes during a severe attack until the symptoms have resolved. If the pain isn't decreasing, then a stone may be caught in the ducts, which requires immediate medical attention.

Having the Gall to Keep It

Although gallbladder attacks often subside on their own, they will recur, so you should take steps to prevent them. When gallbladder symptoms are recurrent, medical doctors commonly recommend surgery to remove the gallbladder (known as cholecystectomy). Although surgery is necessary in some instances (if the gallstones are lodged in the bile ducts, or if the gallbladder is about to burst), gallbladder removal may not always be the answer. Surgery may lead to other issues down the line, such as reduced ability to digest fats, painful inflammation at the gallbladder bile duct site, weight gain (especially around the waist), abdominal distention, flatulence and diarrhea. Without the gallbladder, bile made by the liver can no longer be stored and concentrated between meals. Instead, the bile flows directly into the intestine as the liver produces it. If you have your gallbladder removed, you must choose healthy fats such as algae oil, organic coconut oil, organic olive oil, raw nuts and seeds (well chewed or made into a butter), and molecularly distilled fish oil.

The great news is that by following the Hot Detox you can reduce your chances of developing gallstones in the first place.

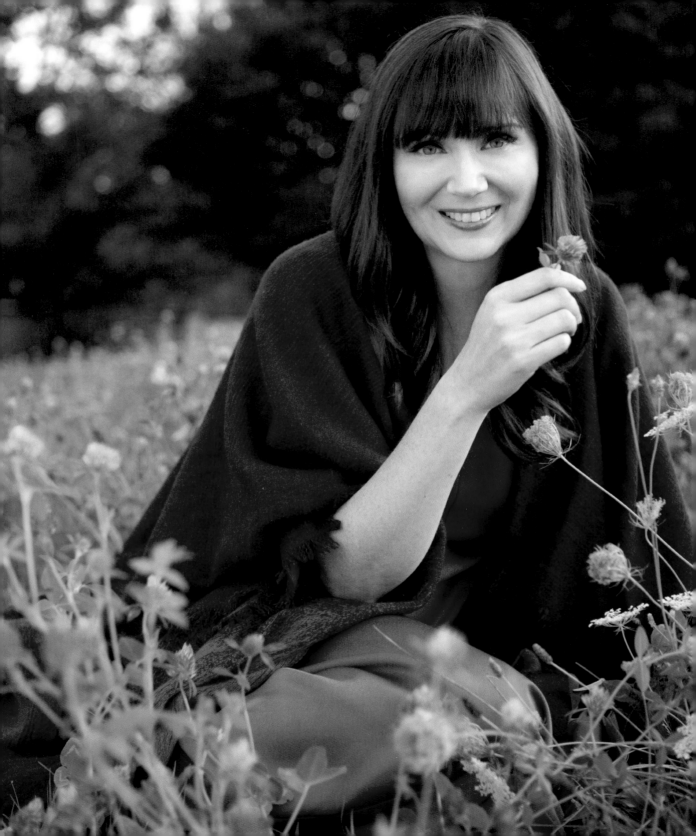

Love Your Lymph

Nothing is impossible.
The word itself says I'm Possible.
—Audrey Hepburn

Your lymphatic system is like a city's curbside garbage and recycling collection system. Can you imagine all the trash that would accumulate in the streets without it? The same is true in your body, where the lymph removes any toxin that gets into or is produced by your body and reroutes it to the organ that can best evacuate it. Whatever doesn't belong in our organs and tissues gets picked up in the lymphatics and flagged as an "invader." Because the lymphatic system is made to act as a filter, it isn't specific to any particular toxins. The lymphatic system is also a vital part of the immune system, working like a highway to carry your immune troops. The network of lymphatic vessels sits alongside the blood vessels in your body. Unlike the circulatory system, in which the heart pumps the blood, the clear lymphatic fluid has no pump and relies on the movement of your muscles to flow. For this reason, it is easy for your lymph to stagnate, and for toxins to accumulate. Fortunately, you can get the lymph fluid moving with some simple boosts, including a clean diet, some helpful herbs and enjoying your favorite exercise.

Food Kung Fu

In traditional Chinese medicine, lymphatic congestion is viewed as an accumulation of damp phlegm in the body. Food and herbs (e.g., bitters) that drain phlegm and dampness are therefore encouraged, while damp-forming foods such as dairy, fried and processed foods, bananas and sugar are avoided. The Hot Detox follows this effective principle. It reduces cold and damp foods and focuses on bitter and warming foods. I'm talking to you, cherries, peaches, ginger, kale, dandelion and cinnamon!

Flow from the Gut

Did you know that the mucosal lining in our gut contains most of our lymphatic tissue? It is so extensive that it even has its own name: the gut-associated lymphatic tissue. This is why a healthy diet and optimal digestion are important for a healthy lymph system. While there are no specific studies showing that certain foods or diets help cleanse the lymph, anti-inflammatory foods rich in antioxidants can be beneficial.

What are some of those foods that contain antioxidants? You guessed it—leafy greens! Leafy greens, such as spinach, kale, Swiss chard, and collard greens, are all high in antioxidants. They are important for any type of detox you are doing, including a lymphatic cleanse.

Fabulous Fat

Eating a diet high in healthy and essential fatty acids and low in saturated fatty acids is also important. Animal fats have been shown to affect the composition of lymph lipoproteins (the molecule responsible for transporting fatty acids within the body). Stay away from fried and processed foods and increase your intake of nuts, seeds and small fish.

Super Selenium

Selenium is an important mineral for the detoxification pathway and improving the immune system. In fact, studies have shown that it induces Phase 2 of the detox pathway through up-regulating an enzyme (glutathione S-transferase) known to detoxify carcinogens from the body. In addition, selenium enhances the immune response through increasing cytotoxic lymphocytes, which are immune cells able to destroy tumor cells. It also has been shown to have a direct effect on reducing lymph accumulation in those who have had lymph nodes removed.

Lymph Liberators

The Hot Detox program incorporates all the food suggestions above, but if you want to deepen your lymph cleanse then here are four top plants that increase lymphatic flow:

- Cleavers (*Galium aparine*): One of the best lymphatic system tonics available, it helps increase lymphatic circulation and reduces lymph node swelling and congestion. Dosage is 0.14–0.27 ounces (4–8 milliliters) of a 1:5 tincture 3 times per day.
- Burdock (*Arctium lappa*): Contains phenolic acids and quercetin, which help improve many of the organs involved in detox, including the lymph system.

How the Lymphatic System Removes Toxins from Your Body

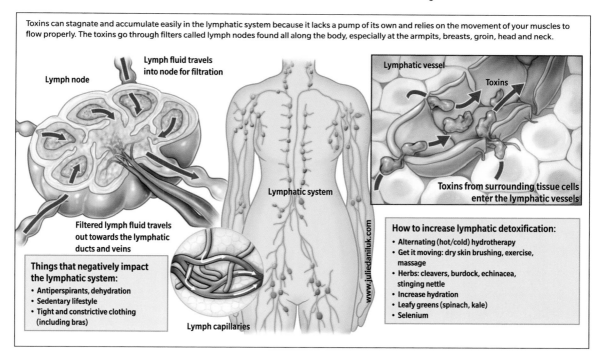

Toxins can stagnate and accumulate easily in the lymphatic system because it lacks a pump of its own and relies on the movement of your muscles to flow properly. The toxins go through filters called lymph nodes found all along the body, especially at the armpits, breasts, groin, head and neck.

Lymph fluid travels into node for filtration

Lymph node

Lymph node

Lymphatic vessel

Toxins

Lymphatic system

Toxins from surrounding tissue cells enter the lymphatic vessels

Filtered lymph fluid travels out towards the lymphatic ducts and veins

www.juliedaniluk.com

Things that negatively impact the lymphatic system:
- Antiperspirants, dehydration
- Sedentary lifestyle
- Tight and constrictive clothing (including bras)

Lymph capillaries

How to increase lymphatic detoxification:
- Alternating (hot/cold) hydrotherapy
- Get it moving: dry skin brushing, exercise, massage
- Herbs: cleavers, burdock, echinacea, stinging nettle
- Increase hydration
- Leafy greens (spinach, kale)
- Selenium

Dosage is 0.07–0.14 ounces (2–4 milliliters) of a 1:5 tincture 3 times per day. Do not take this if you have an allergy to plants in the Asteraceae family.

- Purple coneflower (*Echinacea angustifolia*): This herb is really good at enhancing and balancing the immune system. It stimulates natural killer cells to fight off cancer cells, decreases edema and is anti-inflammatory. Dosage is 0.03–0.14 ounces (1–4 milliliters) of a 1:5 tincture 3 times per day. Do not take purple coneflower if you have an allergy to plants in the Asteraceae family or if you are taking immunosuppressive drugs.
- Stinging nettle (*Urtica dioica*): High in vitamins and minerals (vitamin A, beta-carotene, vitamin C, iron), this

herb is both gentle and stimulating on the lymph system, supporting drainage. Dosage is 0.03–0.14 ounces (1–4 milliliters) of a 1:5 tincture 3 times per day.

Note: The dosages suggested here are for a 150-pound adult. Speak with your naturopathic doctor or herbalist to see if these choices are right for you.

Down with Grime

We all know that brushing our teeth and hair is important, but did you know that it is also incredibly important to brush our skin? Dry skin brushing is a traditional yogic healing practice that stimulates the lymphatic system just under the skin so that it moves more efficiently to help your body get rid of toxins. A detailed method for dry skin brushing can be found on page 76.

Wash Your Troubles Away

A popular water therapy (hydrotherapy) technique to assist in lymphatic flow is to alternate between hot and cold water. This can be done in a shower or a bath, or anywhere that offers easy cleanup. Soak your feet in a bucket of hot water (as hot as you can handle) for 7 minutes and then move to a bucket of cold water for 1 minute. Repeat this cycle three to five times. You can also use the shower to alternate hot and cold water to your legs and arms only. You always want to end on the cold phase. Learn more about hydrotherapy in the skin section on page 75.

Bust a Move

Lymphatic circulation occurs when we contract our muscles. It's actually quite simple: exercise and you will increase your lymphatic circulation. On average, lymph flows at a rate of 100 milliliters per hour at rest and approximately five times faster during the first 10 to 15 minutes of exercise. One of the best forms of exercise for moving lymph fluid is jumping on a trampoline. Save your joints while defying gravity! Bouncing on a large exercise ball while working at your desk is also a fabulous way to multitask your health efforts. And yoga flexes your muscles in a way that is highly beneficial for detoxification. Make sure to download the free Hot Detox yoga flow from www.JulieDaniluk.com.

Touch for Health

A massage therapist can give you a lymph drainage massage. The touch will often be very light to moderate (just enough pressure to stretch the skin). You may experience sensations as lymph fluids begin to move (tingling, coolness in fingers and toes, digestive noise), but the treatment should never elicit pain or discomfort.

A gentle or lymphatic massage has long been used to increase lymphatic flow and decrease lymphedema (accumulation and stagnation of lymph in the body, causing swelling). Lymphatic flow has been shown to increase following a massage in both animal and human studies. Lymphatic pumping techniques have also been shown to increase lymphatic movement through larger lymphatic channels.

It is easy to forget about your lymphatic system until something goes wrong. Not only is the lymphatic system important in fighting bacteria, viruses and other infectious agents, it also destroys old, abnormal and cancerous cells. When it is sluggish and not functioning optimally, it can completely miss identifying cancer cells. According to the Canadian Cancer Society, two out of five Canadians are expected to develop cancer during their lifetimes. Loving your lymph through detoxification can go a long way to help the immune system fight off cancer cells before they get out of hand. By enhancing lymphatic flow, we reduce harmful inflammation, eliminate toxins and sustain our juicy vitality!

Be Kind to Your Kidneys

The kettle is up to its neck in hot water yet it still sings.
—Anonymous

Now let's shine the spotlight on another important organ in detoxification: the kidneys. When your bowels are backed up, the burden falls on the kidneys to eliminate a lot of the toxins in your body. If you're having trouble with digestion and detoxification, you might notice that your urine has a foul smell and is a darker color. This is a good indicator that it is more concentrated with toxins. You may also experience a metallic taste in your mouth and bad breath.

The kidneys are two bean-shaped organs, each about the size of a fist. They are located on each side of the spine, partially protected by the lower ribs. Each kidney contains about 1 million nephrons, and each nephron contains a cluster of capillaries called a glomerulus. Think of a glomerulus as a strainer—it keeps the big molecules inside (blood cells and important nutrients like protein) but allows smaller molecules to escape (fluid, sodium, urea, etc.).

Your kidneys do a lot, but their most important job is to clear waste and toxins out of your body. They work like your local water treatment plant, removing toxins from the town water while retaining important minerals. Waste is created during regular bodily processes such as digestion and self-repair. These waste products end up in the bloodstream and must be filtered out by the kidneys to keep you healthy. Blood enters the kidneys via the renal artery and the waste is filtered from it. The waste and water filtered out of the blood produces urine, which exits the kidneys through the ureters. Urine then gets stored in the bladder until it is about halfway full, when your body tells you to go to the bathroom to pee.

Your kidneys work hard to keep a balanced level (called homeostasis) of fluid, electrolytes and key nutrients in your bloodstream. Every day, the kidneys are responsible for filtering up to 5,072 fluid ounces (150 liters) of blood to produce about 68 fluid ounces (2 liters) of urine that carries away waste products. In addition, the kidneys make three of their own hormones:

1 Renin helps control blood pressure through the balance of sodium (salt) and water.
2 Erythropoietin acts on the bone marrow to make new red blood cells. Many people with kidney disease have anemia caused by a shortage of new red blood cells, which leaves them very tired.
3 Calcitriol helps the body absorb calcium in the intestines. Without calcitriol, the body steals calcium from the bones, which can lead to osteoporosis.

Your kidneys are simply extraordinary organs. They not only help you detoxify but they metabolize critical vitamins. For example, your kidneys help activate the vitamin D that you synthesize in your skin through sunlight exposure. Unfortunately, the high-sugar-consumption diet in North America is making the kidney's job incredibly difficult. Each year the average North American consumes 150 pounds of added sweeteners, like high-fructose corn syrup and cane sugar. This puts massive stress on our kidneys because high blood sugar damages the small arteries and capillaries in them. This is why all the recipes in the Hot Detox are free from refined sugar and low on the glycemic index. (The glycemic index is a system that measures how fast a particular carbohydrate affects blood sugar level over a specific period of time. To learn more about the glycemic index, please check out my first book, *Meals That Heal Inflammation*.)

Restoring Your Kidneys with the Hot Detox

With the tremendous work your kidneys do in every moment to keep your body balanced, it's time to show your kidneys some love by eating a whole-food diet high in fruits and vegetables.

Curcumin, the active compound found in turmeric root, protects the kidneys from the damage caused by drugs, chemicals, heavy metals, diabetes and kidney surgery. Curcumin also reduces inflammatory factors in the kidneys, leading to a decrease in inflammatory damage. It is one of the only known natural substances to regenerate kidney function.

To best reap the proven healing benefits of turmeric root, grate 1 tablespoon of fresh root onto your food before eating. This can be done up to three meals a day. You will notice that I sneak turmeric powder into unusual places such as the Hot Detox breakfasts, but not to worry, turmeric is not the spicy part of curry. It is as mild as cinnamon. I suggest you make the Turmeric Spice Latte on page 145. It's divine!

How the Kidneys Remove Toxins and Waste from Your Body

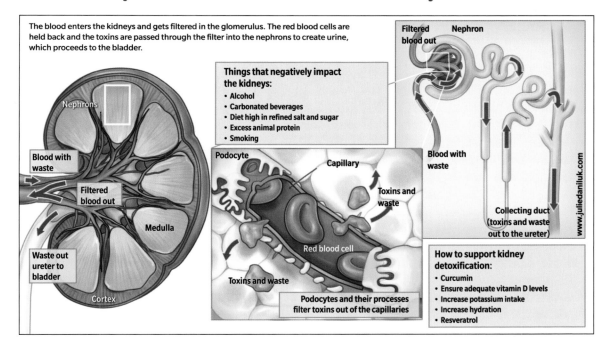

The blood enters the kidneys and gets filtered in the glomerulus. The red blood cells are held back and the toxins are passed through the filter into the nephrons to create urine, which proceeds to the bladder.

Nephrons

Blood with waste

Filtered blood out

Medulla

Waste out ureter to bladder

Cortex

Things that negatively impact the kidneys:
- Alcohol
- Carbonated beverages
- Diet high in refined salt and sugar
- Excess animal protein
- Smoking

Podocyte

Capillary

Toxins and waste

Red blood cell

Toxins and waste

Podocytes and their processes filter toxins out of the capillaries

Filtered blood out

Nephron

Blood with waste

Collecting duct (toxins and waste out to the ureter)

How to support kidney detoxification:
- Curcumin
- Ensure adequate vitamin D levels
- Increase potassium intake
- Increase hydration
- Resveratrol

www.juliedaniluk.com

One of the best foods for kidney *qi* is asparagus. It's a diuretic (produces more urine) that soothes the urinary system, increases the cellular action of the kidneys, helps to break up uric acid and is one of the five vegetables highest in glutathione. Another is tart cherry juice. Both of these foods are great for reducing gout, arthritis and kidney disease through reducing uric acid levels. Uric acid can crystallize into kidney stones and attack joint tissue.

Resveratrol, the beautiful purple pigment in grapes, berries, red-skinned peanuts, purple cabbage and purple onion, is anti-inflammatory and known to protect the heart and brain. This powerful antioxidant also helps "rustproof" your kidneys against free radicals. The recommended daily dosage to protect the kidneys for someone weighing 150 pounds is about 0.01 ounces (250 milligrams).

Your Internal Pressure Gauge

The kidneys have a major influence on blood pressure, and keeping it balanced is crucial for their own health and the health of other internal organs and tissues. Arteries also play a large role in maintaining healthy blood pressure. Picture your arteries as tubes that get inflated and deflated in a gentle rhythm every time your heart beats and pushes blood throughout your body. When you have elevated blood pressure, your arteries overinflate and become "overpressurized," which can lead to damage and micro-tears in the arterial walls. Thus, not only is high blood pressure a leading

Avoiding Contributors to Kidney Disease

The benefits of detoxification come about not only from what you add to your diet (e.g., burdock root), but equally important, what you take out. As you can see from the list below, items you remove when on a cleanse can contribute to kidney disease.

- Alcohol. At a certain dose, alcohol becomes a poison. Binge drinking ages the kidneys and is hard on the nephrons.

- Caffeine. Consuming caffeine strains your kidneys by raising stress hormones and blood pressure, and may even exacerbate chronic kidney failure. Caffeine may increase the risk

of kidney stone formation through an increase in calcium excretion.

- Carbonated beverages. Drinking two carbonated beverages a day has been linked with increased risk of chronic kidney disease and increased formation of kidney stones.

- Animal protein. The purine content of animal protein increases uric acid, which can increase the risk of developing kidney stones.

- Other contributors to kidney disease are smoking, obesity, diabetes and high blood pressure.

cause of stroke and heart attack, but it also damages the blood supply leading to and inside the kidneys. The arteries and capillaries in the kidneys can be compared to filament light bulbs. If the electrical current is too high, the filament will break and the light bulb will burn out. Similarly, high blood pressure can damage the tiny arteries and capillaries in your kidneys, decreasing kidney function.

The Hot Detox program can help you keep your blood pressure at a healthy level. When the weather is cool or seasons are changing, embark upon this 21-day cleanse to reduce sodium and increase potassium, eliminate refined sugars and boost the omega-3 fats in your diet. Over time, your blood pressure should balance out and stabilize.

Let the River Flow

The Hot Detox program is the perfect way to support your kidney function. Soothing

beverages, soups and stews ensure you get the hydration and nutrients you need to let the toxins flow out of your body. The solutions suggested below are the core of the program, so make a cup of tea and tune in.

Hot Detox Solution #1: Good Hydration

Kidneys require good hydration to work optimally. The commonly repeated saying is to drink eight cups of water a day, but this is just an approximate number for the average adult. It will not, and does not, suit everyone because we are all unique, and drinking too much or too little water can tax the kidneys. You can figure out your individual sweet spot for hydration by dividing your body weight (in pounds) in half. That number is the amount of ounces of liquid you should drink in a day. The good news is that broth, coconut water, vegetable juice, herbal tea and fruit-flavored water all count, so you don't need to strictly consume pure water.

Although it's important to hydrate, don't drink too much at one time. It is better to sip your liquids evenly throughout the day rather than chugging down a liter of water in the evening like a camel. We've all done this at one point or another—you forget to drink water all day and so you hurry and drink it down quickly. This is hard on the kidneys because they can't process all that water at once. Instead, carry a glass water bottle with you and sip delicious liquids throughout the day. Hydration is especially important for people who struggle with edema and have weak kidney function. To test your kidney function, ask your doctor for a eGFR test to measure how well your kidneys filter your blood to remove waste and excess fluid. If the number comes back under 60, it means your kidney function is compromised and needs to be monitored regularly.

Hot Detox Solution #2: The Joy of Juicing and Blending

Juicing and blending vegetables is a great way to help improve kidney function. Juicing not only hydrates but can help to dramatically increase our potassium, which in turn will help balance our sodium levels. Sodium and potassium have a beautiful relationship in the body, as both are needed for proper fluid balance, muscle and cardiac function, and nerve impulses. These minerals need to stay in balance for optimal health.

Before industrialization, humans ate whole foods naturally high in potassium and low in sodium, achieving a ratio of seven parts of potassium to one part sodium. However, in the modern diet, we often consume approximately three times more sodium than potassium, as we are no longer eating potassium-rich produce the way nature intended. Instead, we consume processed foods containing high levels of refined sodium chloride. This throws off the potassium-sodium ratio, and can impair kidney function. Consuming too much salt can also result in the body retaining more water to dilute this excess sodium, as the body cannot function with a high concentration. Retention of water leads to fluid leaking between the cells, causing swelling (edema). This doesn't mean we should never eat salt—but we should avoid refined sodium chloride that comes in fried, packaged and processed foods. The Hot Detox suggests pink rock or gray sea salt, which gives you as many as 60 trace minerals in addition to sodium. Eating healthy salts assists you in maintaining a natural balance of minerals.

We are going to balance our sodium levels and help out the kidneys by reaching for specific juices. Some of my favorite items for juices include celery, parsley and cilantro. Carrot and beet are also very beneficial because their beta-carotene is an important phytonutrient for the kidneys that reduces free radical damage.

When juicing, always remember that your juices should be 50 percent juice and 50 percent water to prevent a spike in your blood sugar. You can reduce the glycemic index of your juice by adding lemon, apple cider vinegar or up to one tablespoon of omega-3 oil. Try to wash your produce under some warm water before juicing or blending to avoid the chill.

Hot Detox Solution #3:
Let the Sun Shine In

A great way to improve kidney function is by ensuring adequate levels of vitamin D. Studies show that vitamin D decreases inflammation, decreases fibrosis in the kidneys and restores kidney function. In addition, a deficiency in vitamin D can be connected to kidney disease. This is because the kidneys help to activate this vitamin. When they are not functioning properly, they cannot activate as much vitamin D. The recommendation for vitamin D was once as low as 40 international units per day, but doctors now recommend at least 2,000 IU and up to 5,000 IU if someone is ill.

Hot Detox Solution #4:
Extending the Fuse

In traditional Chinese medicine, the kidneys are your source of vitality. When you are in great health physically, mentally and emotionally, the relaxed parasympathetic yin state is in balance with the sympathetic yang state. The kidneys are incredibly important to the regulation of the body's energy (*qi*), and we have to increase our kidney function to have that verve, that energy, that drive—or what I like to call juicy vitality.

Interestingly, the adrenal glands sit on top of the kidneys. Your adrenals make your stress hormones: adrenaline (aka epinephrine), noradrenaline (aka norepinephrine) and cortisol. All your pep comes from your adrenal glands. Because your adrenal glands are physically attached to your kidneys, if your adrenals get worn down by stress, your kidneys can be affected. Conversely, if your kidney function is sluggish, your adrenal glands may get exhausted. I find it truly amazing that traditional Chinese medicine linked the kidneys to energy and vitality for thousands of years, and today science demonstrates that the adrenal glands are the body's energy spark plug. Another key factor in energy production is that the kidneys are in charge of how we utilize iron, which carries oxygen to every cell.

Our body's stress response is well adapted for dealing with short-term stress. If a lion chases us, our body undergoes physiological changes to stay and fight or run away—commonly known as the fight or flight response. When we look at our full email inbox, sit in a traffic jam or think about taxes, we turn on those physiological stress responses. These responses are a problem when they are activated over the long term. It is exhausting for the adrenal glands, and terrible for your health.

The whole point of relaxation is to reduce this stress response. What is your method of relaxation? You can improve kidney energy by indulging in what you love and what relaxes you, whether it's painting, photography, journaling, walking, reading, listening to music or anything that calms down your nervous system. If you're upset or having a bad day, calling up a friend who is an amazing listener is so good to do.

Energy-moving exercises such as yoga flows (see the Hot Detox online program for a good one) are great rejuvenating techniques. Qigong and tai chi are also wonderful ways to increase the vitality of your kidneys with low-impact, conscious movement. Meditation is another key way to nourish and restore not only the kidneys, but your adrenal glands as well.

Exercise the Breath with Lung Detoxification

Breath is the bridge that connects life to consciousness, which unites your body to your thoughts.
—Thich Nhat Hanh

Few people consider the lungs an important organ for detoxification, yet they are. Think about your lungs' major function: breathing. As you breathe in air, they are primary points of contact with the outside world. Lungs bring oxygen to every cell in the body via the blood. They also remove the carbon dioxide waste made by your cells, and regulate the concentration of hydrogen ions in your blood to assist in balancing the pH of your body.

Lungs are like trees. Inside both of your lungs are the bronchial tubes or bronchi, which branch into smaller tubes called bronchioles. Bronchioles end with alveoli, which are like bunches of tiny air balloons covered in a mesh of blood vessels called capillaries. The capillary network is an interchange where your veins transfer carbon dioxide from the blood to be exhaled, while your arteries take in oxygen to carry throughout your body. The spongy elastic lung tissue stretches, the diaphragm relaxes and the muscles between your ribs expand the chest cavity as you breathe in.

Purge the Plate

An important step in cleansing the lungs is to look at what you're eating. Inflammatory foods and certain chemicals can affect the lining of the lungs, leading to increased mucus production. Having a diet filled with things like artificial sweeteners, high-fructose corn syrup, white sugar or genetically modified foods can cause serious inflammation in the lungs, which dramatically affects your breathing. Fortunately the Hot Detox will remove all the negative foods that contribute to lung inflammation.

An allergy to dairy, or other foods such as wheat, corn or nuts, can also increase mucus production and leave you with excessive amounts of mucus in the lungs, reducing your body's ability to eliminate toxins. The Hot Detox eliminates many commonly allergenic foods, but you should completely avoid any foods you already know you are allergic to. From a traditional Chinese medicine point of view, some foods are damp and can lead to an increase in mucus production. Conversely, healing and drying foods can help decrease mucus and free your lungs. Foods such as onion, bone broth and hot teas are all great options to help you thin out mucus and thus help your body detoxify. The Hot Detox is full of delicious recipes that incorporate these amazing foods.

There are several herbal remedies that help to cleanse the lungs as well. Licorice soothes the lungs and fuels the adrenal glands, which significantly boosts energy and helps recovery from chronic fatigue syndrome and adrenal exhaustion. Lobelia has been shown to help with asthma and to clear the airways. Mullein is an anti-inflammatory, an antibacterial and a natural expectorant that has been used for centuries for healing the lungs and digestive tract and for reducing phlegm. Other good herbal remedies include angelica, elecampane and coltsfoot, which all act as expectorants to eliminate unhealthy mucus buildup. Foods such as ginger, garlic, thyme and horseradish are also excellent for treating dampness and phlegm and act as expectorants.

Cruciferous vegetables, including broccoli, kale and cabbage, have a positive effect on lung function. As we saw in Chapter 3, sulforaphane is a naturally occurring chemical in cruciferous vegetables that increases the amount of active Phase 2 enzymes in the liver. These enzymes are responsible for neutralizing the harmful toxins we breathe every day that can cause respiratory distress in sensitive people, especially those with respiratory conditions such as asthma.

Lemons and limes are great options for thinning and loosening mucus. They are sour and astringent, causing the superficial layer of the mucous membranes to tighten up and decrease fluid secretion. In the respiratory tract, this reduces the production of mucus and helps loosen the remaining mucus so you can expel it.

Try drinking beet juice, especially when you are exercising. Studies have shown that it helps to increase tolerance of exercise and reduce the demand for oxygen during exercises such as walking or running. These effects can be attributed in part to the beetroot raising nitric oxide levels in your blood.

In general, the foods and herbs in the Hot Detox that soothe the gut lining also soothe the lining of the lungs. In fact,

How Toxins Enter and Exit the Lungs

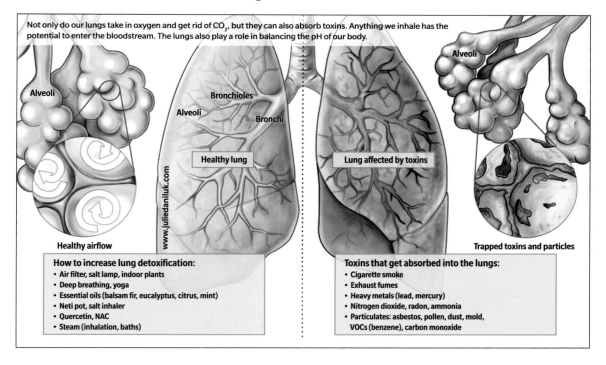

Not only do our lungs take in oxygen and get rid of CO_2, but they can also absorb toxins. Anything we inhale has the potential to enter the bloodstream. The lungs also play a role in balancing the pH of our body.

Alveoli

Alveoli

Bronchioles

Alveoli

Bronchi

Healthy lung

www.juliedaniluk.com

Lung affected by toxins

Alveoli

Healthy airflow

Trapped toxins and particles

How to increase lung detoxification:
- Air filter, salt lamp, indoor plants
- Deep breathing, yoga
- Essential oils (balsam fir, eucalyptus, citrus, mint)
- Neti pot, salt inhaler
- Quercetin, NAC
- Steam (inhalation, baths)

Toxins that get absorbed into the lungs:
- Cigarette smoke
- Exhaust fumes
- Heavy metals (lead, mercury)
- Nitrogen dioxide, radon, ammonia
- Particulates: asbestos, pollen, dust, mold, VOCs (benzene), carbon monoxide

there seems to be an association between gastrointestinal conditions and bronchial hyper-responsiveness. Studies are showing that asthma is more prevalent in people who also have irritable bowel syndrome. The reason for this is still unknown, but there seems to be a connection between an inflammatory state in the bowel (e.g., excess mucus in the bowel) and a similar manifestation in the lungs (e.g., excess mucus in the lungs) via both neuromuscular dysfunctions and inflammatory messengers.

Own Your Breath, Find Your Peace

The muscles in your neck and around your collarbones generally assist with breathing when the function of your primary muscles of respiration is impaired. If your breathing is shallow, it puts strain on these accessory muscles and causes pain, especially in the neck. Deep breathing is a great way to counteract this muscle strain and improve lung detoxification. Yogic breathing exercises, a practice called *pranayama*, train the lungs to increase air capacity, which increases the exchange of oxygen and carbon dioxide from the blood. *Pranayama* also increases respiratory stamina, relaxes chest muscles, expands the lungs, raises energy levels and calms the body in patients with asthma. One study that looked at antioxidants in a group of people trained in yoga for six months found they had higher levels in their bodies than the control group. Multiple scientific studies reveal that yoga practices that use abdominal breathing reinforce diaphragmatic efficiency to increase lung volume during normal breathing and improve lung function overall.

I encourage you to try this *pranayama* exercise: Take a full inhalation of breath for 5 seconds, hold the breath for 5 seconds and then fully exhale for 10 seconds. Repeat nine times. When this becomes easy, increase to a 10 count on the inhalation, hold for 10 seconds, then exhale for 20 seconds. For more great breathing practices, check out www. shambu.co.

If you are not into yoga, any cardiovascular exercise in an oxygen-rich, non-toxic environment is also a great option for the lungs. Cardio increases ventilation and oxygen uptake, and uses sheer force to loosen up mucus from the airways, leading to increases in pulmonary function. Go for a gentle hike, a bike ride, a swim or anything that gets your heart pumping to enjoy the benefits during the Hot Detox—but be careful not to overdo it because cleansing can take some important energy. Consider that exercising in high-traffic areas, or pounding the pavement on busy streets, can expose your lungs to many toxins. Instead, I suggest you practice nature therapy (called *shinrin-yoku* in Japan) by going for a walk on a nature path or hiking trail. Not only will your lungs be more efficient in detoxifying the body, an extra bonus is that unpaved trails are easier on your joints! And let's not forget the many other benefits nature therapy can have, especially on mental health.

Taking It to New Heights

The Hot Detox program is complete with the healing recipes and gentle exercise, but if you feel the need to deepen your lung detox, here are some bonus opportunities.

Knack for Success

N-acetylcysteine (NAC) is a metabolite of the amino acid cysteine. It can be taken orally or inhaled using a nebulizer. Prized for its ability to make mucus thinner so it can be removed easily, it is also an antioxidant, protecting the lungs against oxidative stress and releasing some of that toxin-containing mucus from your lungs. Remember from the liver chapter how NAC is a precursor of the potent antioxidant glutathione? Well, glutathione also has an affinity for the lungs. In addition, NAC is a chelating agent (the Latin root word means "to claw"), which aids in the detoxification of some environmental toxins, such as methylmercury, by clawing on to toxins and moving them out of the body. NAC is a safe supplement, but reported side effects include gastrointestinal upset so discontinue if concerned and consult a holistic medical doctor or naturopathic doctor if you're on medication. Clinical trials have used a dosage of 0.014–0.02 ounces (400–600 milligrams) twice per day (depending on body weight).

Coming Clean

We can enhance the quality of our air through many measures, such as air purifiers. Do not use ozone purifiers, which the American Lung Association warns can harm the lungs. Investing in a high-quality air purifier for your home can go a long way towards making your home a toxin-free zone. Air purifiers fitted with HEPA (high-efficiency particulate air) filters are highly efficient at removing both large and small particles, with a particle removal efficiency of 99.97 percent for particles 1.8 inches (0.3 micrometers) and larger. HEPA filters have been shown to reduce airborne allergens, such as cat dander, mold spores and cigarette smoke. And don't forget your vacuum! It is one of the biggest offenders, allowing dirt to recirculate into the air if it is not equipped with a HEPA filter.

Other simple ways to improve indoor air quality could include enjoying a salt lamp, which creates negative ions that help dirt drop to the floor, or growing more house plants, since they absorb carbon dioxide and excrete clean oxygen. In addition, plants can increase air humidity and remove dust particles. Certain houseplants even act as air detoxifiers. Their leaves can absorb toxins and volatile organic compounds (VOCs) from the air, then translocate them to the plant's roots, where microbes break them down and use them as food sources. Based on an assessment of 50 household plants, the top 10 plants that can remove toxicants from the air and are easy to care for are areca palm, lady palm, bamboo palm, rubber plant, dracaena, English ivy, dwarf date palm, ficus, Boston fern and peace lily. Spider plants, Kimberley queen fern, gerbera daisy and corn plant are other great choices.

The other important step to take is to deal with any sources of allergens and toxins within your house. As we try to clean and purify our air, we need to look at certain things in our home that might contribute to indoor air pollution.

Sack Your Mat

Mattresses off-gas toxins for years, exposing you to those toxins each and every day. Since you spend six to eight hours each day in bed, you can imagine the impact on your lung health. Your mattress and bedspread also trap certain particles like dust mites that can really affect skin. Having a good-quality, certified organic mattress is ideal, but if that is not financially possible, consider putting a dust mite cover on your bed and getting your mattress vacuumed with a high-pressure steam cleaner. This will kill all sorts of microbes and dust mites, and will make a dramatic difference in how you breathe and the condition of your skin. It will even help soothe itchy eyes.

Other substances in our home that release toxins on a regular basis are things like deodorants, detergents, cleaners, candles, chemical air fresheners and anything else that we might inhale. And don't forget your yoga mat! If you use a yoga mat, be sure to choose a good-quality one made from natural rubber to avoid inhaling toxic chemicals. Many yoga mats are coated with phthalates and made from PVC (polyvinyl chloride), and ADA (azodicarbonamide), which can all cause health issues and disrupt hormonal balance. Non-toxic yoga mats are available. For instance, Gaiam sells mats that are free of the six most common phthalates (though they are still made of PVC). Barefoot Yoga and Jade Yoga sell mats made from natural rubber.

By exposing ourselves to these chemicals, we are constantly taxing our lungs. Give your lungs a break by using natural personal care and cleaning products, and switching to natural beeswax candles. You'll immediately notice the difference in the air you breathe!

The Scoop on Pets and Poop

When it comes to air quality, it's important to address not only dust mites but also pet allergies. Many people are allergic to their pets, whether or not they are aware of it. Of course, this doesn't mean you need to get rid of your beloved furry friend. There are things that can be done to help decrease possible allergens. For instance, you can treat your pet's skin with tea tree or lavender oil to reduce the amount of dander. You could also switch your pet to a grain-free or more natural diet because, just like humans, some animals are allergic to their food, which can lead to an increase in dander production. Furthermore, it's best not to let your pet sleep in the same bed as you, or sit on your bed or pillows, especially if you know or suspect you are allergic.

Homeopathic remedies can help you balance your immune system and reduce your allergic reaction to your pet. Increase your quercetin intake by enjoying more onions, apples and foods rich in vitamin C such as berries and citrus. If this still doesn't help and you continue to suffer from terrible allergies that affect your airways, consider plant sterol therapy to help balance your immune system.

Pet waste is a common irritant for people. When cleaning a litter box or picking up your pet's feces, you should wear gloves and maybe even a mask if you have a fragile immune system, respiratory problems or skin conditions of any kind. Handling your animal's feces without rubber gloves is extremely dangerous because the feces can assault your microbiome. If you use plastic bags to scoop, make sure they are free of any holes and thick enough to prevent contamination.

Lastly, think twice before you let your cat or dog lick your face. It might be a loving gesture, but you might be receiving more than love! When you kiss someone, you exchange 80 million bacteria with that person. During the Hot Detox you will work to get your human microbiome back to its optimum condition. Taking on your animal's microbiome is not a good idea.

Keep Calm and Spa On

Powerful yogic and Nordic spa techniques to improve your respiratory system can augment the Hot Detox program. Relax and learn these extra practices at your own speed during or after the formal 10 or 21 days.

Chew the Fat

Oil pulling is an ancient yogic practice first recorded 1,500 years ago in the early Ayurvedic text *Charaka Samhita*. Oil pulling is a way to clean your gums and teeth by rinsing your mouth with oil. Simply swish a tablespoon of sesame or coconut oil around your mouth, flushing it between your teeth for 10 to 15 minutes, and then spit it out. Don't swallow the oil, because it now contains all the microbes, toxins and mucus it collected in your mouth.

Oil pulling therapy has been shown to strengthen teeth, gums and jaws and can prevent bad breath, bleeding gums, dry throat, cracked lips and tooth decay (by killing the streptococcus bacteria that causes cavities). One of the most surprising benefits of oil pulling is tooth whitening. The therapeutic oil works as a solvent, lifting the stains of coffee, wine and tea off your pearly whites.

Net Benefits

The neti pot is like a little teapot with a spout that is the perfect size to fit in your nostrils. The neti pot facilitates *jala neti*, a technique to rinse the sinuses and clear out the mucus that results from allergic reactions or infections. It is a wonderful remedy for reducing reactions to airborne allergens such as pollen, pet dander and mold spores. Rinsing the sinuses washes away the allergens, reducing the swelling, itching, redness and pain. It is also possible to reduce your chances of catching a cold with sinus rinsing, because it washes away bacteria before they can grow into a full head cold.

Here's what you will need for an effective sinus cleanse:

- A ceramic neti pot. I recommend choosing ceramic because salt is corrosive, and plastic or metal can release toxins into the salt water.
- Pure white sea salt, as finely ground as possible, so that it dissolves easily. Avoid table salt, which has added ingredients, and unrefined gray or pink salt, which can contain fine sand that will not dissolve and could potentially lodge in the sinuses.
- Distilled or boiled water at body temperature. Test the temperature by putting a drop on your forearm or taking a sip. If it feels comfortable, you're good to go. Avoid using standard tap water as it can be contaminated with chlorine, fluoride, hormones and other toxins.

Follow these steps:

1. Add 1 teaspoon of salt to 2 cups of water. Stir until completely dissolved.
2. Stand over your bathroom sink (or a large bowl). With the warm saline solution ready in the pot, simply lean over and tilt your head sideways. Insert the neti pot spout fully into the upper nostril.
3. Breathe through your mouth while you gently pour the water into the nostril. After a few seconds, the water will begin to stream out of your lower nostril. If some water drains into your throat, it's okay. Simply spit it out. Work on your technique and the angle of your head until the water only flows into and out of the nasal passages. Use half the solution in the first nostril.
4. Raise your head to vertical and blow your nose into the sink. Do not blow forcefully or you can drive the solution up into the sinuses and ear canals. This is not a serious problem, but is not the intended result. Inhale through your mouth and continue to blow out your nose until it is clear. When most of the water has been dispelled, inhale in and out quickly to speed-dry your sinuses.
5. Repeat on the other side using the other half of the solution.
6. Clean the pot and dry for next use.

Use the neti pot up to twice a day when dealing with sinus inflammation (allergies or infections) or as needed. If you cannot use a neti pot or are traveling, consider getting a clean saline mist from a health-food store or drugstore to rinse your sinuses.

Escape the Fuzz

Do you have a white coating on your tongue? This foul deposit is an accumulation of mucus, microbes and toxins that can be reintroduced into the body unless manually removed. In Chinese medicine, a thick coating reflects an excess of dampness and is commonly associated with poor gut function. A white coating can mean that there is excess cold in the body, giving you yet another great indication that the Hot Detox is just what your body needs. When the coating is caused by an excess cold or damp condition, addressing the underlying problem may be the only way to prevent it from coming back (scraping the tongue will simply remove it temporarily). The Hot Detox will be fantastic at helping your body heal itself in a gentle and warming way by reducing cold and damp or greasy foods.

Cleaning your tongue can also slow the growth of plaque on the teeth. Purchase a tongue scraper from a health-food store or simply use a sharp-edged silver spoon. Start from the back of the tongue and move forward, gently scraping the surface of the tongue, taking care not to hurt the sensitive area at its root. Do this in the morning and at bedtime during the Hot Detox.

Free by the Sea

Energizing, healing, mesmerizing and meditative—being by the sea simply makes us feel better. For thousands of years, humans have flocked to the ocean to reduce lung ailments. Breathing in salt air acts as a cleansing agent and treatment for viruses, bacteria and fungus. Today, health practitioners use salt to fight lung infections and provide relief from pollution sensitivities and respiratory inflammation.

If you are unable to get to the ocean, you may want to consider purchasing a ceramic salt inhaler. This device looks like a clay lighthouse with an opening at the top to allow you to inhale the pure unrefined salt. Unrefined salt contains 84 minerals and trace elements needed for optimum health. The bottom of the inhaler contains the salt, which is placed between two porcelain filters.

Place the tip of the salt inhaler into your mouth and breathe in through your mouth. Hold your breath for a brief moment, and then exhale through your nose. Work up to doing this for 10 minutes a day. To avoid contaminating the inhaler with microbes, *do not* breathe into the inhaler.

Essential Oil Therapy

Inhaling essential oils can also be an effective way to assist the respiratory system. The chart on page 70 lists my favorite essential oils and their purifying actions. You can add this to your daily wellness routine as a gentle accent to your cleanse.

To do this, add a few drops of essential oil to water in a humidifier. Spend 10 to 15 minutes per day breathing over the humidifier with a towel draped over your head, until your nose, head and lungs open up and you can breathe easily. If you don't have a humidifier, do the same with a bowl of hot water.

Oil of oregano can be used internally to kill candida, fungus, parasites and bacteria. However, oil of oregano is not recommended for steam inhalation, as it is too potent and may irritate the sinus. Due to its power to kill off some healthy gut bacteria, it is important to reserve this strong internal remedy for when you are sick.

Day Tripping

You might think that a trip to the spa is indulgent and purely for relaxation, but the science around heat therapies may have you looking for the nearest one. The Hot Detox encourages the heat therapies found in health spas because they can dramatically increase your detoxification success.

The most commonly known heat therapy treatment is the dry sauna. Dry saunas have been shown to increase alkalinity and oxygen concentration in the blood. A single sauna treatment can elevate the oxygen concentration in blood by 53.3 percent and increase blood pH by 0.8 percent. This more alkaline state allows your immune system to better fight disease. Saunas also increase your antioxidant protection mechanism via increased nitric oxide production. Antioxidants are critical for detoxification and also reduce the rate at which your body ages. Therapeutic saunas have also been shown to reduce stress hormones, blood pressure, chronic fatigue and even fibromyalgia!

You should leave a dry sauna if the heat becomes uncomfortable or if you begin to feel faint or ill. I prefer saunas that use infrared heaters because they induce sweat at much lower temperatures (see Chapter 7 for a fuller discussion). This allows everyone to enjoy a sauna without the risk of overheating.

Another popular heat therapy is the steam room. The health of the respiratory system is improved when you can spend some time inhaling steam. Steam can help you secrete the mucus that carries away allergens and toxins, and on top of that, high air humidity helps break up the mucus and make it easier to release. This improves lung function and decreases airway inflammation.

What is so great about adding humidifying air to your heat treatment is that it can help minimize heat loss in the respiratory tract. For people with reactive airways, bronchoconstriction develops when heat is lost in the respiratory tract. When the airways cool down, smooth muscles are affected and react through a reflex that leads to constriction. Increasing the heat and humidity of the air helps prevent bronchoconstriction and allow for maximum airflow rates when you breathe.

Breathing hot, humid air also improves the osmotic gas exchange in the lungs, improving blood detoxification. Adding steam to your sauna treatments has also been shown to be beneficial. A study of wet sauna treatments showed an increase in the concentrations of circulating catecholamines, which relax the bronchial smooth muscle. Translation: You can breathe easier!

Remember that as the Hot Detox program heals your gut, your lung tissue will also improve, resulting in deeper detoxification.

Wake Up and Smell the Healing

Essential oil	Action and indications
Juniper berry (*Juniperus communis*)	• Purifies and detoxifies • Stimulates digestion • Antiseptic • Diuretic • Enhances elimination Increases circulation in the kidneys • Increases the elimination of uric acid and toxins
Helichrysum (*Helichrysum italicum*)	• Stimulates liver cell function • Chelates (claws and carries away) chemicals and toxins • Detoxifies • Anti-inflammatory • Increases blood circulation • Protects and regenerates tissues through scavenging free radicals
Lemon (*Citrus limonum*)	• Antiseptic • Improves microcirculation • Increases white blood cells and immune function • Encourages the elimination of wastes • Decreases constipation • Tonifies the kidney and liver
Grapefruit (*Citrus paradise*)	• Antiseptic • Detoxifies • Diuretic • Helps cleanse the skin, kidneys, lymphatic system and vascular system
Fennel (*Foeniculum vulgare dulce*)	• Improves digestion • Stimulates the circulatory system and respiratory system • Antiseptic • Cleanses the tissues and helps with the elimination of toxins • Tonifies the kidneys, liver and spleen

Essential oil	Action and indications
Patchouli (*Pogostemon cablin*)	• Anti-inflammatory • Antiseptic • Improves digestion • Clears fluid retention by increasing urination • Helps with the process of elimination of toxins
Peppermint (*Mentha piperita*)	• Anticarcinogenic • Antiseptic • Supports digestion • Stimulates the gallbladder • Increases and stimulates perspiration • Anti-inflammatory
Lavender (*Lavendula angustifolia*)	• Anti-inflammatory • Antitumoral • Antiseptic • Prevents the buildup of excessive sebum on the skin • Promotes cell regeneration and renewal
Orange (*Citrus aurantium*)	• Anti-inflammatory • Increases circulation • Decreases fluid retention through increasing urination • Encourages the elimination of wastes
Eucalyptus (*Eucalyptus spp.*)	• Anti-inflammatory • Antiseptic • Mucolytic (dissolves or breaks down mucus) and expectorant • Increases the blood's oxygen supply so that more oxygen can be delivered to cells
Balsam fir (*Abies balsamea*)	• Strong antimicrobial • Mucolytic and decongestant • Antispasmodic • Anti-inflammatory • Helps stimulate the respiratory system and immune system

7

Love the Skin You're In

*The finest clothing made
is a person's own skin.*
—Mark Twain

Your skin is the largest organ of your body. You have up to 18 square feet (two square meters) of skin, and it is approximately 0.12 inches (three millimeters thick). This outer layer is the cover that protects your internal muscles, bones, ligaments and organs. What we touch and place on our skin is absorbed into the body, making it one of the largest areas for toxin absorption.

In the past it was thought that the skin worked simply as a barrier to block toxins from entering the body. But in the last decade we have started to understand how permeable the skin really is. Some drugs administered to the surface of the skin can be absorbed more efficiently than when taken orally. So if the skin can absorb medications more effectively than swallowing, what is happening when you put on lotions or cosmetics that are full of toxic chemicals? Or when you dye your hair, handle gasoline or use toxic cleaning products without protective gloves?

Fortunately, the skin is also one of the places that the body is best able to get rid of toxins. Your skin detoxifies primarily by sweating. Science has shown that the body releases certain toxins through sweat more easily than through bowel movements or urine. The human body has 4 million sweat glands, or about 650 sweat glands per square inch of skin. This means 650 opportunities per square inch to sweat out impurities! You can help the skin do its job properly by keeping it in tiptop shape.

The Hot Detox program supports skin detoxification beautifully. The warming foods in the cleanse will help you break a sweat to wick away toxins through your skin. The orange produce speeds up the flipping of skin cells, all the cooked greens provide hormone balance, and the red fruits and veggies help you make more collagen. The suggestions outlined in this section are not all essential requirements of the Hot Detox program, but try to add in as many as you feel comfortable with. The science is clear that moving toxins out through the skin is one of the fastest ways to help stubborn inflammatory symptoms such as skin conditions, weight gain and even memory loss.

Moving to Move Toxins

Muscle contractions during exercise rapidly elevate internal temperature, which is followed by an increase in sweat rate. Moreover, exercise reduces cardiovascular-related death by 50 percent and decreases incidence of type 2 diabetes and specific cancers (in particular breast cancer by 20–30 percent and colon cancer by 30–40 percent). How is this possible? Sweating has been shown to increase production of special heat-shock proteins, which activate the immune system, specifically macrophages, and are therefore important in cancer prevention. Heat therapies also increase activity of natural killer cells,

which are tumor antigens that directly result in the death of tumor cells.

Your body regulates heat generation and preservation to maintain an internal temperature between 97.8 degrees to 99 degrees Fahrenheit (or 36.5 to 37.2 degrees Celsius). When body temperature tips above this range, the hypothalamus (often called the body's thermostat) in the brain responds by increasing the sweat rate to encourage our body to cool off. When you sit in a sauna or in a hot room for yoga, your body doesn't have the chance to reach equilibrium so it just keeps sweating. Sweating for half an hour is an opportunity to expel substantial toxins.

Make sure to bring an electrolyte beverage, such as coconut water with a pinch of sea salt or my Ginger Recovery Drink (page 138) to any activity that makes you sweat. Sweating drops your body's salt content, which can cause your blood pressure to plummet. Those with low blood pressure who exert themselves in a hot yoga class or try to stay in a sauna too long risk passing out.

Feel Hot to Look Hot!

Science shows that yoga performed in a hot environment demands 10 to 40 percent more energy. For every degree Celsius it goes up in the studio, a person's energy consumption goes up by 0.5 percent! Hot yoga can improve body tone, lower cholesterol, reduce weight and exert a therapeutic effect on physiological and psychological processes. Hot yoga is even associated with faster return to sleep after waking up in the middle of the night. Pairing hot yoga techniques with the Hot Detox program is a complementary way to increase results, but please take it easy so you don't overexert yourself.

Yogic postures can have a profound detoxifying effect when performed consistently. The compression applied to an organ during a posture forces blood and other fluids out of the region. Upon releasing the posture, fresh vital fluids then return to the area. Each posture also affects the nervous system. When the nerves are free to function, the organs of detoxification will be quick to follow. Enjoy the Hot Detox yoga flow created by Yogi Shambu in the Hot Detox online program.

Sweat Today, Smile Tomorrow

Some doctors specializing in chronic illness caused by environmental factors have measured their patients' sweat and concluded that sweat indeed removes toxins from the body. Studies are showing that toxic metals, phthalates and bisphenol A (BPA) are eliminated in sweat much more efficiently than in urine or any other method of detox. (Chelation therapy is possible for heavy metals like mercury, but it is very invasive and comes with possible risks and adverse effects such as hair loss, headaches and liver damage. I prefer a gentler and more natural way—to sweat it out!) Anyone struggling with hormonal imbalances can benefit from ridding the body of these harmful substances.

Heavy metals can cause damage to our memory. With an aging population, this is a growing concern. Detoxing these metals out of the body is a great way to protect and improve memory. In fact, one of my clients was frightened that she was starting to

Sugar Daddy

One of the most important factors for skin health is to stop eating refined sugar, including products that contain high-fructose corn syrup. The Hot Detox program is a great way to break your refined sugar habit for good by finding new recipes that bust your cravings. Eating sugar causes a reaction called glycation, in which the sugar in your bloodstream attaches to protein or fat and forms harmful molecules called advanced glycation end products (AGEs). The more sugar you eat, the more of these AGEs you develop. If you accumulate a lot of AGEs in your system, they begin to damage surrounding proteins, such as the collagen and elastin that keep your skin firm and elastic. So sugar literally ages you on a cellular level, making you look older!

experience memory loss. After consulting with Bryce Wylde, Associate Medical Director of the P3 Health Clinic in Toronto, high levels of cadmium were found in her blood. We started her on the Hot Detox and after 21 days, her memory returned!

Mercury and cadmium contamination may alter the gastrointestinal absorption of essential nutrients, which can lead to nutritional deficiencies and inflammatory bowel disease. Cadmium prevented my client from colonizing good bacteria in her gut, and the result was gastrointestinal inflammation. As she needed thyroid support as well, we were careful to detox her slowly and safely, as some toxins released from fat tissue during weight loss, caloric restriction or exercise may suppress thyroid function. If you suffer from hormonal imbalances, it is important to check your hormone levels with a functional medical doctor or qualified

Toxic Compounds and Minerals Released in Sweat

- Chloride, chromium, iron, magnesium, manganese, potassium, sodium, and zinc are lost in sweat and need to be replaced. Copper is often elevated in the body and therefore does not need supplementation.

- Amphetamines, methadone

- Phthalates

- Bisphenol A (BPA)

- Aluminum, antimony, arsenic, cadmium, lead, nickel, mercury, thallium and tin

- PCBs (some, but not all polychlorinated biphenyls)

health professional before undertaking heat therapies. Taking the gentle path to support metal detoxification will allow you to avoid a healing crisis.

All Gain, No Pain

If you want to speed up sweating without the need to move a muscle, then heat therapy can raise your body temperature rapidly. Sauna therapy can increase antiaging growth hormones, dilate your lungs, relax your muscles, increase oxygen consumption and aid with fat metabolism. Sauna use increases your metabolic rate and circulation by 5–10 percent and your cardiac output by 60–70 percent, which allows you to burn more calories per hour. Beyond the mental health and immune benefits of reducing heavy metals in the body, many people use sauna therapy for weight loss.

Sauna use is also shown to increase performance in endurance athletes.

However, you need to make sure you are using a high-quality and healthy device. Many saunas are made cheaply with glue, toxic wood finishes and poor-quality metal coils, which can do the body more harm than good, as heating up glue, polyurethane and metal in a small confined space is toxic. Instead, choose a quality sauna built with untreated sustainable wood and medical-grade heaters, such as the models made by Sauna Ray in Canada.

Infrared saunas are much better than old-fashioned wood-burning saunas for several reasons. First, wood sauna temperatures can be difficult to regulate and have been known to go as high as 212°F (100°C). A sauna that's too hot or dry can cause your lungs to hurt and your skin to itch. Second, an infrared sauna can be up to 30 degrees cooler yet create a more profuse sweat than a wood-burning sauna. This is because the heat from the infrared unit penetrates the body in a way that triggers a sweat response in the body. An infrared sauna is therefore safer if you are concerned about blood pressure, have chronic fatigue or an aversion to heat therapy. You get the benefits of profuse sweating without the danger of overheating.

Infrared saunas penetrate up to five millimeters into our tissues and seem better able to detoxify bismuth, cadmium, chromium, mercury and uranium. They enhance mobilization of fat-soluble xenobiotics, dramatically eliminating toxins that cause hormonal imbalance.

I think one of the best features of sweating is it increases production of enkephalin, a neurotransmitter that reduces the perception of both emotional and physical pain. So when you work up a sweat, you are better able to cope with injuries that come your way!

Full Steam Ahead

A steam bath (also known as a steam or mist sauna) has been shown to be better than a standard dry sauna for the elimination of arsenic, aluminum, cobalt, copper, nickel, lead, antimony, tin and thallium. Heat stress is higher in a dry sauna, and there is a higher increase in heart rate. Noradrenaline levels increase in both dry and mist saunas, but are higher in a dry sauna. Sweat rate and volume has also been shown to be higher in a dry sauna than in a steam bath, so you may want to steam a few minutes longer to get the same benefits, but many people find the higher humidity more comfortable.

The trouble with steam baths is they can be a hotbed for mold growth. Be sure to use one of the essential oils on page 70 to disinfect mold and protect yourself by spraying the steam bath down before using.

Good Things Come to Those Who Sweat

Thankfully, there is a movement of health-minded folk who are beginning to understand that perspiration is a critical way to expel toxins from the body. For example, having a high level of toxins in the body can affect the heat regulatory mechanisms of the autonomic nervous system. This results in a failure to sweat readily. Normally, the rate and composition of sweat is controlled by the anterior hypothalamus in the brain. When toxins disturb the hypothalamus, it

can be difficult for some people to sweat and eliminate. With heat therapy treatment, these people tended to normalize and were eventually able to sweat and eliminate the toxins. Skin brushing, nutritional changes, supplements and ample hydration can all help you to begin to sweat more effectively.

Join the Polar Bears!

A short exposure to cold water produces dilation in the vascular system that increases the blood flow to underlying tissues and organs. Some practitioners of hydrotherapy also believe submerging your body up to your neck in cold water can increase circulation to the thyroid gland. When you return to a warmer temperature, a secondary reaction of vasodilation increases blood flow to the skin and extremities.

Enjoy a heat therapy for 5 to 15 minutes, followed by a cold plunge up to the neck for 60 seconds. Rest or repeat the cycle for up to an hour. Do not submerge the head during the cold plunge or you may experience headaches and ear pain. If you are using a lower-temperature infrared sauna, you can increase the heat therapy time to 30 minutes and then take a cold shower afterwards to produce vasodilation and wash off the toxic sweat. Return for another round if desired. If you have a weak heart, be sure to check with your doctor before beginning this practice.

Contrast hydrotherapy (using hot followed by cold water) is shown to improve muscle soreness and help maintain muscle strength after exercise. It also helps lower creatine kinase levels (a marker of muscle damage) up to 48 hours after exercise. The perception of recovery was found to be superior after contrast water therapy even before there was actual evidence of physical recovery.

Studies also show significant increases in blood flow from baseline during each warm water phase of contrast therapy. Significant fluctuation (vasodilation and vasoconstriction) of lower-leg blood flow was observed, as contrast therapy created a "pumping" effect in the vascular system. This pumping of blood into and out of the tissues can profoundly increase detoxification.

Float Your Boat

Have you ever had the joy of feeling weightless? Although I am all for a nice hot bath, I have found that soaking in a local Epsom salt floatation center is even better due to the strength of the magnesium sulfate—you float, weightless, on top of the water. Incredibly, an open-faced tub filled with ten inches of water can contain up to 1,200 pounds of high-grade Epsom salt. As you float in the tub, your body experiences a lack of stimulation, which switches off your fight-or-flight stress response and returns you to a relaxed, parasympathetic response. It is the closest you can get to returning to the womb.

Floating in an Epsom salt bath increases magnesium and sulfate in the body. Your entire body chemistry changes, and you experience decreased muscle tension, blood pressure and heart rate. Blood vessels dilate, increasing cardiovascular efficiency and the supply of oxygen and nutrients to every single cell in your body. Studies indicate that floating reduces the levels of stress and stress-related neurochemicals, such as

Reasons for Decreased Sweating	
Medications	• Anticholinergics • Opioids • Clonidine • Barbiturates • Alpha-2-receptor antagonist • Alcoholism
Nervous system	• Diabetes mellitus • Multiple sclerosis • Demyelinating conditions

adrenocorticotropic hormone and cortisol. At the same time, magnesium supports the brain to release natural feel-good chemicals such as endorphins, serotonin and dopamine, which in turn reduce the symptoms of stress, anxiety and even migraine headaches. Magnesium sulfate floats also accelerate recovery following strenuous physical activity, exercise or injury, as they aid in muscle relaxation and lactic acid clearance.

As an extra bonus, Epsom salt provides usable sulfate to increase phenol sulfur-transferase, an enzyme that facilitates the important sulfation detoxification pathway. To learn more about the benefits of floating, watch my video lessons as part of the Hot Detox online program.

Brush to Look Plush

You brush your hair and your teeth, so why not brush your skin? Beyond sweating, exfoliation is one of the most beneficial ways to detoxify the skin. It helps by increasing blood flow to the skin and unclogging your pores so that sweat and toxins can be more easily eliminated. Using a loofah in the shower is helpful, but dry skin brushing is even more effective.

Dry brushing removes dead skin accumulation, improving the appearance of skin as well as opening blocked or clogged pores, allowing the skin to breathe. What's extraordinary about skin brushing, though, is that it does more than just exfoliate. It helps to increase circulation, meaning we are also working on cleansing our lymphatic system. This helps to eliminate cellular water because the lymph is responsible for collecting all of the toxins from your tissues and transporting it over to the blood.

When dry brushing, make sure you have your own dry skin brush. Your skin has thousands, or millions, of microbes running over it, and skin infections may be transferred from person to person. When choosing a dry skin brush, avoid plastic and look for natural bristles, which are the most gentle and effective for the skin. The brush should not scrape the skin, but be effective enough to exfoliate.

To effectively brush your skin, begin by making small gentle circles with the brush. Draw the brush, using this circular motion, over the surface of the skin towards the heart. Start at the fingertips and venture up the arms, always brushing towards the heart. Make sure to get the front of the arm, the back and under the armpits to massage the lymph nodes.

On your torso, circle around each breast as you dry brush. You'd be surprised how many lymph nodes and lymphatic vessels lie around the breasts. Don't forget your back (a long-handled brush will be helpful for this step). You can even skin brush your neck (very gently due to the large amount of lymph here), again tracing towards the heart. Use less pressure on your neck to prevent stressing this delicate skin.

Finish with your legs by starting at your toes and making gentle little circles up your feet and legs, all the way back to your heart. This moves your lymph fluid and helps increase circulation to the skin, encouraging the elimination of metabolic waste.

The only parts of your body that you don't want to dry brush are the sensitive areas of the genitals and nipples. When you've completed the whole body, rinse off in the shower. You'll be amazed what regular dry skin brushing will do for your skin's appearance and circulation.

Dry brushing before bathing is a great way to slough off dead skin and wash it down the drain. A session can be as quick as 2 minutes or as long as 15 minutes, depending how much time you have. Simply do as much as you can as often as you can. Daily brushing is best, but even three times a week is good. Any amount that you can commit to is wonderful self-care. A good way to remind yourself to do it is to hang your dry skin brush where you'll see it in your bathroom. If you're brushing your teeth and you spot the brush, you can take the few minutes to go through the process.

By cleansing the skin, we help take the burden off our lymphatic, digestive and elimination systems. It's a real act of self-love—a moment of body awareness that is quite meditative. I encourage my clients to recite positive affirmations to themselves while skin brushing, such as "Thank you, body, for working today. Thank you for my hands that cook my food, thank you for my legs that carry me to my family, and thank you for my eyes to see beauty in the world." As Louise L. Hay might say, "Reciting positive loving messages can 'detox' our negative thought patterns."

Bye-bye, Cellulite!

A great benefit of skin brushing that is often overlooked is the elimination of the fatty deposits beneath the skin. By disturbing them with lots of dry skin brushing, the look of cellulite can be diminished. It's not a promise, but we do know that the only way to decrease cellulite is to manually break it down. Once it is trapped in the skin, cellulite is hard to get rid of, so give extra energy to scrubbing down these areas of your body, like your thighs.

Other Ways to Flake Off

While detoxifying, avoid using excessive soap as it can reduce your ability to produce vitamin D. Your skin requires the cholesterol in your skin oils to make vitamin D, and soap removes these oils. Leaving the natural oils on the skin is also important for detoxification and internal moisture. People who use a lot of soap often have terrible dry skin irritations because they are stripping their skin of natural beneficial oils. Use soap for the armpits and genital areas, but stick to exfoliation and skin brushing for the rest of your body, using soap only when absolutely necessary.

Not a fan of dry skin brushing? A salt scrub (see page 79 for a recipe) will exfoliate dead cells and allow the skin to breathe and detoxify. Scrub the skin in a circular motion with a scoopful of salt scrub for a few minutes to allow the oil to absorb, then rinse with warm water. Your skin will feel moisturized, exfoliated and fragranced with a healthy natural scent. The salt removes dead skin and opens pores to allow for more efficient detoxing. Plus, you'll feel like a million bucks afterwards! I love how invigorating salt scrubs are and how the skin is so beautifully buttered up.

Remember to try oil pulling and tongue scraping (in Chapter 6), too, as these techniques also improve the skin. By removing toxins from the mouth, you improve the vibrancy of the skin.

Protect Your Skin Ecology

Did you know you have more than a pound of bacteria on your skin? The skin has a microbiome of its own that contains over a thousand different types of microbes. Keeping a balance of good bacteria ensures our skin stays beautiful. The superficial layers of the skin are naturally acidic (pH 4–4.5) due to the lactic acid that skin bacteria produce in sweat. A number of studies suggest that an overgrowth of negative bacteria can be a root cause of acne, dermatitis and even rosacea. A great way to naturally balance the bacteria of the skin is to use a probiotic mask once a week. Simply break open one capsule of probiotic (look for a high-potency, broad-spectrum product) and mix it into ½ teaspoon of organic coconut oil to make a paste. Massage this paste into your face and leave it on for 30 minutes to 4 hours. Rinse gently. Some probiotic strains have been studied and shown to have specific functions. *Streptococcus thermophilus*, for instance, can increase production of ceramide (important to maintain the skin barrier and prevent skin conditions) when applied topically, whereas *Bifidobacterium longum* can decrease inflammation of the skin.

How to Make a Salt Scrub

1 Start with a two-cup widemouthed glass Mason jar with a tight-fitting lid. Do not use a plastic container as it can leach toxins.

2 Fill the jar halfway with a healthy salt. Coarse sea salt, Epsom salt, or kosher salt are all good options. Epsom salt contains magnesium, which has relaxing properties, but sea salt is less expensive.

3 Add your choice of healthy oil until the jar is almost full. Coconut, avocado, rosehip, sesame, macadamia and olive oil are all good choices. Coconut oil is great for people with skin problems as its strong antibacterial effect helps with skin infections. Do not use baby oil (i.e., mineral oil), which is a petroleum by-product. Mix the salt scrub with a spoon until uniform.

4 Stir in 30 drops of an essential oil that suits your detox needs. Examples include lavender (relaxing), peppermint (energizing), orange, lime or lemon (mood-enhancing), sandalwood (anti-inflammatory) or vanilla (aphrodisiac). Or you can try cooking extracts such as vanilla, almond, peppermint and coconut. The extracts are basically the delicious essence that is edible and the essential oil is the concentrated volatile compounds that evaporate and impart intense aroma.

Stress Less for Healthier Skin

Not only do our bodies have a central stress response system called the hypothalamus-pituitary-adrenal (HPA) axis within the nervous system, but the skin, being exposed to environmental and physical insults every single day, has its very own HPA axis as well. In fact, the skin can produce its own stress hormones. Emotional and psychological stress have been linked to skin conditions such as psoriasis, dermatitis, acne, alopecia, itchy and red skin, and aging.

The stress hormone cortisol can harm your skin. Cortisone creams (which have a similar chemical structure to cortisol) can thin your skin and cause premature aging, but so will stress. Keeping your stress levels under control is key to battling the premature aging of your skin.

Now that you know how amazing your body is at getting rid of toxins when given a chance, are you all fired up to start the Hot Detox? Part 2 will cover off all the practical steps you can take in order to detoxify yourself head to toe. In just 21 days, you will be feeling and looking up to 10 years younger! If you take on only 3 or 10 days, you can also see huge benefits. You can just do another 10-day cleanse when you can. Not only are a number of the detox practices easy but many of them are also fun, so enjoy the ride and reap the benefits.

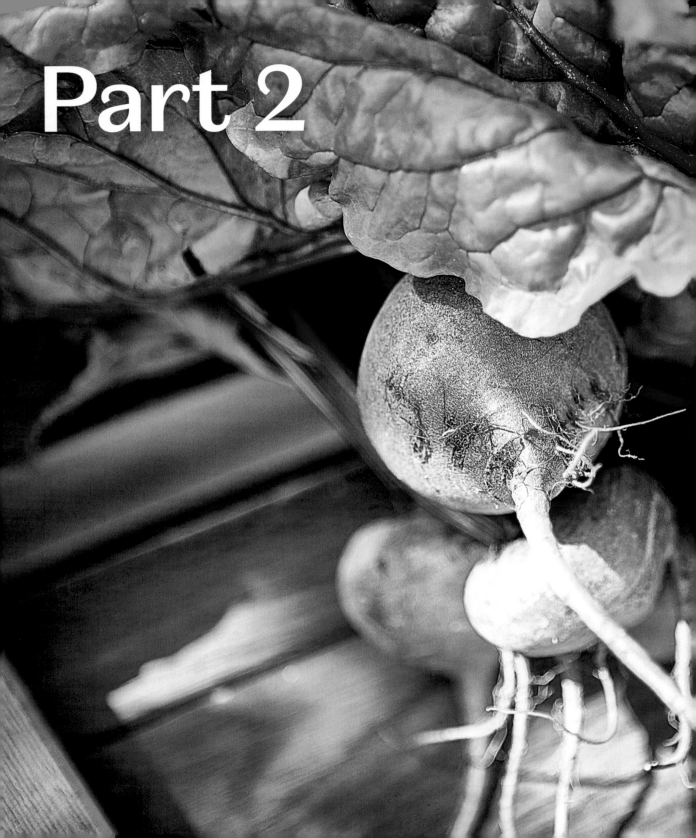

Part 2

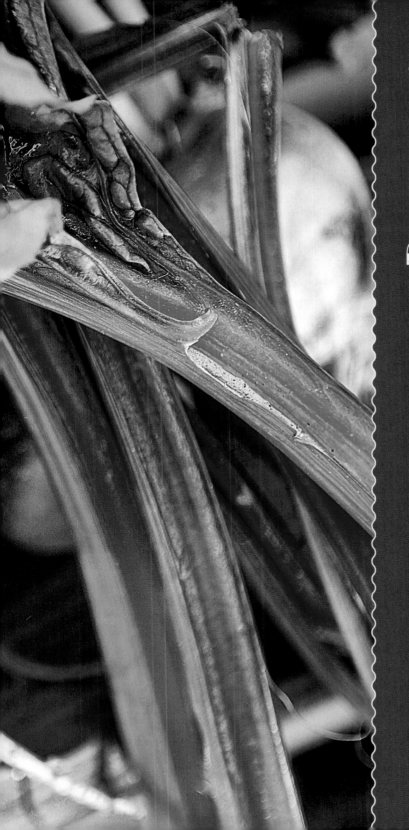

The Hot Detox Plan

"You have turned my life around. I was diagnosed with rheumatoid arthritis in 2007 shortly after the birth of our second daughter. I had difficulty walking, and my hands were swollen and painful. While the prescriptions initially helped my pain symptoms, I have now completed the 21-day program several times and had wonderful results.

Since your programs, I've run two full marathons in 2013 and 2014 as well as several half marathons, 10Ks and 5Ks. My CRP (C-reactive protein) levels that measure my inflammation have gone from an initial 15 down to being 1.8 — my lowest result yet! The program works! Thank you for everything, Julie!"

— Kelly S.K.

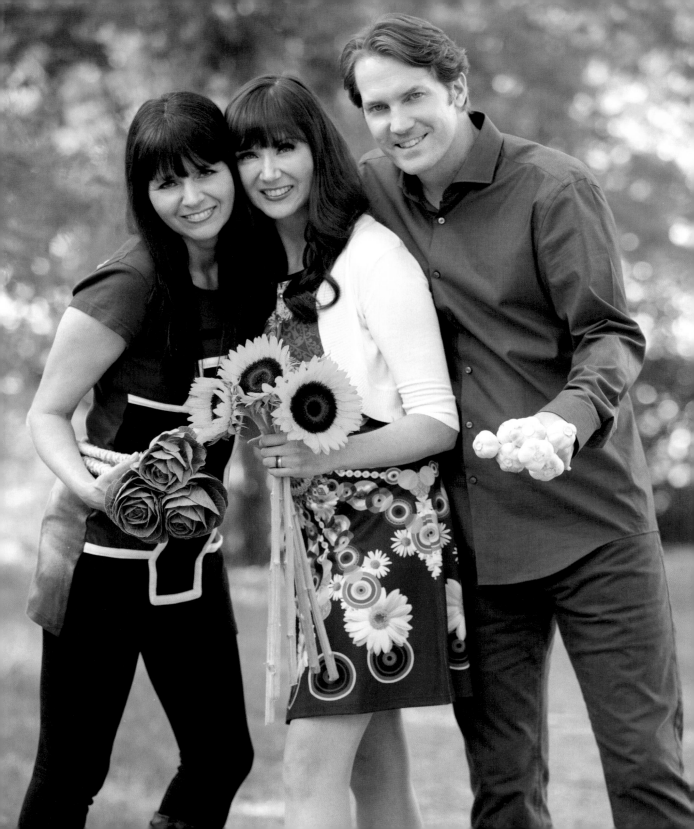

8

Getting Started

*You don't have to be great to get started
but you have to start to be great.*
—Les Brown

etting up powerfully for a detox program reduces fear, hunger and resistance. If you are fully prepared, the journey will be more comfortable and you will have a much greater chance of completing it. Take the time you need to understand why you are cleansing, the benefits you will experience and the keys for success by reading this chapter entirely. I promise that after your body gets over its regular routine of coffee, dairy, sugary snacks and gluten, your energy will be more stable and even-keeled, and you will feel fantastic.

The Hot Detox is an all-natural method of giving your system the time and conditions it needs to remove impurities and rebuild a healthy body. As described in Part 1, the Hot Detox is a food-based program influenced by the ancient healing wisdom of Ayurveda and traditional Chinese medicine. It is designed to bring the body into balance over 21 days, but I break it down into three phases to make it approachable and doable. There are also 3-day and 10-day versions of the plan in case you want to try out the Hot Detox but feel that 21 days is more than you can commit to right now. I suggest you fully commit for 21 days—it's only 3 weeks of your life! What have you got to lose besides pain, inflammation and a life of digestive discomfort? Many of my clients have found such relief that they choose to do a longer 42-day cleanse by doing two programs back-to-back. This really gives your system a thorough detox!

> I had no interest in food or cooking, and when I was on my own, I ate very poorly and had cravings for cookies and ice cream. I started to have some major intestinal problems that lasted for months. I started reading your book out of curiosity and couldn't put it down.
>
> So I started cleaning out my cupboards and buying different food. I started losing weight that first week, about 2 pounds, and it has continued at that rate very consistently since then. It is now 12 weeks, and I am down 24 pounds! I am so happy with the results as far as the weight loss goes, but also with being able to decrease or discontinue some of my medications. I also gradually tapered off my Pantoloc for reflux. I have enjoyed trying all sorts of new foods, like Hemp Hearts, maca and turmeric. Because I live alone, I will cook a full recipe and freeze what I don't eat right away in individual portion-size containers. On my lower energy or busy days I can just pull something out of the freezer.
>
> Besides the weight loss, I have been enjoying more energy, more mentally alertness and the ability to cope better with stress. What's not to like? The results speak for themselves. I am enjoying cooking again for the first time in years, and enjoying the flavor of food, without refined sugar or high levels of salt and saturated fat. When I look back, it's hard to believe how easy and smooth the process was for me.
>
> I can't say enough good things!
> — Karen M.

Luck Favors the Prepared

The beginning of the cleanse might just be the most important part. It's like any adventure: you need to get ready before you set out. If you were going to climb a mountain, you wouldn't just wake up one day and do it. You would prepare yourself physically and mentally, and also make sure you had all the equipment necessary to successfully reach the top and enjoy the journey. The Hot Detox is similar: if you're not properly prepared for the cleanse, the climb might become too steep and you could end up losing your grip. Since preparation is key to success, that's what you need to tackle first.

In the days leading up to the cleanse, focus on getting everything you need to prepare your delicious healthy meals. These are the six main kitchen tools you will need to get going on the Hot Detox:

1 A good-quality blender to prepare smoothies and blended soups, for example
2 A food processor, if you can afford it, for speed grating and chopping and making dips
3 A vegetable peeler and/or box grater so you can thinly slice (ribbon) and grate vegetables (especially if you do not have a food processor)
4 A wooden cutting board (plastic cutting boards breed the wrong kind of microbes)
5 Two excellent knives: a chef's knife and a paring knife, preferably stainless steel or ceramic
6 Glass canning or Mason jars in both pint and quart sizes, which can multitask as both water bottles and food storage

If you cannot afford a blender or a food processor, borrow one from a friend or watch for good deals on appliances, as these appliances often go on sale. If you love kitchen gadgets, a dehydrator that makes crackers, wraps and cookies at a low temperature will preserve the maximum nutrition of your detox creations. But don't worry, the recipes always give you an oven method in case a dehydrator is out of your budget.

The next main thing you need to do to prepare for this journey is to go grocery shopping for the healthy foods that you'll be enjoying on the cleanse. (For a sample detailed shopping list, visit www.JulieDaniluk.com.) Keep in mind that if you cannot afford a recommended superfood, or if it is just not a fit for your life (though I encourage you to try new things), there are always substitutions to ensure that you can do this cleanse no matter your tastes or financial situation. In fact, you might find that the recipes are less expensive than eating at a fast food restaurant. You just might save some money on this cleanse!

Now that you have the tools you need to start the cleanse, take a few days before starting the program to properly set yourself up. I want you to be really gentle with yourself, but I also want you to start trying new recipes as soon as you are inspired. This is to get yourself used to what you will be eating: remember, during this phase you're climbing to base camp and acclimating. You're adjusting to healthy tastes, and the biggest thing you have to acclimate is your tongue. This is why you should try some new recipes during this preparation phase. Your tongue is used to two predominant tastes: sweet and salty. During this preparation phase and during the 21 days of the program, your tongue may need to become accustomed to three more tastes: sour or astringent, bitter, and spicy.

Try Before You Buy

Try a small amount of a new ingredient before committing to buying a lot of it. For example, before you buy a whole bunch of horseradish, do you like it? Can you buy a tiny amount and taste it with a main dish before you start the cleanse so that you don't over-purchase something you don't like? What about ginger, which is a key component to the Hot Detox? If it's too strong a taste for you at first, try adding some honey to help you get used to it. Cilantro is another important ingredient for the Hot Detox, but a lot of people are genetically predisposed to think it tastes strange. If you're not already used to eating it, buy a small bunch of cilantro to make sure you like it. Cilantro is powerfully detoxifying, helps you drop heavy metals and is very healing, so you owe it to your body to give it a try. Of course, if you don't like it, you can substitute parsley, but you should figure that out during this preparation phase.

A big part of psyching yourself up to do a cleanse is to remind yourself that there are always ways around things that you don't like. I'm not going to ask you to do something you hate—that's counterproductive. It would train you to dislike your food, which would turn you off doing a cleanse or trying new things ever again. It's important that you not only love how you're feeling but also love the ingredients you're using, so let's make sure that happens by figuring out your likes and dislikes ahead of time.

Be Keen on Green

During this preparation phase, I also want you to try incorporating more green foods into your diet. At the apex of the Hot Detox, you will be enjoying 7 to 10 servings of vegetables and 2 to 3 servings of fruits every day. Keeping an open mind throughout the preparation phase will help you get there. Your stomach also needs to get used to eating more fiber, and you need to make sure it can actually digest raw vegetables. If you experience a sore stomach or loose stools after eating raw vegetables, then you need to stick to cooked or steamed vegetables on the cleanse, as cooking softens the cellulose and makes it easier to digest and absorb. Blending can also be an option as it helps rip the fiber apart enough to allow you to pull out all the goodness from the produce without any stress on your bowels. Testing in the preparation phase will help you know how to prepare your meals throughout the program.

What Will You Be Eating during the Hot Detox Program?

All the foods you'll consume on the Hot Detox program will be prepared in certain ways so that they are both a warm temperature and contain warming ingredients when you enjoy them. While other detox programs focus on smoothies with frozen banana or raw green salads, the Hot Detox brings the goodness and benefit of warming foods into your diet with warm smoothies thickened with avocado or hemp seed, warming teas, incredible spiced stews and cooked vegetables. The Hot Detox menu also relies on spices and warm preparation techniques to accelerate the detoxification process. These ingredients and techniques help heal and restore your gastrointestinal tract and digestive processes so that you can enjoy eating without distress.

Prepare in Bulk and Freeeeeeze!

Let's face it: there will be busy days when you just won't feel like cooking. The solution is to prepare in advance. I have to acknowledge that according to both Ayurvedic and traditional Chinese medicine theory, eating food that has been previously frozen is not ideal because freezing energetically cools the food in a way that is hard to rebalance. Saying that, I had to make the Hot Detox easy for people who work 40 to 50 hours a week! I just ask that you completely rewarm frozen food. It is better to eat rewarmed healthy food than junky food prepared with sugar, flour and harmful oils. When you have some downtime, I suggest making soups and stews in large quantities to freeze. This will save you time and energy, and you will have a wonderful meal waiting for those on-the-go days.

Buy containers that will not break when frozen (bottles with narrow tops, for example, tend to break as the contents freeze and expand). Look for something safe like wide glass containers with a safe lockable lid. Avoid plastic containers, as residue can end up in your food.

Freezing can also help you save money by stocking up on produce when it's in season. With some know-how and a good freezer, you can preserve everything from apples to zucchini. Freezing storage time for most fruits and vegetables is six months to a year, depending on how new your freezer is. Make sure to store foods at or below 0°F (−18°C), with little temperature fluctuation to avoid freezer burn.

Berries may be frozen in a single layer on a cookie sheet first, then immediately stored in bags or containers. Vegetables must be blanched, since this will destroy the enzymes that cause loss of color, flavor, texture and nutrients. To blanch, simply immerse prepared vegetables in a large amount of salty boiling water for a short time, depending on the kind of vegetable and size—an average of three minutes. Then immediately drain and refresh in ice water. Dry well and pack in freezer bags, removing as much air as possible.

Whatever you choose to freeze, be sure to put a date on the container so you know how old the food is when you go to eat it.

A Good Time Is the Right Time

The last thing to consider during the preparation phase is: Is this the right time for you to be starting this cleanse? Evaluate your life for any situations or events that might stop you from getting the most out of the Hot Detox. It's not a good idea to start this cleanse if it will overlap with an important wedding, major holidays or vacations, the birth of a baby in the family or a stressful transition at work. Look ahead on your calendar for potential hitches like parties or your regular night out with the girls/guys, and make changes where necessary to avoid awkward situations and overwhelming temptations. You may experience some symptoms on the cleanse (see page 99), so set yourself up powerfully by finding a 21-day window without massive demands on you. If that window doesn't exist, start a 3- or 10-day Hot Detox instead, and do it more frequently.

That said, you might be a person who wants to start this cleanse regardless of other priorities or demands. I have done cleanses during the most stressful periods of my life because my brain sharpens up, I feel more positive and I have more energy. For example, when I had a serious accident that resulted in a very painful injury, the first thing I did was start this cleanse. I needed my body to recover as quickly as possible, and I wanted to have the maximum amount of anti-inflammatory nutrients from produce and superfoods strengthening my body. I ate no added sugar or grains so that my brain could better cope with the stress of the terrible injury I was up against.

This might be a good approach for

you, or you might be the kind of person who needs a lot of comfort foods when convalescing. When you go swimming, do you stick your toe in and creep in slowly because you can't stand change? Or are you a person who just jumps in and gets it over with? If you're that kind of "dive in" person, you might be able to handle this cleanse regardless of what is happening in your life. If you're a "toe in" person, be loving and gentle with yourself— take this at your own pace. If you feel ready when you finally take the plunge, you will be 100 percent enrolled! You should enjoy discovering new exciting foods instead of feeling like you're entering a detox prison.

Once you evaluate your life and current situation, draw a line in the sand. Set a date for when you are going to start the cleanse and stick to it. This is the last step in the preparation phase before jumping into Phase 1, so make sure you are committed and ready to go.

> After successfully completing the 3-day detox and feeling fabulous, my husband, myself and 19-year-old university student, athletic, busy, active daughter decided to do the 21-day detox. I must let you know that I have been attending physiotherapy for a rotator cuff injury since January. I had been taking an anti-inflammatory medication for a chronic back injury as well as for helping the shoulder. However I had to stop this medication due to out-of-control, bleeding, infected eczema on my hands. The new, raw skin is now trying to heal. Coincidently, or not ... the day after completing the anti-inflammatory detox, my physiotherapist and myself noticed a 100 percent improvement in my rotator cuff! I don't believe it's coincidence at all, but rather eating food to get rid of inflammation.

> Thank you. This is what my body has been craving for!
> — Debbie D.

To Bean or Not to Bean

At this time, you also have a decision to make. You can do the full cleanse as a vegetarian/vegan, or you can do it as an omnivore, meaning you'll include eggs, poultry and fish in Phase 1 and Phase 3. There are benefits to both methods, and neither way is wrong. The choice depends on you and what your body needs. If you're already a vegetarian or vegan, or if you want to take this cleanse to the highest level quickly, you can do the entire cleanse as a vegan cleanse, including the first nine days. The main benefit of a vegan cleanse is the elimination of potential toxins from animal-sourced foods. You'll be avoiding the small amounts of heavy metals that are found in fish, and any antibiotics in convention-ally raised chicken. A vegetarian or vegan cleanse can also be a cheaper and deeper cleanse, but I personally find a lower-carb omnivore diet has the fastest results for weight balance and autoimmune issues.

Is Kale the New Beef?

If you choose a vegan cleanse, be very care-ful about your caloric intake because you're not going to have the nutrient density of animal proteins. Vegetarians have to be careful to avoid deficiencies in vitamin B12, iron, zinc, omega-3 and even protein. Making smart choices with vegetarian protein sources can help you avoid this problem. For example, you can double up on things like Hemp Hearts, pumpkin seeds, kale, beans, spirulina and lentils. A lot of people complain about exhaustion on a cleanse, and it's often because they don't have macronutrient balance or enough calories to keep them sustained. Note that if you choose not to eat fish on the cleanse, you should include a preconverted omega-3 fat source, such as NutraVege (www.ascentahealth.com), derived from algae. Look for a dose of at least 1,000 milligrams of combined EPA (eicosapentaenoic acid) and DHA (docosahexaenoic acid) fatty acids.

Something else to consider when deciding whether to do the cleanse as a vegan is whether you have digestive distress with certain foods. A vegan cleanse relies heavily on legumes as a protein source and gluten-free grains, but not everyone can properly break down these complex foods. If you have an intolerance to disaccharides, you may need to avoid beans, legumes and grains to heal your gut lining. Similarly, if you have inflammatory bowel disease (IBD) or irritable bowel syndrome (IBS), you might find it easier on your digestive system to do the cleanse as an omnivore. Avoiding the recipes that contain grains and legumes will relieve the digestive lining from the stress of breaking down difficult carbohydrates. You might find huge digestive relief from eating this way, and even relief from any mental health symptoms you may experience. Eliminating grains and sweeteners has helped my clients and family attain a happy digestive tract and, in turn, a positive frame of mind.

Whether you do this cleanse as an omnivore or a vegan, you will still be able to achieve awesome success. The choice completely depends on whether you are a good vegetarian or a better omnivore. I like to say there are 7 billion diets for 7 billion people. You will find the menu that is best for you. This cleanse is your chance to feel it out and even try to eliminate grains from your diet. If you choose to do it purely as a vegan or vegetarian, this is a great opportunity for you to try some new delicious vegetarian recipes and check how well you tolerate legumes.

The Chicken and the Egg

The benefit of doing the cleanse as an omnivore is that you will be able to better manage your blood sugar and get all the nutrients you need to keep up with an active lifestyle. If you're a person who has a very busy schedule and lots to accomplish, including animal-sourced foods in your cleanse will allow you to better cope with stress and also have more energy for day-to-day life.

When it comes to choosing animal protein, look for the cleanest available. Choose healthy small fish and organic, free-range chicken and eggs if those are affordable for you. These decisions will make a big difference. Most farmed fish are raised in an environment treated with fungicides, which are dreadful for the human body. However, there are certified organic fish farms starting up that are free of harmful chemicals, so be on the lookout for sustainable options near you. Conventional meat is raised with many toxins and pesticides, and on top of that, the feed is often genetically modified. Large amounts of antibiotics are used on factory-farmed animals to keep them alive, often under brutal conditions. To avoid problems associated with these additives, either choose to eat certified organic animal proteins or choose to do a vegan cleanse. Either of these options is healthy and will allow you achieve a beneficial cleanse.

Preparing Friends and Family for Change

When you're doing the Hot Detox, let your friends and family know so that they can be better prepared to support you. Tell them you're serious about making healthy changes and explain the symptoms that you are coping with. If you ground your decision in something real, they are more likely to have compassion. You can also invite a family member or friend to do the Hot Detox with you! You are much more likely to succeed with live support. If you don't have enrolment from friends or family to participate in the Hot Detox with you, then consider someone you can text or email for mental and emotional support.

Your Base Camp Checklist

As you acclimate at base camp, remember the five key tasks of this preparation phase:

1 Get used to enjoying lots of produce by testing how well your stomach can tolerate the amount of fiber provided by different fruits and vegetables.
2 Get your tongue used to all five tastes: sour, bitter, sweet, salty and spicy.
3 Prepare some baked goods and soups ahead of time so you can save time when you need it.
4 Test out your taste buds with different or unusual ingredients, and make sure you like a new ingredient before you buy a lot of it. If you don't like an ingredient, explore substitutions or try to get used to it.
5 Map out all the health-food stores close to you. Get to know what they stock. Do you need to shop at two stores to get what you need? What specialty store has the extra ingredients that will spice up your cleanse and make sure it stays really fun and delicious?

With those five things accomplished, you are ready to enter Phase 1 of the Hot Detox. Enjoy the journey!

The Hot Detox

Kid, you'll move mountains. Today is your day!
Your mountain is waiting. Let's get on your way!
—Dr. Seuss

Now that you have assembled the tools to ascend Detox Mountain, you need to start climbing! Soon you'll be pushing for the summit, where your mind clears and your digestion optimizes. You'll be powerfully nourished and left fortified. You will feel rejuvenated and experience a new sense of commitment to your long-term vitality.

The menu plans for each phase cover both the 21-day and 10-day options. If you only have time for a 3-day detox, simply follow the menu for Phase 2. The menu plans are just a guide, so relax and enjoy the discovery of new ingredients as your budget and time allow.

The menu plans include as many healthy recipes as possible. Feel free to halve recipes or double them to adapt the menu to your lifestyle. If you are busy or just aren't able to make something, you can repeat the recipes that you enjoy. You can easily repeat the morning beverage of choice. Later in the chapter, you'll also find a menu plan for those who have less time to cook and don't mind repeating a few dishes. I have included many of the detoxifying superfoods as optional ingredients because the recipes work without fancy additions, but please add them in when possible. I encourage you to stretch your palate—you may find a new favorite!

What's on the Hot Detox Plan

These guidelines outline exactly what foods will detox your body and what foods you should avoid to assure success. The green-light foods contain powerful nutrients that assist the organs in detoxification. The yellow-light foods are to be eaten with caution because they may be inflammatory if you are sensitive to them. The red-light foods are known to be inflammatory and/ or toxic, and you should avoid them for the entire cleanse. My wish is that the Hot Detox inspires you to stay away from the red-light foods for good because you love new favorite treats.

If you suffer from inflammatory bowel disease (IBD) and find that your symptoms do not subside on this program, you may have to eliminate some of the foods on the safe list. These vary by individual, but most high-fiber carbohydrates, such as whole grains and starchy vegetables; complex carbohydrates, such as The Hot Detox Bread (page 168); and whole nuts or seeds can cause problems. During a flare-up, I suggest you puree everything when possible, eat warm soups and avoid eating large or heavy meals. Cook foods thoroughly to improve digestibility. To heal severe intestinal inflammation, you may want to try avoiding all sugars and starchy carbohydrates (beans, grains and root vegetables).

On the Menu: Green Light

Vegetables — 7 to 10 servings per day

Vegetables are rich in vitamins, minerals, phytonutrients and fiber, and generally low in sugar. They reduce inflammation, support digestion, improve regularity of bowel movements and minimize spikes in blood sugar. Select a range of colors, with at least 50 percent being brightly colored or dark green, preferably certified organic and local. They can be fresh or frozen.

Eat vegetables steamed or lightly cooked for easy digestion, especially if you have IBS or a sensitive stomach. You can eat unlimited servings of green or non-starchy vegetables because they contain lots of fiber that sweeps away toxins. Green sprouts and tender greens are best raw, as garnishes.

Healthy Options
Artichoke, beetroot, carrot, cabbage, cauliflower, celeriac root, celery, kohlrabi, Jerusalem artichoke, jicama, kudzu root, kale, leek, mushrooms, mustard, okra, onion (including green onion and scallion), parsnip, pumpkin, rutabaga, shallot, squash, string beans, sweet potato, taro root, turnip, yacon root and yam are warming or neutral and help balance cooler vegetables listed below.

These healthy cooling vegetables should be cooked or combined with warming spices/foods: asparagus, bamboo shoot, bell pepper, broccoli, cucumber, eggplant, most leafy greens (arugula, bok choy, collard, dandelion, lettuce, rapini, sorrel, spinach, Swiss chard, watercress, wild greens), radish, sea vegetables (including seaweed and kelp), snow pea, spirulina, sprouts, tomato and zucchini.

Omnivore proteins: Poultry, eggs and fish — 0 to 9 servings per week

If possible, eat organic, cage-free poultry (0 to 6 servings per week) and organic or free-range omega-3 enriched eggs (0 to 9 per week).

Focus on sustainably caught and certified organically raised fish (2 to 6 servings per week), using *SeaChoice Canada's Sustainable Seafood Guide* as a resource. Fish are rich in anti-inflammatory omega-3 fats. If you don't eat fish, take a filtered fish oil or algae supplement (2 to 3 grams per day).

Fish is always best eaten fresh; dried, frozen and canned are acceptable substitutes when fresh isn't available. If you eat salted dried fish, make sure to thoroughly soak and drain it several times before cooking to decrease the amount of salt. If you can source it, sun-dried, unsalted fish is a good choice. Minimize consumption of canned foods. They are heated at extremely high temperatures for sterilization and may contain high amounts of salt as well as toxins (such as plastics and heavy metals) leached from the can.

After Phase 3 of the cleanse, you can test out wild game such as venison, bison, buffalo and elk.

Healthy Options
- **Poultry:** chicken, Cornish hen, emu, quail, partridge, turkey
- **Eggs:** from free-range omega-3 enriched hens
- **Fish:** anchovy, Arctic char, black cod (sablefish), halibut, herring, mackerel, wild ocean salmon, sardine, trout
- **Mussels and scallops** are fine if you tolerate shellfish and if sustainably harvested.

Vegan proteins — 0 to 3 servings per day

Nuts and seeds (1 to 3 servings per day) are best eaten raw, as they're rich in anti-inflammatory fats, healing minerals, vitamin E and protein. Soaking or sprouting increases their digestibility.

Beans (0 to 3 servings per day) are rich in folic acid, magnesium, potassium, and soluble fiber. They have a low glycemic index and help support cardiovascular health by decreasing LDL cholesterol. Eat them well cooked; in soups, salads and curries; or pureed into spreads or dips.

Healthy Options
- **Nuts:** almond, Brazil nut, cashew (fresh only), chestnut, coconut,* filbert/hazelnut, walnut, macadamia nut, pecan, and nut butters made from these nuts
- **Seeds:** chia, flax, hemp, perilla, pumpkin, sacha inchi, sesame and sunflower seeds, and their butters
- **Legumes:** adzuki, black-eyed, common beans (varieties include anasazi, black, black turtle, borlotti, cannellini, caparrone, cranberry, great northern, green, haricot, mottled, navy, pinto, pink, red and white kidney, romano, runner, shell, snap, string, yellow, white and white navy), garbanzo, Lima, mung, pigeon, all lentils, and all peas

Fruits — 1 to 3 servings per day

All fruits are rich in soluble and insoluble fiber, as well as antioxidants. Choose a

---

*Coconut isn't a true nut; it's a fruit. People who have tree nut allergies can often tolerate coconut.

range of colors; organic whenever possible. Count a smoothie as 2 fruit servings.

Healthy Options
- **Warming fruits** include avocado, cherry, coconut, date, guava, hawthorn, kumquat, longan, lychee, mandarin peel (dried), mango, nectarine, peach, raspberry.
- **Neutral fruits** include apricot, cranberry, fig, grape, olive, papaya, pineapple, plum.
- **Cooling fruits** include apple, banana, bilberry, blackberry, blueberry, cantaloupe, citrus fruits, currant, elderberry, gooseberry, kiwi, mango, monk fruit, mulberry, passion fruit, pear, persimmon, plantain, rhubarb, strawberry, watermelon. Cook cool fruits or combine them with warm spices on the Hot Detox.

Wood mushrooms — 0 to 2 servings per day

Not only are they generally hypoallergenic, but many mushrooms also enhance immune function and help fight intestinal yeast infections including candida.

Healthy Options
Chaga, enoki, king oyster, maitake, oyster, reishi, shiitake, snow ear, wild mushrooms, wood ear and most Asian mushrooms.

Oils and fats — 2 to 10 servings per day

Oils are best eaten raw and stored in a cool, dark place. Raw healthy oils, especially omega-3s, lubricate your cells and have powerful anti-inflammatory properties. Avoid frying any oil.

Healthy Options
Eating healthy oils daily gives every cell in your body an "oil change" and supports tissue healing.
- Whole-food sources of healthy fats include avocados, nuts, seeds and dark leafy greens.
- For medium-temperature cooking, organic coconut oil is ideal (it breaks down in the gut into a product that kills yeast). Cold-pressed virgin olive, avocado and grape seed oils are also good for low temperature sautéing, whereas organic cold-pressed flaxseed, hemp, fish, algae, camelina, chia and sesame oils can be used in cool food applications such as smoothies and dressings.
- Organic ghee (clarified butter) is a healthy choice when eaten in moderation by people who aren't sensitive or allergic to dairy.
- Omega-3 fats are highest in coldwater fish, some algae, ocean krill, enriched eggs, seeds (chia, flax, perilla and sacha inchi) and walnuts.

Culinary herbs and spices — unlimited servings

Used since ancient times to support digestion, prevent food spoilage and support probiotics. Most are either directly anti-inflammatory or help prevent inflammation by improving digestion and strengthening your immune system. Herbs and spices can be eaten raw or dried, in tea form or as flavorful ingredients in any recipe.

Healthy Options
Anise seed, basil, bay leaf, cardamom, chive, cilantro leaf/coriander seed, cinnamon bark,

clove, cumin seed, curry leaf, dill leaf and seed, fennel seed, fenugreek, garlic, ginger root, marjoram, mint, nutmeg, oregano, parsley, rosemary, sage, savory, star anise, thyme and turmeric

Salad dressings and condiments

Avoid white vinegar in salad dressing. Avoid cheap balsamic vinegar as it is often sweetened with sugar.

Use lots of spices and garlic in dressings for their anti-inflammatory and antifungal qualities.
- **Acids:** freshly squeezed lemon or lime juice and apple cider vinegar
- **Oils:** olive, avocado, flax, sesame or hemp
- **Mustard** made with apple cider vinegar and naturally fermented pickles makes a great condiment.

Sweeteners

Stevia, dates and small amounts of raw honey may be used as sweetening agents in beverages and foods as necessary to make the transition to natural sweetness. Honey is both antibacterial and antifungal. Monk fruit is intensely sweet but does not elevate your blood sugar, so it is beneficial for those who want to balance blood sugar.

Healthy Options
Stevia, honey, monk fruit and dates

Beverages

Drink 6 to 12 glasses daily of liquid, depending on body weight and activity level.

Herbal teas hydrate, cleanse and heal so enjoy freely.

Healthy Options
- Pure filtered or spring water, stevia-sweetened lemonade, diluted vegetable juices, fresh diluted fruit juice
- **Teas:** burdock root, chai, dandelion leaf and root, green tea, fruit including citrus peel, hibiscus, holy basil (tulsi), lavender, mint, peppermint, rose, rooibos and sumac

Dairy alternatives

Many health-food stores offer sugar-free varieties of non-dairy yogurt or kefir containing live bacterial cultures, or make your own yogurt (on page 158).

Healthy Options
- **Milk:** unsweetened almond, coconut, sesame, and cashew or hemp
- **Yogurt or kefir:** coconut-, nut- or seed-based

Consume Cautiously: Amber Light

Gluten-free whole grains — up to 2 servings per day for women, and 3 servings per day for men

Broad-leaf seeds are considered pseudo-grains that are easy to digest (amaranth, quinoa, kasha/buckwheat). Other gluten-free grains are grasses and a bit tougher to digest (black, red and brown rice, wild rice, sorghum, teff and millet). Make sure any bread item is gluten-free and yeast-free (unleavened). 1 serving = ½ cup cooked.

Rotate different grains to avoid developing an allergy. Soak in spring water before cooking to increase digestibility. Choose well-cooked whole grains that digest slowly to avoid spiking blood sugar. Avoid grains if you have IBS.

Nightshades

Potatoes and eggplant contain an alkaloid called solanine that can increase joint and bowel inflammation if you are sensitive to it, so they are eliminated for the course of the Hot Detox. Watch for pain when you reintroduce them. Other nightshade plants with specific alkaloids are as follows: capsaicin in sweet and hot peppers, tomatine in tomato and nicotine in tobacco. Because these alkaloids are different, some people are sensitive to potatoes but not tomatoes. If you suffer from pain, test each type of nightshade and see if your inflammatory condition improves. You can avoid pain by using the tasty substitutions in this book.

Avoid the Following: Red Light

Refined and concentrated sugars

Quick-acting carbohydrates such as sucrose, high-fructose corn syrup, fructose, molasses, maple syrup, maple sugar, maltose, lactose, glucose, turbinado sugar, cane juice, raw sugar and Sucanat are all forms of sugar that can cause inflammation. Limit the use of maple products and molasses if you notice a sugar sensitivity. Avoid chewable supplements as they are sweetened with sugar. Look out for hidden sugar in packaged foods.

Condiments and sauces

Ketchup; Worcestershire, steak, barbecue and chili sauces; shrimp- and wheat-based soy sauces; sugar pickles, horseradish, mincemeat; white vinegar and commercial salad dressing containing poor-quality oils and additives

Coffee and black tea

The caffeine in coffee and tea can contribute to adrenal exhaustion. It also speeds Phase 1 of the liver detox pathway, causing a backlog of toxins waiting to be processed in Phase 2, so it is best to avoid coffee on the Hot Detox. Swap black tea for green tea, white tea or yerba mate and drink them to reduce coffee withdrawal headaches.

If you must drink coffee, then only drink organic fair-trade coffee without cream or sugar.

Dairy

Avoid milk and cheese, particularly moldy cheeses such as Roquefort, Gorgonzola, brie and blue cheese. Also avoid conventional processed cheeses such as American cheese slices or the one found in instant macaroni and cheese.

Food dyes

Studies show that artificial colorings, which are found in soda, fruit juices and salad dressings, may contribute to behavioral problems in children and lead to a significant reduction in IQ. Animal studies have linked other food colorings to cancer. The worst offenders include Blue #1 and Blue

#2 (E133), Red dye #3 (also Red #40, a more current dye) (E124), Yellow #6 (E110) and Yellow Tartrazine (E102).

Artificial additives and preservatives

Avoid monosodium glutamate (MSG commonly causes headaches), trans fats (which compete with omega 3 for absorption), sodium sulfite (a source of sensitivity) and sulfur dioxide (E220). Butylated hydroxyanisole (BHA) and butylated hydroxytoluene (BHT) are preservatives found in cereals, chewing gum, potato chips and vegetable oils that affect the neurological system of the brain and alter behavior. BHA and BHT are also oxidants, which form cancer-causing reactive compounds in your body.

Wheat and gluten grains

Gluten is a protein in grain that is very difficult to digest and can cause sensitivity symptoms such as headaches, joint pain, IBS, acne, ADHD and dark circles under the eyes. Avoid gluten-containing grains (barley, kamut, contaminated oats, rye, spelt, triticale and wheat) and foods containing them (pasta, malt, cereals and candy). Breads, pastries and other yeast-raised baked goods are exceptionally hard to digest due to the hybridization of grains in the last 20 years.

White button mushrooms

Many commercial mushrooms are grown on manure and may harbor pathogens that can infect or irritate your gut.

Alcohol

Alcoholic beverages such as wine, beer and all hard liquor (whisky, brandy, gin, rum, vodka) are laden with yeast and taxing to the brain and liver.

Processed nuts

Avoid rancid nuts and seeds, as they're pro-inflammatory and extremely damaging to the liver and cardiovascular system. Nuts and seeds that have been processed (including presliced or chopped) or cooked (especially at high temperatures) are more likely to contain damaged oils. Only eat fresh pistachios and cashews. Avoid peanuts because they're a common allergen and are almost always high in inflammation-causing molds.

Carbonated beverages

Soda contains 9 teaspoons of sugar per can and is very inflammatory to the brain. Artificial sweeteners are even more dangerous and best avoided.

Pickled and smoked meats

Hot dogs, corned beef, smoked fish and luncheon meat contain nitrates that are dangerous for human health.

Packaged and processed foods

Canned and boxed packaged and processed foods usually contain refined sugar, toxic dyes, flavor enhancers, additives and preservatives that tax your liver. Look for added ingredients by reading the label.

The Hot Detox Phase 1: Less Is More

This first part of the 21-day cleanse lasts for 9 days, or 4 if you are choosing the 10-day option. This phase is where you start to climb the mountain. During this time, you're going to work on breaking the addiction to refined sugar and eliminating potential inflammatory allergens such as gluten-containing grains and flour. You're also going to get rid of anything that plays havoc with your taste buds, such as artificial flavors and sweeteners. This phase will help prime your digestive system to receive and absorb the amount of nutrition you'll ultimately be eating.

> Julie, your nutritional advice has been life changing. You opened my eyes to what I was doing to my health. I was eating 6,000 milligrams of sodium a day — yikes! In just a short 10 days I posted a blood sugar of 5.9 after lunch, which is amazing for me ... half what it was the week before starting your program. My blood pressure is normal with no medication. I knew there had to be a better way. Thanks for showing me.
> — Licio P.

The Two Commitments of Phase 1

As you jump into Phase 1, here are my two commitments to you: Phase 1 is going to be delicious, and it's going to satisfy you because it's going to give you choices.

Eating delicious food is strategic as well as self-satisfying. If you lose pleasure in eating food while on the cleanse, you may not last. You'll run out of steam. The food needs to be tasty, and I assure you it will be.

If you don't like the way some foods taste, experiment and play with these recipes to make them enjoyable for you. That's the beauty of figuring out a menu that works for you — you can have fun with it! If you are used to restaurant food, add extra unrefined sea salt while your taste buds adjust to the new flavors. Keep lemon juice on the counter as a condiment and add it to anything that needs a spike of sour deliciousness. Drop some unpasteurized honey into a smoothie to make your taste buds soar. Customize the recipes and play with the sweet, sour and salty tastes so that you can tolerate bitterness and learn to appreciate spiciness.

Think of it this way: the spiciness and bitterness are the medicine, and the sweet, sour and salty are the delivery system to get it down. The old saying is "A spoonful of sugar makes the medicine go down." For the Hot Detox, we'll say, "A spoonful of honey, a spoonful of lemon juice or a pinch of salt will make the medicine of that bitter rapini and that spicy ginger go down." That might not flow off the tongue as easily, but it will change your life!

Second, you will stay satisfied on this cleanse. There are no set amounts of food in the program because everyone needs different amounts of food depending on body size and genetic makeup. If you are a 200-pound male, you require one-third more food than a 120-pound woman. That's why I need you to use your intuition and eat to fullness. Don't be scared of certain dishes that contain nuts and seeds because the fats in those foods will help you manage your weight. Throw away the calorie counter. Aim for food satisfaction and nutrient density, and the rest will follow.

Rules to Detox By

This plan is meant to help de-stress and detoxify your body so you can operate at your optimum.

- Drink 6 to 10 glasses of purified warm water or herbal tea daily, depending on your body size.

- Commit to eating 7 to 10 servings of vegetables. Cook well if needed.

- Prepare meals in advance so it's easy and convenient to stay on the plan.

The Hot Detox Phase 2: Summiting the Mountain with a Deep Detox

Over the first 9 (or 4) days, you slowly climbed Detox Mountain. Phase 2 is the summit. You're at the peak! This is the period of deep cleansing with a liquid, vegan meal plan for 3 days. Here we eliminate all animal products and enjoy easy-to-digest liquid soups, teas and warm smoothies that give your digestive system a rest. You'll also be eating less heavy fats so that you can give your liver a holiday, and increase bitter herbs and teas to boost support of your detoxification organs. Your lymph will get a little extra tender love and care. Your kidneys will be flushed because of the increase in fluid consumption, especially detox teas that will help them work optimally. All your detoxification organs will be thriving during this period of deep cleansing.

At this point, you will have to make sure that you are getting enough calories. Increase portions to suit your appetite and body size. This 3-day, liquid, vegan cleanse

is low in calories. Living on seeds like Hemp Hearts and lots of produce, you may lose five to eight pounds during Phase 2. Be sure to keep drinking—have something in your hand almost all the time, like tea or a smoothie or soup, so that you never feel hungry or light-headed. Also make sure you add enough high-quality salt to avoid low blood pressure.

Detox Symptoms and Solutions

While you will be enjoying amazing benefits internally, you might also begin to experience some detoxification symptoms at this point. This is completely normal. Just like climbing a mountain, any altitude sickness at the summit is worth it. Watch for the symptoms discussed below, but don't worry if you experience them. Some mild symptoms are a completely normal part of the detoxification process.

Dr. Zoltan Rona, MD, reports, "There are really no good tests to see if a liver or kidney flush is complete, but most people can tell it's time to stop by the way they feel. Symptoms such as fatigue, headaches, abdominal discomforts and skin problems should all be improved. Headaches and weakness may be early signs of detoxification and are not a reason to stop any cleanse. A cleanse should be stopped if more serious symptoms occur, such as vomiting, fever, or severe abdominal pain." Because this program is designed to be gentle, I anticipate you won't experience harsh detox symptoms. The secret to getting through milder symptoms is self-compassion—go easy on yourself.

Headache. Headaches are often due to dehydration, so drink more liquid throughout the day. As you detox your liver, the circulating toxins and shifting of hormones can also lead to headaches. Lemon-flavored magnesium powder works to reduce the muscle spasms that cause headaches. Alternatively, headaches can be caused by lack of caffeine, if your body was used to it. Yerba mate, green tea or white tea is permitted and will provide a small amount of caffeine to take the edge off—the hair of the dog that bit you.

Light-headedness. A lack of calories or low blood pressure can result in light-headedness. Check in with yourself to see if you need a snack. If so, definitely reach for seeds (such as pumpkin or hemp), avocado or some protein to stabilize your blood sugar and help you feel good and satiated.

Your blood pressure may drop if you are accustomed to consuming restaurant food, which supplies 5,000 to 7,000 milligrams of daily sodium. You will be consuming as little as 1,500 milligrams on the Hot Detox because the recipes enhance flavor without excessive sodium. If you become light-headed or you notice that your blood pressure is a bit low, enjoy more unrefined Himalayan or Utah pink salt and your blood pressure should stabilize. Licorice tea is also a good way to balance adrenal function and blood pressure if needed.

Fatigue. This common symptom of cleansing can be addressed with power naps. You might feel fatigued because of your lack of caffeine, in which case herbs can give you energy without causing more toxicity. Schisandra berries and maca root can both give you a lift while continuing to cleanse your liver.

Bloating and gas. Bloating and gas often result from the digestive system being unaccustomed to getting so much fiber from produce. If you have digestive troubles, avoid cold shakes and drink things at room temperature. Puree your legumes in a soup. Even though foods are liquid, chew to produce more enzymes. Before meals, drink lemon juice to help digestion.

Loose stools or diarrhea. Loose stools may be a sign you are overwhelming your system with too much fiber. Or you may have had a big dump of bile from your gallbladder, because this cleanse helps create bile, which moves the toxins out of your body. This is a common sign of detoxification. Stay hydrated and ease off heavy fiber (raw produce or grains) and legumes.

A strong cup of ginger tea will reduce discomfort, and a strong cup of green tea can stop diarrhea as the tannins work to tighten up the bowel. Probiotics balance your bowel function and can also be used for diarrhea. You may want to consider activated charcoal if it continues. Slow down and return to an easier part of the cleanse if digestive discomfort is ongoing, and seek the help of a naturopathic doctor to address underlying issues like bowel infections and IBS.

Constipation. Occasionally people get plugged up with too much fiber, which stops food from moving along the digestive tract. If you have constipation, stay hydrated and reach for soothing foods that will help to move the fiber along, such as ground chia or flaxseeds, dandelion or mustard greens, and apple cider vinegar. Other great solutions include whole-plant aloe vera juice or sunflower lecithin added to your smoothies. Or try a yoga pose where you pull your legs to your chest (www.shambu.co). Rubbing castor oil on your belly can alleviate some of the pain and move things downwards. You could also try taking digestive bitters that contain gentian root before meals.

> I was diagnosed with psoriatic arthritis and was on a 17-month waiting list to see a rheumatologist. I had tried many different supplements and health experts and nothing was working. I was in extreme pain and inflammation. My hands and fingers were swollen and felt like they were on fire. This kept me awake most nights. I felt like the tin man — stiff, sore and grumpy. I was getting very little sleep and was still working full-time.
>
> After following your book, I started feeling better. I kept a food diary for a whole year to uncover my trigger foods to ensure I would never, ever feel like I used to. I finally did get into the rheumatologist armed with your book, my food diary and feeling great. Since I felt so great, I didn't need any drugs. I haven't needed any drugs for almost 3 years because I have been following your anti-inflammatory "Live-It" and no longer need to see the rheumatologist.
>
> My motto is "Real Food Is Medicine." I spend time each week meal planning, cooking real food and encouraging as many people as I can to eat real food. I have recommended your book to so many people.
>
> Thank you for giving me my life back!
> — Roxanne A.

Enjoying the View

Phase 2 is when you get to revel in the progress you have made. You will most likely have moments of intense joy and clarity at this stage because there's a euphoria that comes with cleansing your body of toxins and allergens. Your body will be efficient and so nourished that, even though you might experience some detoxification symptoms, you'll also experience extreme lucidity. It's like reaching the summit on your climb up the mountain — you might have a sprained ankle or trouble breathing, but the expansive view gives you a change in perspective. Here above the treetops, you can oversee the full scope of your life. Some people experience epiphanies about what to do in other areas of life. Greater clarity of mind and body may cause us to question what else needs to be eliminated or nourished in our lives. This is why I cleanse during periods of stress. I want to have my greatest mental awareness and be able to handle whatever is thrown my way.

Don't be surprised if you want to lengthen the time that you spend sitting on the summit. Some people choose to do two back-to-back Phase 2s and extend the liquid cleanse to six days because they feel so euphoric. This is okay because even though Phase 2 is a light liquid menu, there's enough nutrition to maintain good health. You're getting essential fatty acids, protein, good carbohydrates and almost all your vitamins and minerals. If you suffer from a vitamin B12 deficiency, you may want to add a supplement on the longer vegan cleanse, because it is the only vitamin that is not covered. So if you're loving the experience here, feel free to extend your stay.

· ·

Try to enjoy fermented foods every day to rebuild your microbiome. Choices include Cashew Coconut Yogurt, Ginger Kimchi, Probiotic Cheese, Pretty Purple Sauerkraut, umeboshi plums or Beet Kvass.

The Hot Detox Phase 3: A Walk into Happy Valley

As you enter Phase 3, which is the final 9 (or 3) days, you once again have a decision to make about whether to do the last phase as a vegan, a vegetarian or an omnivore. Are you a bit hungry after Phase 2? Do you want to introduce animal foods again? Maybe you're comfortable being vegetarian and including eggs in your diet, but you want to avoid flesh foods like fish or chicken. You may also choose to stay purely vegan on this last phase. Omnivore, vegetarian or vegan? It's really up to you because all three paths have their benefits!

In Phase 3, you're going to work on rebuilding, rehydrating, relaxing and renewing your body. You'll be doing more experiments with powerful superfoods. You've been on this cleanse for 2 weeks now, and it's time to add in some more exciting foods if you're ready. Maybe you want to try some acai powder, an unusual herb like maca or the exotic schisandra berry? These exciting superfoods can offer more variety and nutrients.

In Phase 3, I also encourage you to try out any recipes you may be resisting. Are you willing to try fermenting your own foods? Can you make your own coconut yogurt? Can you make your own sauerkraut? If you haven't already, prepare some of the more advanced recipes. These will add some great life skills to carry into the future. I call this anti-inflammatory lifestyle a "Live-It" because you can enjoy it as a way of life rather than falling off a diet.

This last phase is all about powerful nourishment and really priming your brain to focus on positive foods that bring you mental clarity and balance. When you come off the cleanse entirely, this will leave you fortified. You'll be reintroducing powerfully nutritious solid foods. You're also going to keep eating grounding foods like cinnamon, ginger and good fats. If Phase 3 is done correctly, the nourishing foods you enjoy will make you feel rejuvenated and energized, with a new sense of commitment to your long-term vitality.

> My husband and I did your 21-day detox in September. We are a middle-aged couple with lots of inflammation, and my husband is celiac. We benefited in so many ways. It was amazing! You designed it so well. We could shop and prepare meals with your help. I crave the feeling of being inflammation-free now that I have felt being pain-free first-hand. My brain fog is gone and my joints are free from pain. I lost some weight, which I have not been able to do for 15 years. Even my 22-year-old joined us on our journey … which amazed me.
>
> We are continuing to eat as clean as we can and enjoy making the anti-inflammatory foods part of our daily lives. Thank you so much.
> — Roxanne G.

Happy Valley

With your newfound energy and rested digestive system, you're ready for the slow march into Happy Valley. Now that you're ready to descend from the summit, remember to take it slow. Many people topple off the mountain as they come back down because they pick up speed too quickly. As you start including other foods back into your diet, you might be tempted by "old food friends" or you many want to include more complex foods right away. However, you've just done three days of a liquid cleanse, and you have to wake up your digestive system slowly to solid food again. Do not eat wildly complex foods right away, and don't rush back into eating a large amount of food. Start off by eating smaller quantities to let your digestive system get back into the swing of digesting solid food. Chew well. Sit down to eat and really enjoy the nourishment you are taking in.

Being disciplined when you come out of a liquid cleanse is very important. Just as you take some moments to allow your body to come to an equilibrium after an intense workout, the actions you take after a liquid cleanse allow the digestive system to settle into its more efficient functioning.

Taking It to the Streets: How to Dine Out on the Hot Detox

From rich restaurant meals to fast food and on-the-go snacks, the lure of convenience foods can be especially strong while on the Hot Detox, and you may notice you have cravings for food you wouldn't normally want. So what are you to do?

The key is to be prepared. Keep fruit, vegetables and nuts on hand for "in case of emergency" food cravings. If you are going out for a nice meal with friends, consider taking a seasoning packet or small jar of detox salad dressing with you, so you can order your menu item without sauce (e.g., cream sauces, commercial salad dressings, BBQ sauce and teriyaki sauce). Always carry a water bottle as you may be mistaking your hunger for dehydration.

I have completed a 40-day cleanse while traveling for work and found my mind was razor sharp because I did not have to fight foods that caused inflammation. Brain fog is often a result of eating sugar, rancid oils, deep-fried foods, antibiotic-fed meat, dairy, or other inflammatory foods. By packing a third of my luggage with food, I was able to avoid the pitfalls of restaurant meals and emerged looking and feeling younger than when I started! Make sure to eat every few hours to maintain excellent energy levels.

How to Conquer Your Cravings

Eat some protein. You may have noticed that I suggest a lot of Hemp Hearts (unshelled seeds) in the Hot Detox recipes. Sources of vegan protein (such as hemp, sunflower, pumpkin and sesame seeds) have the ability to release satiety hormones faster than fat or carbohydrates and cause you to feel fuller while eating less. A study published in *Nutrition Metabolism* indicates that increasing your protein intake by 30 percent can reduce total caloric intake by approximately 450 calories per day.

Fill your hands after 8:00 p.m. Take up a nighttime hobby like knitting that requires you to use your hands. When late-night cravings take hold they are usually in the form of high-fat, high-sugar foods. Recent studies show that American adults consume up to 64 percent of their total calories at night! Try satisfying those cravings with low-sodium vegetable soups, which fill the stomach and induce satiety.

Call in the troops. Having a supportive friend that you can call when you're in trouble is important. Social support has been shown to bring awareness to the nutritional content of food.

Snack Away!

Let's face it, the biggest reason people give into cravings so easily is that the foods they crave are convenient and cheap. Here is a quick list of healthy snacks to prepare, carry or order for thoughtful travel.

- Vegetable soups and chicken broth

- Organic seed bars sweetened with dates or honey

- Enamel-lined cans of Eden organic beans — they offer 6 grams each of fiber and protein in a ½-cup serving

- Freeze-dried organic berries — they never go bad and are never out of season

- Organic fruit crisps made without sugar or oil

- Roasted sweet bell pepper strips or artichoke hearts in a glass jar

- Sun-dried tomatoes packed in olive oil — these tender gems are an easy add-in to salad

- Healthy detox dips such as hummus, guacamole, white bean dip and tapenade

- Wash and go — serve dip with carrots, red bell peppers, celery stalks. Be careful to avoid raw vegetables if you suffer from IBS or IBD. Avoid peppers if intolerant to nightshades.

- Trail mix of fresh nuts plus juice-sweetened cranberries or goji berries

- Austrian pumpkin seeds, which don't have hulls

- Hemp Hearts — rich in omega-3 fatty acid, these help your skin retain moisture

- Garlic-stuffed green or jumbo black Californian olives

- Organic sugar-free applesauce — try a ½ cup serving of cinnamon or berry flavor with added flax powder or slippery elm powder

- Nut or seed butter on celery. See tip on page 162 for Chai-Spice Butter.

Breathe deeply. When we are low on energy, we usually crave simple sugars to give us a quick boost. Deep breathing, called *pranayama*, is an ancient Indian technique to energize your system (see page 63).

Bring on the veggies. Filling up your stomach with nutrient-dense, low-calorie, low-sodium vegetable juice before meals will initiate feelings of fullness and give your body the nutrients it needs.

Spice up your life. We are hard-wired to want flavor because, in nature, different plant flavors mean that we are getting a broad range of nutrients. Trick your senses into satisfaction by eating spicy foods instead of salt and sugar. You will also experience many of the medicinal benefits of the herbs, such as boosting your metabolism and decreasing inflammation.

Eat fat to lose fat. If you're craving fatty foods, try taking a teaspoon of fish oil and wait 15 minutes. Not only will the fish oil satisfy your cravings for fat while supporting a healthy metabolism, but it will help to regulate hormones, which will control your cravings in the long run—especially cravings that are premenstrual symptoms. Keep enjoying the medium chain triglycerides (MCT) in all the coconut recipes, as they break down to beta-hydroxybutyrate (BHB), which fuels the brain and turns off your cravings for carbs completely. For more information on ketones, check out the Hot Detox online course at www.JulieDaniluk.com.

An apple a day keeps the cravings away. The pectin fiber in apples absorbs water and creates bulk in the stomach. This slows the release of glucose into the bloodstream and keeps you satiated for an extra hour or two. By helping prevent your blood sugar from spiking, the slow release will help you avoid a blood sugar "crash" that leaves you craving more sugar or food. Because apples are cooling in traditional Chinese medicine, sprinkle apple slices with ginger or cinnamon or, better yet, bake or stew apples to warm them up.

Get down with vinegar. Vinegar can help cut cravings in three important ways.

1 Vinegar helps keep food in the stomach for longer, which reduces the hunger hormone, called ghrelin. This in turn improves digestion, and helps you feel full faster and for a longer time.
2 Vinegar helps prevent spikes in blood sugar following a meal and lowers the glycemic index of a food.
3 Vinegar has been shown to increase the metabolism of fat by the liver, which can last up to 3 hours after a meal.

Remember to choose raw unpasteurized apple cider vinegar to gain the appetite-suppressing benefits of the nutrients contained.

Brush your teeth. A residual taste in your mouth can trigger the craving for more food. A minty-clean, fresh-breath taste will discourage you from consuming danger foods. Rinsing your mouth with water can be just as effective.

Avoid the Stomach Slap-back!

You can't keep insulting your stomach without your stomach eventually slapping you back. What I mean by this is that if your stomach doesn't respond well to a certain type of food, whether dairy, fried foods, wheat or whatever, it's not going to function well if you keep eating them. You have to love your stomach. Eat foods that feel good and nourish you, and treat yourself occasionally. Trust me, you can find new nourishing foods that quickly become favorites, making it easy to "break up" with the naughty foods forever. My coaching here is that if a certain food really doesn't jibe with your digestive system, avoid it.

Shake it off. Stress is usually our number-one trigger for giving in to cravings. Practicing meditation and stress-relieving techniques has been shown to decrease cravings for sugary foods and lower cortisol levels. Cortisol is a hormone created by our adrenal glands that is triggered and released by stress. When we were cavemen, we needed quick energy in the face of stress to escape from potential harm. This is why many of us crave sugar when we are stressed, even when we are not being chased by a bear.

Go nuts. Drinking a glass of water and eating one ounce of nuts (equivalent to 6 walnuts or 12 almonds) can extinguish cravings and dampen your appetite by changing your body chemistry and controlling hunger hormones.

The Hot Detox 21-Day Plan

	Day	Morning beverage	Breakfast	Morning snack with tea of choice
Phase 1	1	Ginger tea	Squeaky Clean Granola *with* Coconut Cashew Yogurt	Super Guac *with* Detox Olive Crackers
	2	Burdock tea	Pommy Paleo Pudding	Carrot Cake Smoothie
	3	Dandelion Root Koffee	Paleo Pumpkin Bagels *with* Probiotic Cheese *and/or* Berry Chia Jam	Shamrock Butter *with* celery or carrot sticks
	4	The Hot Detox Tea	Antioxidant Smoothie Bowl	Beet Kvass
	5	Hot Apple Toddy	Hot Detox Flax wrap *with* Probiotic Cheese *and/or* Chia Berry Jam	Joint-Healing Gell-O
	6	Chai tea	Faux-tmeal Breakfast	Raw or roasted zucchini slices *with* Olive Tapenade
	7	The Hot Detox Tea	Meals-That-Heal Seed Bar	The Red Devil
	8	Warm ACV and Honey Drink	Blueberry Seed Soak *or* Detox Frittata	Shamrock Butter *with* celery and carrot sticks
	9	Gut Booster Juice	Pumpkin Spice Smoothie Bowl	Super Guac *with* Detox Olive Crackers
Phase 2	10	Hot water with lemon and a few drops of stevia if desired	Tiger Spice Smoothie	50 Shades of Green
	11	Ginger Recovery Drink	Joint-Healing Gell-O *or* Vegan Lemon Gell-O	Smooth Feeling
	12	The Hot Detox Tea	Pumpkin Pie Smoothie	Detox Rocket

Lunch	Afternoon snack with tea of choice	Dinner	Day	
Detox Kichadi *with* Ginger Kimchi *or* Chicken with Sugar Snap Peas and Fresh Herbs	Bone Broth *or* Vegan Broth *with* vegetables*	Dijon Chicken or Lentil Soup	1	
Asian Salad Bowl *and* Asian Onion Soup		Lazy Cabbage Rolls *or* Detox Kichadi	2	
Beet Bop Salad *with* Tea-Time Eggs		Mediterranean-Style Skillet Chicken *with* steamed greens and choice of dressing *or* Power Protein Vegan Bowl	3	
Sweet Potato and Asparagus Salad *and* 1 hard-boiled egg topped with 1 tsp Instant Pesto		Sautéed Comfort *or* Hemp Burgers	4	Phase 1
Fast Lentil Salad *or* Broccoli Wasabi Dip *with* celery or carrot sticks		Pineapple Chai Chicken *or* Detox Kichadi	5	
Cauliflower Crust Pizza *or* Garlic Roasted Asparagus	Bone Broth *or* Vegan Broth *with* vegetables*	Detox Frittata *and* stir-fry of mixed greens with 2 Tbsp Sunny Anti-inflammatory Dressing	6	
Onion Lentil Dip *and* Salad Soup		Super Shepherd's Pie	7	
Kale Squash Soup *or* Comforting Chicken Soup		Detox Nut Butter Stew *topped with* Pretty Purple Sauerkraut	8	
Sunny Sunflower Pâté *with* roasted or raw veggies		Savory Carrot Cashew Bake *with* Garlic Roasted Asparagus	9	
Fast Carrot Soup	The Bitter Truth *and* Bone Broth *or* Vegan Broth *with* vegetables*	Golden Milk *and* Garlic Cauliflower Mash	10	
Quick Cauliflower Soup	Oh-So-Hardcore Detox Drink *and* Bone Broth *or* Vegan Broth *with* vegetables*	Turmeric Spice Latte *and* Butternut Squash Puree	11	Phase 2
Kale Squash Soup	Deep Green Dream *and* Bone Broth *or* Vegan Broth *with* vegetables*	Nettle Tea *and* Spiced Sweet Potato Mash	12	

*Stir in vegetables of choice (e.g., sprouts or baby greens) to add extra nutrition and variety.

The Hot Detox 21-Day Plan (continued)

	Day	Morning beverage	Breakfast	Morning snack with tea of choice
Phase 3	13	Digestive Gripe Water	Detox Flush Pudding	Anti-inflammatory Powerhouse
	14	The Hot Detox Tea	Banana Pecan Muffin	Citrus Chaser
	15	Cinnamon tea	Hot Detox Bread *with* Detox Marmalade	Joint-Healing Gell-O
	16	Dandelion Root Koffee	Apple Breakfast Bars	Berry Bliss Shake
	17	Hot Pommy	Cran-Almond Muffin	Detox Macaroons
	18	Raspberry tea	The Early Riser *or* Carrot Cake Bars	Tomato-Free Soup
	19	The Hot Detox Tea	Berry Bliss Shake	Raw or cooked snap peas
	20	Schisandra tea	Extreme Ginger Bake	The Green Hornet
	21	Cranberry tea	Hulk Flourless Pancakes	1 peach or ½ an avocado

Lunch	Afternoon snack with tea of choice	Dinner	Day
Artichoke Skordalia *with* Fasolakia Lemonata (Lemon Green Beans)	Bone Broth *or* Vegan Broth *with* vegetables*	JFC Coleslaw *and* Hemp Burgers *with* Whole Roasted Garlic	13
Pressed Radish Salad *with* Broccoli Lentil Soup		Sesame-Crusted Fish *with* Messy Gingered Sweet Potatoes	14
Fennel Ginger Salad *and* Sesame-Crusted Fish		Detox Curry *and* Coco Quinoa *and* steamed greens with Detox Dressing	15
Gentle Healing Dal *with* Baba's Sautéed Cabbage	Bone Broth *or* Vegan Broth *with* vegetables*	Wild Fish Cakes *with* Hemp Mayo *and* Roasted Leeks with Olives and Garlic	16
French White Bean Dip with Mint *or* Beet Cashew Dip *with* Hot Detox Bread *or* Hot Detox Flax Wrap *and* sprouts		Chicken with Sugar Snap Peas and Fresh Herbs	17
Roasted Squash and Dried Cherry Salad		Turkey Loaf *with* The Green Goddess	18
Lynn's Quick Borscht *with* Hot Detox Bread		Delish Fish *or* Zucchini Kasharole	19
Salmon Niçoise Salad		Chicken Tikka *with* Roasted Squash and Dried Cherry Salad	20
Garlic Cauliflower Mash *with* Garlic Dandelions Greens		Herbed Halibut *with* Fasolakia Lemonata (Lemon Green Beans)	21

Phase 3

*Stir in vegetables of choice (e.g., sprouts or baby greens) to add extra nutrition and variety.

The Hot Detox 10-Day Plan

	Day	Morning beverage	Breakfast	Morning snack with tea of choice
Phase 1	1	Chai tea	Faux-tmeal Breakfast	Raw or roasted zucchini slices *with* Olive Tapenade
	2	The Hot Detox Tea	Meals-That-Heal Seed Bar	The Red Devil
	3	Warm ACV and Honey Drink	Blueberry Seed Soak *or* Detox Frittata	Shamrock Butter *with* celery and carrot sticks
	4	Gut Booster Juice	Pumpkin Spice Smoothie Bowl	Super Guac *with* Detox Olive Crackers
Phase 2	5	Hot water with lemon and a few drops of stevia if desired	Tiger Spice Smoothie	50 Shades of Green
	6	Ginger Recovery Drink	Joint-Healing Gell-O *or* Vegan Lemon Gell-O	Smooth Feeling
	7	The Hot Detox Tea	Pumpkin Pie Smoothie	Detox Rocket
Phase 3	8	Digestive Gripe Water	Detox Flush Pudding	Anti-inflammatory Powerhouse
	9	The Hot Detox Tea	Banana Pecan Muffin	Citrus Chaser
	10	Cinnamon tea	Hot Detox Bread *with* Detox Marmalade	Joint-Healing Gell-O

Lunch	Afternoon snack with tea of choice	Dinner	Day	
Cauliflower Crust Pizza or Garlic Roasted Asparagus	Bone Broth or Vegan Broth with vegetables*	Detox Frittata and stir-fry of mixed greens with 2 Tbsp Sunny Anti-inflammatory Dressing	1	Phase 1
Onion Lentil Dip and Salad Soup		Super Shepherd's Pie	2	
Kale Squash Soup or Comforting Chicken Soup		Detox Nut Butter Stew topped with Pretty Purple Sauerkraut	3	
Sunny Sunflower Pâté with roasted or raw veggies		Savory Carrot Cashew Bake with Garlic Roasted Asparagus	4	
Fast Carrot Soup	The Bitter Truth and Bone Broth or Vegan Broth with vegetables*	Golden Milk and Garlic Cauliflower Mash	5	Phase 2
Quick Cauliflower Soup	Oh-So-Hardcore Detox Drink and Bone Broth or Vegan Broth with vegetables*	Turmeric Spice Latte and Butternut Squash Puree	6	
Kale Squash Soup	Deep Green Dream and Bone Broth or Vegan Broth with vegetables*	Nettle Tea and Spiced Sweet Potato Mash	7	
Artichoke Skordalia with Fasolakia Lemonata (Lemon Green Beans)	Bone Broth or Vegan Broth with vegetables*	JFC Coleslaw and Hemp Burgers with Whole Roasted Garlic	8	Phase 3
Pressed Radish Salad with Broccoli Lentil Soup		Sesame-Crusted Fish with Messy Gingered Sweet Potatoes	9	
Fennel Ginger Salad and Sesame-Crusted Fish		Detox Curry and Coco Quinoa and steamed greens with Detox Dressing	10	

*Stir in vegetables of choice (e.g., sprouts or baby greens) to add extra nutrition and variety.

The Busy Person's Hot Detox Plan

	Day	Morning beverage	Breakfast	Morning snack with tea of choice
Phase 1	1	Warm ACV and Honey Drink	Blueberry Seed Soak	Super Guac *with* Olive Crackers
	2	Burdock tea	The Early Riser *or* Banana Pecan Muffin	Berry Bliss Smoothie
	3	Hot water with lemon and a few drops of stevia	Detox Flush Pudding	Joint-Healing Gell-O
	4	Chia Chuck Berry	Faux-tmeal Breakfast	Tomato-Free Soup
Phase 2		If doing a 10-day cleanse, follow the yellow liquid menu for 3 days (see Phase 2 on pages 110–111).		
Phase 3	5	Nettle tea	Pommy Paleo Pudding	Raw or cooked snap peas
	6	Cinnamon tea	Lemon Gell-o *and/or* Banana Pecan Muffin	Broccoli Wasabi Dip *with* celery and carrot sticks
	7	Rosehip tea	Pommy Paleo Pudding	Super Guac *with* veggies

The Busy Person's Way to Cleanse

If your time is crunched and you can only spend a few minutes making a meal, repeat dishes more frequently and stick to the easy recipes. Take some time to make Hot Detox Bread (page 168) or Paleo Pumpkin Bagels (page 178) before you start so you can include some extra high-fiber choices that will stick to your ribs.

I've outlined a menu plan here that requires less prep time. Just follow these healthy choices for 9 days, do the 3 days of Phase 2 and then come back to this menu for another 9 days. If you're doing the 10-day cleanse, then do easy recipes like these for 4 days before Phase 2 and then return to this menu for 3 days after Phase 2.

Remember, you don't need to follow this menu plan precisely. If you want to use up leftovers or you have found a favorite recipe you prefer to repeat, do what works for you!

Lunch	Afternoon snack with tea of choice	Dinner	Day	
Gentle Healing Dal *or* Dijon Chicken or Lentil Soup *with optional* Paleo Pumpkin Bagel	Bone Broth *or* Vegan Broth *with* vegetables*	The Early Riser	1	**Phase 1**
Fast Lentil Salad *or* Broccoli Wasabi Dip *with* Hot Detox Bread	Bone Broth *or* Vegan Broth *with* vegetables*	Lazy Cabbage Rolls	2	
Lazy Cabbage Rolls *with optional* Paleo Pumpkin Bagel	Bone Broth *or* Vegan Broth *with* vegetables*	Detox Kichadi *or* The Hot Detox Soup Mix	3	
Detox Kichadi *or* The Hot Detox Soup Mix *or* Dijon Chicken Soup *with optional* Paleo Pumpkin Bagel	Bone Broth *or* Vegan Broth *with* vegetables*	Dijon Chicken or Lentil Soup *with* JFC Coleslaw	4	
If doing a 10-day cleanse follow the yellow liquid menu for 3 days (see Phase 2 on pages 110–111).				**Phase 2**
French White Bean Dip with Mint *with* veggies *or* Hot Detox Flax Wrap *or* Asian Onion Soup *with optional* Paleo Pumpkin Bagel	Bone Broth *or* Vegan Broth *with* vegetables*	Broccoli Wasabi Dip *and* Asian Onion Soup	5	**Phase 3**
Fast Carrot Soup *topped with* seeds *with* Detox Bread	Bone Broth *or* Vegan Broth *with* vegetables*	Chicken Tikka *with* steamed greens and choice of dressing	6	
Quick Cauliflower Soup *with* JFC Coleslaw (or Stir-fry)	Bone Broth *or* Vegan Broth *with* vegetables*	Lazy Cabbage Rolls	7	

*Stir in vegetables of choice (e.g., sprouts or baby greens) to add extra nutrition and variety.

The Hot Detox 3-Day Plan

Day	Morning beverage	Breakfast	Morning snack with tea of choice
1	Hot water with lemon and a few drops of stevia if desired	Tiger Spice Smoothie	50 Shades of Green
2	Ginger Recovery Drink	Joint-Healing Gell-O *or* Vegan Lemon Gell-O	Smooth Feeling
3	The Hot Detox Tea	Pumpkin Pie Smoothie	Detox Rocket

I did Julie's 3-day detox after seeing her on the *Marilyn Denis Show*. I had been living with pain for many years, both from back issues even after surgery, and arthritis pain in my hands, feet and back. For several years I have been taking 4 to 6 Tylenol and Advil almost every day just to function and keep moving. On the evening of the third day of the 3-day detox my joints were less swollen. I could remove rings that I had not been able to take off for several years! I have hardly taken an Advil or Tylenol since! I was sold.

So when your 21-day detox was offered, I was in.

I have been insulin-dependent diabetic since 1986, and wondered how this program would work for me. Because this program is based on food instead of just juice fasting, I did very well. I monitored my blood sugars often to see where I was — ate plenty of snacks and felt grounded and full.

Thank you, Julie — my lifestyle has improved immensely.

— Barbara B.

Lunch	Afternoon snack with tea of choice	Dinner	Day
Fast Carrot Soup	The Bitter Truth *and* Bone Broth *or* Vegan Broth *with* vegetables*	Golden Milk *and* Garlic Cauliflower Mash	1
Quick Cauliflower Soup	Oh-So-Hardcore Detox Drink *and* Bone Broth *or* Vegan Broth *with* vegetables*	Turmeric Spice Latte *and* Butternut Squash Puree	2
Kale Squash Soup	Deep Green Dream *and* Bone Broth *or* Vegan Broth *with* vegetables*	Nettle Tea *and* Spiced Sweet Potato Mash	3

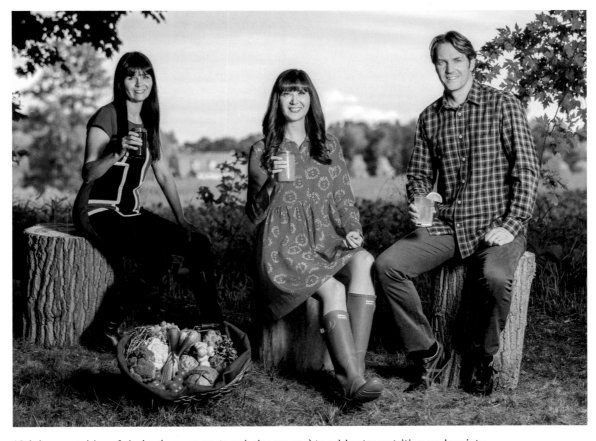

*Stir in vegetables of choice (e.g., sprouts or baby greens) to add extra nutrition and variety.

Three Key Rules for after a Cleanse

1 Avoid all junk food, such as white sugar, white flour and soft drinks. Avoid all sugars, such as chocolate, molasses and maple syrup.

2 Include liberal amounts of nutritious food from a broad diversity of choices. Aim for 7 to 10 servings of vegetables (a serving is ½ cup of cooked or 1 cup raw).

3 Feature low-carbohydrate vegetables, seafood, lean meats and eggs. If following a vegan menu, eat plenty of beans and lentils, seeds and mushrooms to supply a steady stream of protein. Enjoy more starchy vegetables, such as yams, sweet potatoes and squash, or gluten-free grains at each meal.

Post Hot Detox: How to Sustain the Heat

After Phase 3, the Hot Detox cleanse is officially over. You've gone through the preparation and the 21-day journey, and now you're ready for the reintroduction phase: the post detox. Do not come off this cleanse harshly by eating junk food or inflammatory foods. You may have come down off the mountain, but please don't slide into the valley! When people break a cleanse with pizza, deep-fried food, burgers, cookies, pastries, bread or other standard crave foods, they can experience a massive reaction or a super-cortisol (stress) response to eating toxic foods. Avoid doing this at all costs. Now is your chance to keep some of these warming principles in your day-to-day life.

You now have an opportunity to learn more about your body and what you can tolerate. You've been off most allergens and toxic foods for 21 whole days. Give yourself the gift of reintroducing foods slowly so you can see whether they work well in your body. For example, if you want to try dairy in the reintroduction phase, try sheep and goat milk first to see if you can tolerate other animal dairy besides cow. If you tolerate those well, then try cow's milk. Or, if you decide to go back to grass grains, don't jump straight to wheat. Introduce gluten-free grains first, such as teff and millet. If you want to return to eating gluten, then start with some sprouted kamut or spelt to see how well you tolerate them. If you eat gluten right away, you'll never know if you tolerate spelt or kamut better because you've already maxed out your system with wheat. Maybe you should eliminate wheat and gluten altogether, and this is the opportunity. The key is to take it slowly, and use the reintroduction process as an investigative method for how specific foods make you feel.

I encourage you to keep cooking the healthy recipes from the cleanse in your day-to-day life. You can also dig into *Meals That Heal Inflammation* and *Slimming Meals That Heal* for 250 extra recipes that will help you create an even more delicious Live-It plan: an inflammation-busting way of eating for an entire lifetime.

Reintroducing Foods Back into Your Life

After day 21 of the Hot Detox, it is time to test foods you haven't eaten for a while to see if you are sensitive, intolerant or allergic to the foods you used to eat every day. Reintroduce one new test food at a time so

Accelerated Food Reintroduction Testing Schedule

Day 22	Day 23–25	Day 26	Day 27–29	Day 30
Eat 3 portions of dairy and check for reactions.	Avoid test food. Watch for symptoms such as sinus problems, dark circles under eyes, bloating or stomach upset. Consider these statistics: Only 50 percent of people of European descent, 25 percent of Africans, and 5 percent of Asians can digest dairy. If no negative reaction, then proceed with caution.	Eat 3 portions of sucrose-based sweetener.	Avoid test food. Watch for itchiness, rashes, joint pain, fatigue, brain fog, bloating, irritability, low self-esteem. If you want to test yourself on sugar and sugar-containing foods, be warned you may feel a huge rush and think you feel fine, but pay attention to the crash. If no negative reaction, then use in small amounts with caution.	Test 1 gluten grain (e.g., barley, oats or rye). Watch for joint pain, fatigue, brain fog, bloating, weight gain, depression or anxiety. Minimize exposure for long life.

you can tell exactly what is at fault if you feel bloated or tired. You will be tempted to jump back onto the foods you've missed, but be patient. You may want to go back to eating old choices, but I encourage you to keep exploring new and more health-supportive alternatives.

With the reintroduction of certain foods, you might notice some physical changes, such as congestion, itchiness, swollen tongue, irritability, bloating, dark circles under your eyes, fatigue, hives or an infection in your ears, nose or throat. These typical signs of an allergic reaction to food are the answers you have been looking for! Keep in mind that it's possible to experience almost any symptom with any allergen. The reaction you experience will depend on your body, the food you're allergic to

and how strongly your body reacts to it. Use a food journal to keep track of what you eat, and record any symptoms that are out of the ordinary. Stop eating a food once you've confirmed that you're sensitive or allergic to it, and keep it on your list of foods to avoid for 3 to 6 months, after which you can test it again.

When testing these foods, be careful not to confuse euphoria and excitement with food tolerance. Your desire to have these foods back in your diet can cloud your judgment, and so can your body's physiological reaction to them. We often crave the foods that we are unable to tolerate; these foods can mask our symptoms and make us feel better in the short term. These feelings of bliss increase our desire to reach for that food again.

You Can't Test the River with Both Feet!

You would never jump into fast-flowing water with both feet, would you? Without testing the depth of the water first, you could get swept away. The same goes for the wild world of food. I want you to journal, journal, journal! This is the best way to know how food is affecting you. I suggest you stick your toe into uncharted territory by testing mild trigger foods and then build from there.

First, put back in any fruit or veggies that you think may not agree with you. You may notice that bananas, oranges, eggplant and tomatoes are tougher to digest, so if you kept them out for this cleanse, now is the time to try adding them back in your diet one at a time. Potatoes and eggplant contain an alkaloid called solanine that can increase joint and bowel inflammation if you are sensitive to it. Watch for pain when you reintroduce them and avoid it by using the tasty substitutions in this book.

When you finish experimenting with vegetables and fruits, try cultured dairy. Studies have shown that foods containing milk and dairy from small animals such as sheep or goats are easier to digest than cow's milk and can be healing to the digestive tract. Goat and sheep yogurt or live-cultured soft goat cheese can help provide the digestive tract with probiotic bacteria, which knock out problematic yeast overgrowth. People with European or East Indian heritage may tolerate small amounts of cultured dairy products and ghee. High-fat cheese and milk from cows are less ideal because they are difficult to digest and contain certain fats that can trigger inflammation. At the end of your dairy experiments, try older cow cheeses and really watch for symptoms. Dairy can cause constipation and mucus, so be careful to write down in your journal how you feel.

An anti-inflammatory diet is free of all wheat gluten. If you feel you must reintroduce gluten grains, I suggest you begin with oats, as they are technically free of wheat gluten as long as they are processed in a separate gluten-free facility. Next, introduce barley and then rye, which are relatively low in gluten. Spelt and kamut are close relatives to wheat and contain high amounts of gluten. Wheat has been hybridized and is the hardest grain of all to digest. To keep your joints mobile, your gut happy and your inflammation down, I recommend that you reduce the amount of gluten you consume for life.

Use the chart on page 117 as a guide on how to best reintroduce potentially inflammatory foods back into your diet. Note that I don't suggest eating these foods if you are confident you are sensitive to them. I am just giving guidelines in case you really want to test them. People with serious inflammation should follow the stricter guidelines outlined in *Meals That Heal Inflammation*.

More Tips on Food Reintroduction

After the detox is complete, try some wild game or lean cuts of naturally raised, grass-fed beef and bison. How does red meat feel in your system? If good, move on to trying smoked meats and fish if you would like, but remember these are unhealthy. Be careful to check for symptoms such as headaches and bloating the day after eating them. These include sausages, hot dogs, corned beef, pastrami and pickled tongue.

To test yourself for a dairy allergy, introduce cultured sheep and goat products such as yogurt and kefir; then try soft cheeses and ghee (clarified butter). I don't recommend reintroducing cow's milk due to allergenicity, but if you really want it, select lactose-reduced cheeses and well-fermented yogurt from organic, grass-fed, naturally raised animals.

If you really want to add corn back to your diet, please consider buying organic corn to avoid genetically modified varieties. Corn is high on the glycemic index and can cause allergic reactions.

When faced with a breakdown, I want you to ask yourself, "What do I really crave?" Then go underneath that food craving to listen to your inner voice. The inner voice will tell you what you really want. Do you want joy, happiness and peace? Healing foods will always lead you to your true desire!

I send you love and good energy, today and always.

Part 3
The Recipes

Recipe Icons

- Gluten-free
- Free of soy and its derivatives
- Free of dairy and its derivatives
- Free of eggs and egg products
- Free of peanuts and tree nuts
- Contains low-alkaloid nightshades (e.g., ripe tomatoes, red bell peppers, goji berries)
- **V** Free of animal products and their derivatives

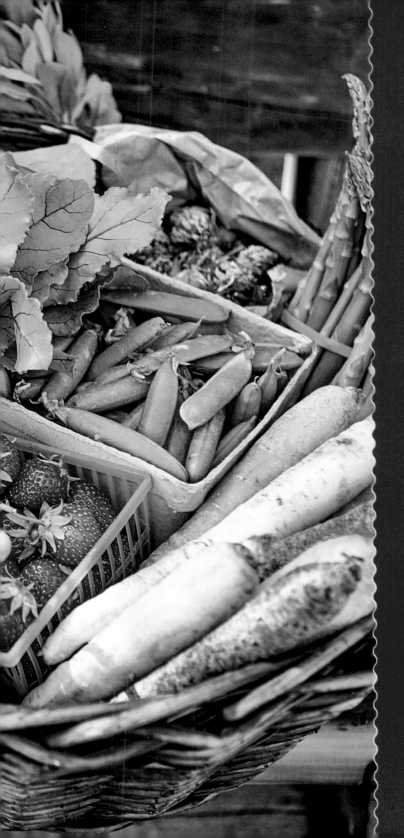

Fast Detox Meals and Special-Occasion Treats

"Just wanted to send a personal note thanking you for the 21-day detox. It had so much information to kick-start my weight-loss journey. I have lost 32 pounds now and feel great. I'm sleeping better, and I have way more energy. My knees don't ache anymore, and I have much more flexibility."

—Lora J.

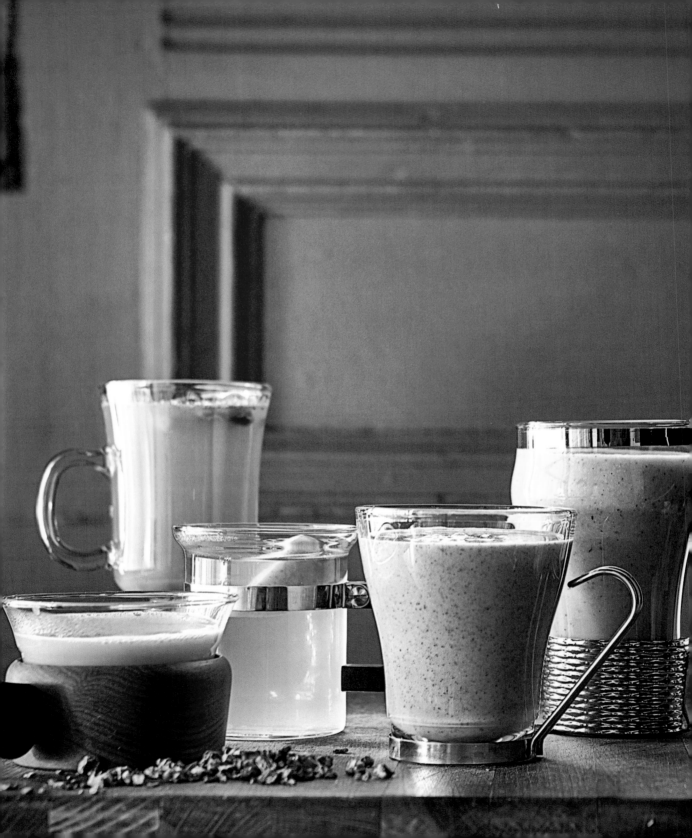

10

Liquid Healing

Making Your Own Nut and Seed Milks

Empower yourself with this formula and make your own nut- or seed-based milks! Aside from saving you money, it will also reduce your exposure to BPA-lined packages and potentially inflammatory additives.

A few popular nuts and seeds (almonds, Brazil nuts, hazelnuts, pecans, macadamia nuts and sesame seeds) need straining to achieve a smooth texture. This is easy to do. Straining with a nut-milk bag (sold at health-food stores) is best, although cheesecloth or a fine-mesh sieve will work too. Softer nuts and seeds (cashews, coconut, Hemp Hearts and sunflower seeds) do not need to be strained, provided they are well soaked and you own a high-powered blender. Avoid making milk with walnuts, as they go rancid quickly and can taste bitter.

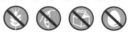

1 cup	raw nuts or seeds of choice
2 cups	filtered water, for soaking the nuts or seeds
4 cups	filtered water, for the milk
pinch	pink rock or gray sea salt

optional sweetener and flavorings

1–2 Tbsp	raw liquid honey or coconut nectar (see Tip) *or* 2–3 medjool dates, pitted
1 Tbsp	pure vanilla extract or raw cacao powder

optional detox boosters

1 Tbsp	ground chia seeds (to thicken the milk, if desired)
½ tsp	ground cinnamon

buttermilk option

1 Tbsp	raw apple cider vinegar or organic lemon juice

Be sure to hold down the lid of the blender while blending, as the pressure can build up inside. If you have a less powerful machine, avoid burning out the motor with this heavy mixture by blending it in short stretches.

To make a nut- or seed-based "cream," simply use half the amount of water — 2 cups instead of 4 cups — and keep the rest of the recipe the same.

You can find coconut nectar or syrup (which comes from the coconut tree blossom) at health-food stores.

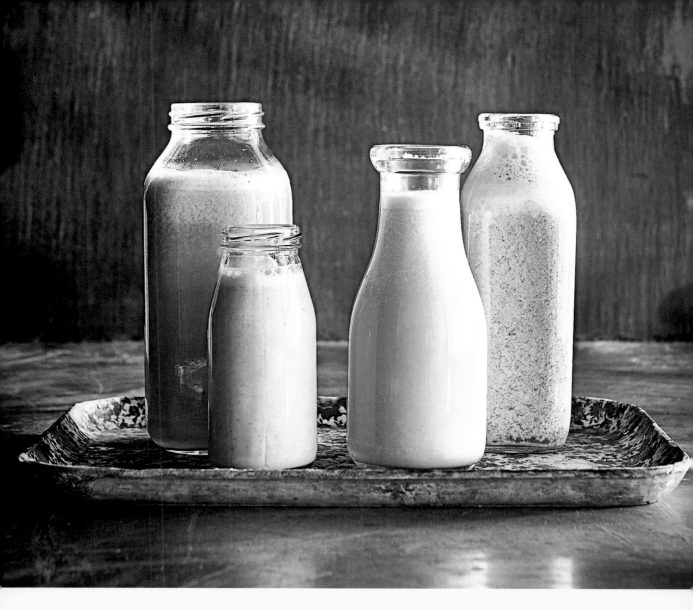

1 Soak the nuts or seeds in 2 cups water for 2 to 4 hours. Drain and rinse.

2 In a blender, place 4 cups water, the salt and the rinsed nuts or seeds, and blend on high speed until liquefied.

3 Strain the milk if necessary, pressing to extract as much liquid as possible.

4 If using any of the optional ingredients, return the milk to the blender, and blend them in well.

5 Transfer to Mason jars for storage.

Makes 4 cups. Will keep for 3 to 4 days in the fridge. Shake well before using.

Vanilla Cinnamon Pecan Milk

This nut milk is one of the richest and most flavorful. Once made, you can serve as is, or strain with a nut-milk bag or cheesecloth if you want a smoother consistency. Pecans are a rich source of healthy fats as well as the antioxidants ellagic acid and vitamin E, which protect the body from infections and inflammation.

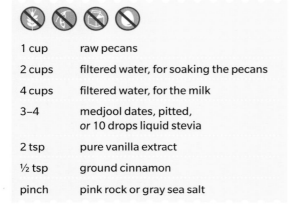

1 cup	raw pecans
2 cups	filtered water, for soaking the pecans
4 cups	filtered water, for the milk
3–4	medjool dates, pitted, or 10 drops liquid stevia
2 tsp	pure vanilla extract
½ tsp	ground cinnamon
pinch	pink rock or gray sea salt

1 Soak the pecans in 2 cups water for a few hours or overnight. Drain and rinse well.

2 Place the pecans, 4 cups water, and the rest of the ingredients in a blender. Blend on high speed for about 2 minutes or until the mixture is extremely smooth.

3 Serve as is, or strain for an even smoother texture.

4 Transfer to Mason jars for storage.

Makes 4 cups. Will keep for 4 days in the fridge. Shake well before using.

 If you strain the milk, save the leftover nut pulp to add to smoothies, porridge or puddings.

Sweet Seed Milk

Seed milk is an inexpensive and healthy milk replacement. Sunflower seeds and Hemp Hearts are little slivers of sunshine, rich in vitamin E, which assists in the liver's detoxing capabilities.

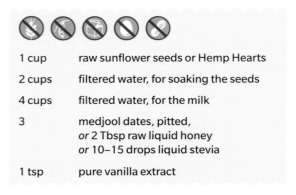

1 cup	raw sunflower seeds or Hemp Hearts
2 cups	filtered water, for soaking the seeds
4 cups	filtered water, for the milk
3	medjool dates, pitted, or 2 Tbsp raw liquid honey or 10–15 drops liquid stevia
1 tsp	pure vanilla extract

1 Soak the sunflower seeds or Hemp Hearts in 2 cups water for a few hours or overnight. Drain and rinse well.

2 In a blender, add the drained seeds, 4 cups water, the dates or honey or stevia (if using), and the vanilla. Blend on high speed until smooth. (If you have a high-powered blender, straining should not be required.)

3 Transfer to Mason jars for storage.

Makes 5 cups. Will keep for up to 4 days in the fridge. Shake well before using.

Coconut Beverage

This beverage is an alternative to 2% milk. Over the years I have been asked for my opinion on various alternative milks. Unfortunately, many store-bought products have ingredients (such as sugar and carrageenan) that many people are sensitive to. Milk substitutes can also be expensive. My sister, a mother of five boys, created this recipe for a homemade coconut beverage that children love — and it's easy on the wallet!

1¾ cups	(14-oz can) organic coconut milk (preferably full-fat)
3 cups	filtered water (if using light coconut milk, reduce to 2 cups)
1–2 tsp	pure vanilla extract
pinch	pink rock or gray sea salt

optional sweetener

1 Tbsp	raw liquid honey or coconut nectar

1 Place all the ingredients in a blender, including the honey or coconut nectar if using, and blend on high speed. Add more water if you want a thinner consistency.

2 Transfer to Mason jars for storage.

Makes 4½ cups. Will keep for up to 4 days in the fridge. Shake well before using.

 Ingredients such as carrageenan are often used to stabilize and thicken alternative milk beverages. Because this recipe is free of stabilizers and thickeners, you'll need to shake it before using.

Coconut Beverage
(Made with Dried Coconut)

This is such an easy and inexpensive version of coconut beverage that you may never buy store-bought again!

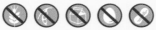

1 cup	unsweetened dried shredded coconut
4 cups	filtered water
1 Tbsp	raw liquid honey or coconut nectar
1–2 tsp	pure vanilla extract
pinch	pink rock or gray sea salt

1 Soak the coconut in the water for 2 hours.

2 Transfer the coconut and soaking water to a blender, along with the remaining ingredients, and blend on high speed until smooth. If you do not own a high-powered blender, you may need to strain out the larger pieces of shredded coconut.

3 Transfer to Mason jars for storage.

Makes 5 cups. Will keep for up to 4 days in the fridge. Shake well before using.

Coconut beverage is my favorite replacement for milk because it looks and tastes the closest to dairy. It's also very energizing!

Juicing and Blending to Boost Immunity

Juicing and blending make it easy to ingest seven to 10 vegetables and 3 fruits a day, which is the best way to detoxify and get immune-boosting nutrients. Using a rainbow of colors is important, not only because it is a feast for the eyes, but also because it delivers the entire spectrum of nutrients we need — from vitamin A to zinc.

Here is a nutrient guide based on color:

- Foods high in vitamin A are most often **yellow** or **orange**, such as carrots, squash and sweet potatoes. They help to repair the skin and digestive lining.
- Foods high in vitamin B tend to be **green**; think asparagus, chard, spinach and green beans. These foods work to nourish the nervous system.
- **Red** foods like berries and red bell peppers are high in vitamin C and are critical for the production of collagen, the protein we use to make skin, joints, tendons and ligaments.
- The foods that have the highest numbers of antioxidants are **blue** and **purple**, such as black-berries, blueberries, Concord grapes, purple cabbage and figs.

Juicing and Blending: What's the Difference?

Juicing extracts the nutrients and liquid from vegeta-bles and fruits, leaving the fiber behind. It's beneficial in three main ways:

1 You can maximize how many vegetables and fruit you fit into your day — up to 30 servings! Few people can eat that amount, but with a juicer, you can reach that level with ease, if needed.

2 When you remove the fiber from the vegetable and fruit, you can more easily absorb the nutrients that are locked inside them. For those fighting an inflammatory illness, juicing ensures you get maximum nutrition without struggling with digestion. My friend Joe Cross (creator of the documentary *Fat, Sick and Nearly Dead*) calls juice "liquid sunshine," and I couldn't agree more!

3 Reducing the fiber allows the digestive system the most complete rest. Fiber can be irritating for some people with IBD (inflammatory bowel disease, such as colitis or Crohn's disease) and is best minimized when experiencing a flare-up.

Blending, on the other hand, purees produce into smoothies with all the fiber left in. Here are the three main benefits of blending:

1 It's a great way to consume more dark leafy greens like spinach, kale and chard. Simply add hot filtered water to green vegetables, lemon juice and seeds, blending to make a warm shake-soup to start your day alkaline and energized.

Safety Tip

 When blending hot liquids, be sure to hold the blender lid down firmly as the heat could cause the lid to pop off.

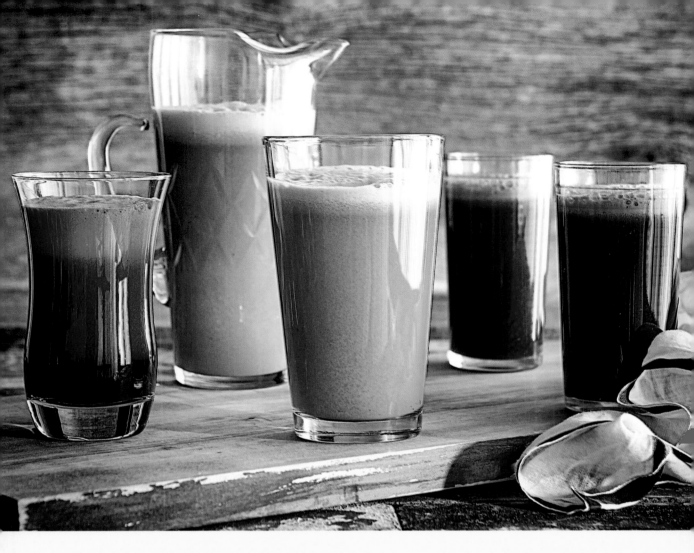

2 You can serve vegetables to picky eaters. If you prefer a more classic smoothie, you can start with fruit and sneak in vegetables to ensure that everyone gets their daily dose of vitamins, phytonutrients and minerals.

3 Blenders really shine when you blend all kinds of superfood powders, nut butters and soothing spices into the mix. The possibilities are vast, and the cleanup is easy. Blenders are also affordable, making blending a great first step for any health seeker.

A masticating juice extractor or juice press fully extracts vitamins, enzymes and minerals from the vegetables. A high-speed centrifugal juicer, on the other hand, produces a low yield, requiring you to process the pulp again; in that case I suggest using a blender. You get all the nutrients with the added benefit of the fiber!

50 Shades of Green

If you have a sensitive tummy, it's best to avoid smoothies with frozen bananas. Hemp Hearts can add creaminess instead. They're a rich source of iron, perfect for keeping your iron levels at an optimal level, and hypoallergenic.

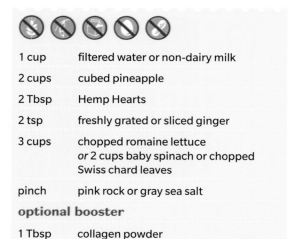

1 cup	filtered water or non-dairy milk
2 cups	cubed pineapple
2 Tbsp	Hemp Hearts
2 tsp	freshly grated or sliced ginger
3 cups	chopped romaine lettuce *or* 2 cups baby spinach or chopped Swiss chard leaves
pinch	pink rock or gray sea salt
optional booster	
1 Tbsp	collagen powder

In a blender, layer the water or non-dairy milk, pineapple, Hemp Hearts, ginger, collagen (if using) and salt. Add the greens last. Blend on high speed for 30 seconds or until creamy.

Makes 3 cups.

 The ginger and pineapple in this drink will help you digest the raw greens.

If you buy organic ginger, there is no need to peel it, which will save you time and deliver greater flavor.

If you can't find collagen powder and don't mind a thicker beverage, replace the collagen powder with gelatin powder (from grass-fed or pasture-raised cows).

Anti-inflammatory Powerhouse

This juice combines the sweetness of apple and carrot, the spiciness of ginger, the sour of lemon and the richness of beet — a fantastic balanced start to the day. The lemon and optional omega-3 oil reduce the beverage's glycemic index, easing cravings. Beets provide iron, folate, potassium, magnesium and vitamin C, which all have anti-inflammatory and detoxifying properties. And beets' betaine hydrochloride eases digestion.

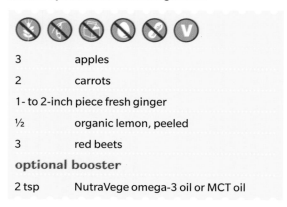

3	apples
2	carrots
1- to 2-inch piece fresh ginger	
½	organic lemon, peeled
3	red beets
optional booster	
2 tsp	NutraVege omega-3 oil or MCT oil

Juice all the produce whole in the order listed, stir the omega-3 oil into the juice if using and serve immediately.

Makes 2 cups.

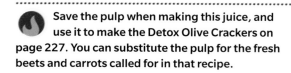 **Save the pulp when making this juice, and use it to make the Detox Olive Crackers on page 227.** You can substitute the pulp for the fresh beets and carrots called for in that recipe.

Berry Bliss Shake

Did you know that wild blueberries help to heal stomach ulcers? They work by building up the defensive barriers of the gastrointestinal mucous membrane and killing off *H. pylori*, the bacteria that causes ulcers.

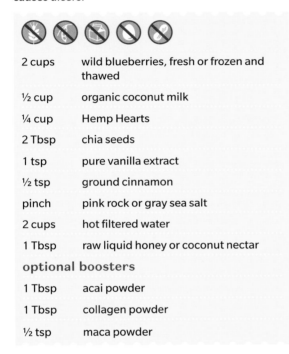

2 cups	wild blueberries, fresh or frozen and thawed
½ cup	organic coconut milk
¼ cup	Hemp Hearts
2 Tbsp	chia seeds
1 tsp	pure vanilla extract
½ tsp	ground cinnamon
pinch	pink rock or gray sea salt
2 cups	hot filtered water
1 Tbsp	raw liquid honey or coconut nectar

optional boosters

1 Tbsp	acai powder
1 Tbsp	collagen powder
½ tsp	maca powder

Place all the ingredients except the honey into a blender, including any of the boosters if using, and blend on high speed until smooth. Add the honey, and blend well.

Makes 4 cups.

I specify pink rock salt or gray sea salt throughout this book because either salt provides more than 60 trace minerals that are helpful for detoxification and the anti-inflammatory process. Regular table salt is refined and may contain sugar. If you can't find unrefined gray or pink salt, use regular sea salt.

The Bitter Truth

This drink is pure medicine; whichever bitter vegetable you end up choosing, it will help flush the liver. Bitter compounds in plants stimulate the production of digestive juices that carry toxins from your liver into your bowels for elimination. Western eaters tend not to like bitter tastes, but in Asia, India and Europe, people seek out bitter flavors. I softened the bitter notes in this recipe with the sweetness of carrot and sourness of lemon.

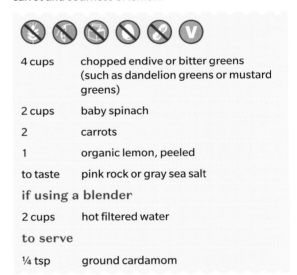

4 cups	chopped endive or bitter greens (such as dandelion greens or mustard greens)
2 cups	baby spinach
2	carrots
1	organic lemon, peeled
to taste	pink rock or gray sea salt

if using a blender

2 cups	hot filtered water

to serve

¼ tsp	ground cardamom

1   If using a juicer, juice the endive or bitter greens, spinach, carrots and lemon. Add the salt.

If using a blender, first grate the carrots. To the blender, add the carrots, endive or bitter greens, spinach and lemon along with the hot water and salt, and blend on high speed until smooth.

2   Pour into a large serving glass, and sprinkle with cardamom.

Makes 1 cup juice or 4½ cups blended beverage.

Carrot Cake Smoothie

The fiber in carrots works like an internal toothbrush, helping to scrub away harmful waste on the insides of your intestines. Did you know that fiber also binds to excess estrogen to balance your hormones? Another great reason to cleanse!

 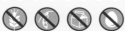

1½ cups	coconut beverage (page 127 or store-bought) or other non-dairy milk, more if needed
1 cup	grated carrots
3–4	medjool dates, pitted, *or* 10 to 12 drops liquid stevia
3 Tbsp	raw cashews or Hemp Hearts
1 Tbsp	chia seeds
1 tsp	pure vanilla extract
½ tsp	ground cinnamon
⅛ tsp	ground cloves
⅛ tsp	ground nutmeg
pinch	pink rock or gray sea salt

optional booster

1 Tbsp	collagen powder

to serve (optional)

to taste	unsweetened dried shredded coconut
pinch	ground cinnamon

1 In a blender, combine all the smoothie ingredients, including the collagen if using, and blend until smooth.

2 Add more non-dairy milk as needed to reach the desired thickness.

3 Pour into serving glasses. If desired, sprinkle with coconut and a pinch of cinnamon.

Makes 2 cups.

 Another great alternative sweetener is monk fruit, known as *lo han guo* in Southeast Asia. In 2009 it was approved for use in North America, but it has been used for centuries in the East to sweeten treats and beverages and aid in digestion. The amount of monk fruit needed to sweeten shakes varies from product to product because it is 150–200 times sweeter than sugar, so start small and carefully add tiny amounts if you want to try this zero-calorie sweetener in the Hot Detox.

Citrus Chaser

All citrus fruit contain the flavonoids hesperidin, quercetin, diosmin, naringin and rutin. These phytonutrients (also known as vitamin P) transport vitamin C into our cells. They also help with liver detoxification and allergy reduction.

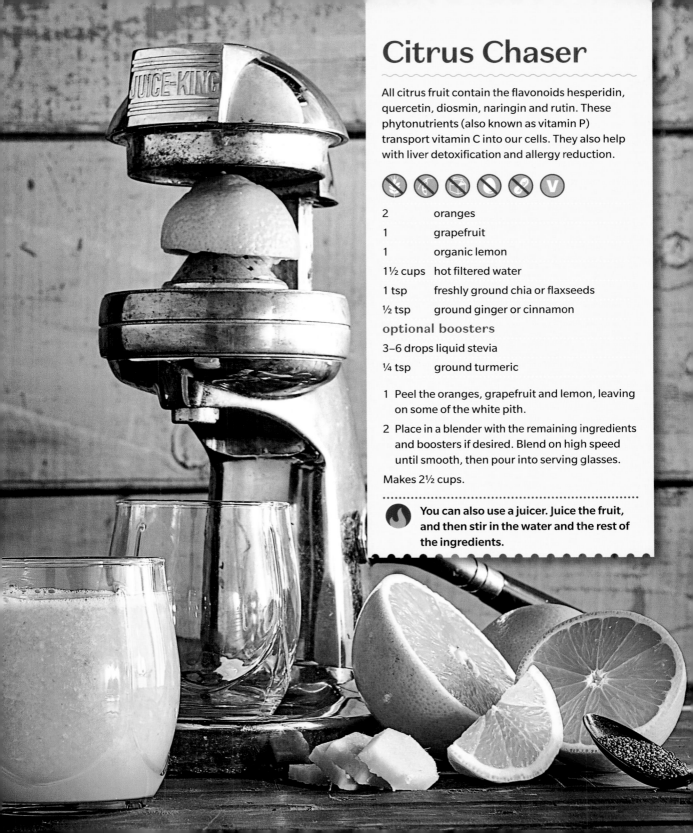

2	oranges
1	grapefruit
1	organic lemon
1½ cups	hot filtered water
1 tsp	freshly ground chia or flaxseeds
½ tsp	ground ginger or cinnamon

optional boosters

3–6 drops liquid stevia	
¼ tsp	ground turmeric

1 Peel the oranges, grapefruit and lemon, leaving on some of the white pith.

2 Place in a blender with the remaining ingredients and boosters if desired. Blend on high speed until smooth, then pour into serving glasses.

Makes 2½ cups.

You can also use a juicer. Juice the fruit, and then stir in the water and the rest of the ingredients.

Chia Chuck Berry

This hot drink is so fun that you shouldn't be surprised if you find yourself doing the twist in the kitchen!

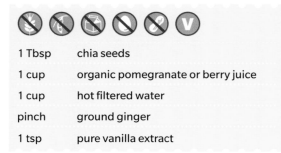

1 Tbsp	chia seeds
1 cup	organic pomegranate or berry juice
1 cup	hot filtered water
pinch	ground ginger
1 tsp	pure vanilla extract

Soak the chia seeds in the pomegranate or berry juice overnight in the fridge. Warm it up gently the next day by adding the hot water and spices. Mix all ingredients together and enjoy!

Makes 2 cups.

Deep Green Dream

This recipe is supersatisfying with its sweet, sour and salty taste. Healthy fats will kill your cravings on the Hot Detox, so enjoy this drink often. Of the green powders, spirulina is my favorite because it contains almost every vitamin and mineral.

½	ripe avocado (about ⅓ cup)
¼ cup	Hemp Hearts
¼ cup	organic lemon juice
2 Tbsp	raw liquid honey or coconut nectar *or* 12–15 drops liquid stevia
1–2 tsp	Hawaiian spirulina powder *or* 1 cup baby spinach
pinch	pink rock or gray sea salt
2 cups	filtered water
optional boosters	
1 Tbsp	collagen powder
1 tsp	maca powder

1   Place all the ingredients in a blender, including the collagen and/or maca if using, and blend on high speed until smooth and creamy.

2   Adjust sweetness by adding more honey to taste.

Makes 3 cups. Will keep in the fridge for up to 24 hours. Shake well before using.

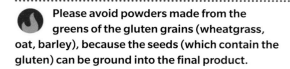

Please avoid powders made from the greens of the gluten grains (wheatgrass, oat, barley), because the seeds (which contain the gluten) can be ground into the final product.

Dandelion Root Koffee

This is a great coffee replacement. You can use dandelion root to detoxify, relieve constipation, soothe an upset stomach and help shed water weight. Tea made from the dandelion root or leaves has been used in traditional Chinese and Native American medicine for centuries. Its mildly bitter flavor stimulates bile flow and can help accelerate your body's natural detoxification process.

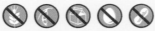

1 cup	filtered water
2–3 tsp	roasted and ground dandelion root

to serve (optional)

1 tsp	raw liquid honey or coconut nectar or monk fruit powder to taste
¼ cup	non-dairy milk
1 Tbsp	MCT oil

You can buy raw or dried root at a health-food store. To prepare raw dandelion root, see the Tip below. If you buy dried chopped dandelion root, roast it at 300°F for 30 minutes or until it reaches a chocolate-brown color. The sweet smell of dandelion roasting in your oven is fantastic! Let it cool, and then grind in a clean coffee or spice grinder.

Boil the water, and combine with the dandelion root in a coffeepot or similar container. Let steep for at least 10 minutes. If desired, sweeten with honey or stevia, and serve with non-dairy milk.

Makes 1 cup.

 For an extra adventure, go DIY! Try to find a pesticide-free dandelion patch. Dig up the deep taproots, and rinse several times under running water to clean off the dirt. Cut the roots into ¼-inch pieces, and roast on a parchment-lined baking sheet at 300°F for 2 hours. Let it cool, then grind in a clean coffee or spice grinder.

Digestive Gripe Water

Fennel and anise seeds have several flavonoid antioxidants, such as kaempferol and quercetin, that remove harmful free radicals from the body, helping to protect you from infection, degenerative disease and various types of cancer. Grinding these spices releases their essential oils.

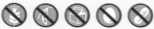

1 tsp	fennel, dill or anise seeds
¼ tsp	baking soda
1½ cups	filtered water, just off the boil

optional boosters

¼ tsp	ground ginger
2–3 drops	liquid stevia *or* 1 tsp raw liquid honey

1 Grind the fennel, dill or anise seeds in a clean spice or coffee grinder, or mortar and pestle. Place in a teapot or covered pot with the baking soda and ginger if using.

2 Pour in the boiling water, cover and steep for 10 minutes. Strain and sweeten if desired, as it cools.

Makes 1½ cups.

 Gripe water has been used since 1850! The fennel, dill and anise seed contains volatile essential-oil compounds (such as anethole and limonene) that soothe digestive troubles. The baking soda is great for heartburn as well.

Detox Rocket

This smoothie puts toxins on a rocket express ride out of your body! The beets increase liver detox, the antioxidants in the berries protect the intermediate phase (see the illustration on page 39), the lemon juice (and optional lecithin) increase bile flow and the coconut water provides energizing minerals.

4 cups	chopped boiled beets (about 4 small beets)
2 cups	unsweetened coconut water
2 cups	organic berries (blueberries, raspberries and/or strawberries)
¼ cup	Hemp Hearts
2–4 Tbsp	organic lemon juice

optional boosters

1 Tbsp	collagen powder
1 tsp	sunflower lecithin powder

Place all the ingredients in a blender, including the collagen and/or lecithin if using, and blend on high speed until smooth.

Makes 5 cups. Will keep in the fridge for up to 2 days. Shake well before using.

Make a batch of cooked beets ahead of time, to add to the Hot Detox recipes in a snap. Place 4 to 5 medium beets (skins on) in a saucepan and add water to cover. Add 1 tablespoon of lemon juice to stop the beets from bleeding. Bring to a boil, reduce heat and simmer until tender, 30 to 40 minutes. Drain, cool slightly and slip off the skins.

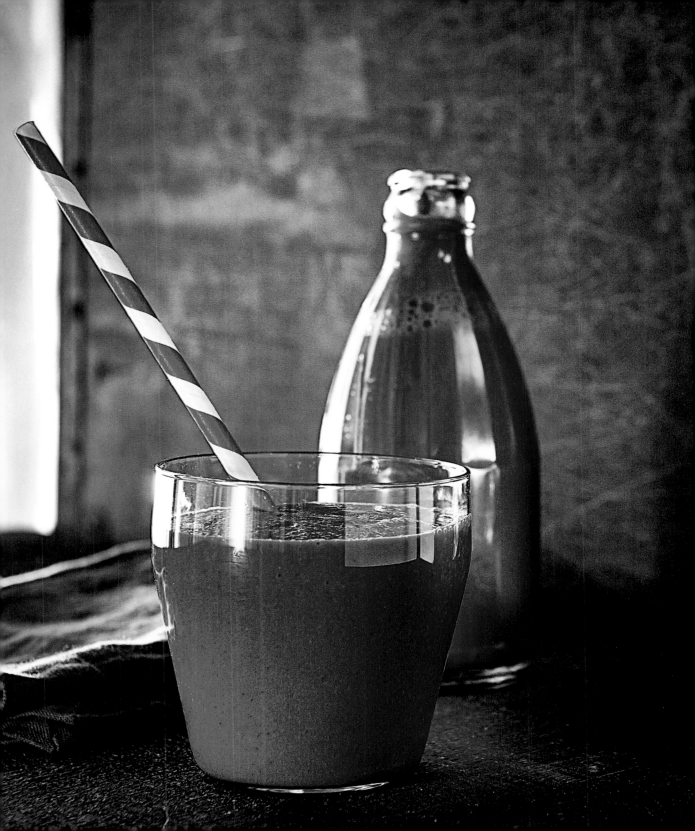

Ginger Recovery Drink

I developed this recipe to replace the popular sports drinks people have when exercising. Take it to your hot yoga class — you may find it increases your energy. The citrus helps with liver detox, the dates provide slow-burning sugars, the ginger reduces digestive gas and bloating and the sea salt replaces electrolytes.

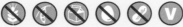

2–3 Tbsp	organic lemon or lime juice
2	medjool dates, pitted and chopped, *or* 8 drops liquid stevia
1 tsp	ground ginger *or* 1 Tbsp freshly grated ginger
pinch	pink rock or gray sea salt
3 cups	warm filtered water

Place all the ingredients in a blender or food processor, and let stand for 10 minutes. Blend on high speed until smooth. Serve warm or at room temperature.

Makes 3 cups.

 When buying fresh ginger, look for a smooth shiny skin, which means it's superfresh!

Golden Milk

Golden milk is served in the Ayurvedic tradition to reduce *vata* in the fall and winter season. Think of *vata* as a wind energy that can make you experience brain fog or feel fearful. This recipe is traditionally made with cow's milk, but many people find dairy to be problematic because it's mucus forming. I use Hemp Hearts or cashews as a creamy and delicious dairy-free alternative.

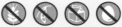

2 Tbsp	Hemp Hearts or raw cashews
2	medjool dates, pitted, *or* ½ banana
⅛ tsp	ground cardamom or cinnamon
⅛ tsp	ground turmeric
1 cup	filtered water, just off the boil
optional boosters	
1 tsp	coconut butter (see Tip; use coconut oil if coconut butter is unavailable)
2 threads	saffron

Place all the ingredients in a blender, including the coconut butter and/or saffron if using, and blend on high speed until smooth. Serve warm.

Makes 1½ cups.

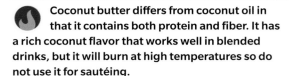 **Coconut butter differs from coconut oil in that it contains both protein and fiber. It has a rich coconut flavor that works well in blended drinks, but it will burn at high temperatures so do not use it for sautéing.**

The Green Hornet

This is a delightful shake with the right balance of creaminess, sweet citrus and a bit of a kick. Swiss chard and beet greens are from the same plant family and contain very detoxifying phytonutrients called betalains, which have been shown to reduce inflammation.

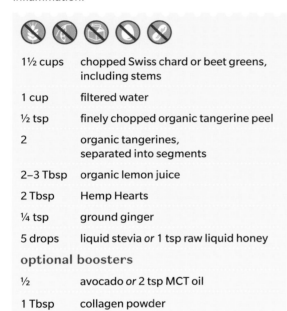

1½ cups	chopped Swiss chard or beet greens, including stems
1 cup	filtered water
½ tsp	finely chopped organic tangerine peel
2	organic tangerines, separated into segments
2–3 Tbsp	organic lemon juice
2 Tbsp	Hemp Hearts
¼ tsp	ground ginger
5 drops	liquid stevia *or* 1 tsp raw liquid honey

optional boosters

½	avocado *or* 2 tsp MCT oil
1 Tbsp	collagen powder

Place all the ingredients in a blender, including the optional boosters if using, and blend on high speed until smooth.

Makes 2 cups.

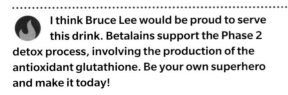 **I think Bruce Lee would be proud to serve this drink. Betalains support the Phase 2 detox process, involving the production of the antioxidant glutathione. Be your own superhero and make it today!**

Gut Booster Juice

This juice is traditionally used to help heal the lining of the stomach. The optional sauerkraut juice balances the flavor, but avoid it if you have an active ulcer.

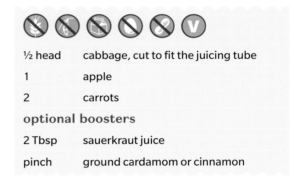

½ head	cabbage, cut to fit the juicing tube
1	apple
2	carrots

optional boosters

2 Tbsp	sauerkraut juice
pinch	ground cardamom or cinnamon

Using a juicer, process the cabbage, apple and carrots. If desired, stir in the sauerkraut juice and/or sprinkle with cardamom or cinnamon.

Makes 2 cups.

 This traditional stomach remedy may seem intimidating at first. Be brave and give it a try!

Heart Blush

Raspberries are very high in vitamin C, a key nutrient to help improve your body's ability to absorb iron. These crimson berries contain high levels of dietary fiber (which makes up approximately 20 percent of their total weight), and in combination with chia or flaxseeds, you have a strong bulking agent for your GI cleanse.

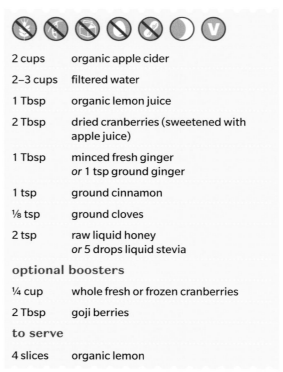

2 cups	organic raspberries or strawberries
1 cup	hot filtered water
2 Tbsp	Hemp Hearts
2 Tbsp	ground chia or flaxseeds, freshly ground if possible
1 Tbsp	coconut nectar or 6–10 drops liquid stevia

optional booster

1 tsp	sunflower lecithin powder

Place all the ingredients in a blender, including the lecithin if using, and blend on high speed until smooth.

Makes 2 cups.

 Sunflower lecithin is optional here but really worth adding. It can increase bile flow and the size of your bowel movements! It has reduced many of my clients' constipation issues.

Hot Apple Toddy

There is evidence that cranberries, ginseng and goji berries can assist in the fight against cold viruses.

2 cups	organic apple cider
2–3 cups	filtered water
1 Tbsp	organic lemon juice
2 Tbsp	dried cranberries (sweetened with apple juice)
1 Tbsp	minced fresh ginger or 1 tsp ground ginger
1 tsp	ground cinnamon
⅛ tsp	ground cloves
2 tsp	raw liquid honey or 5 drops liquid stevia

optional boosters

¼ cup	whole fresh or frozen cranberries
2 Tbsp	goji berries

to serve

4 slices	organic lemon

1 Place all the ingredients, including the boosters if using, in a pot. Bring to a low boil, then cover, reduce the heat and simmer for 10 minutes.

2 Remove the cranberries, ginger and other boosters if you prefer a smooth beverage. Then stir in the honey or stevia as it cools. Serve with a slice of lemon.

Makes 4 cups.

Enjoy the cranberries and/or goji berries in your porridge or applesauce as a midmorning snack.

The Hot Detox Tea

I formulated this tea to create the perfect mix of berry flavor and detox ingredients. The dried herbs, berries and powders can be found at the health-food store or online.

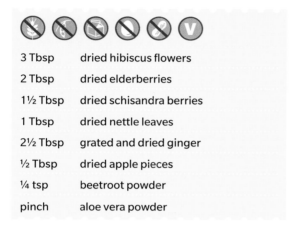

3 Tbsp	dried hibiscus flowers
2 Tbsp	dried elderberries
1½ Tbsp	dried schisandra berries
1 Tbsp	dried nettle leaves
2½ Tbsp	grated and dried ginger
½ Tbsp	dried apple pieces
¼ tsp	beetroot powder
pinch	aloe vera powder

1 Mix all the ingredients together in a bowl.

2 To make tea, bring 4 cups of filtered water to a boil in a pot. Remove from the heat, stir in half of the herb mix (reserve the rest for another time), cover and let steep for at least 10 minutes and up to 2 hours.

3 Pour the tea through a fine-mesh sieve into a Mason jar. Enjoy throughout the day. You can make a second brew by adding another 4 cups of hot water to the ingredients in the pot, with good results.

Makes enough dried tea mix for 8 cups of brewed tea. Unused mix keeps for up to a year.

If you don't feel like mixing this yourself, you can purchase a premade version from Lemon Lily, an organic tea company in Toronto (www.lemonlily.ca). I also have a soothing digestive chai formula and other wonderful tea recipes on my website.

Hot Pommy

A compound found only in pomegranates called punicalagin is shown to cleanse blood vessels. A recent yearlong study of patients with severe artery blockages showed that those who drank just 1.7 fluid ounces of pomegranate juice each day lowered their blood pressure by 12 percent and their atherosclerotic plaque by 30 percent.

1 Tbsp	organic lemon juice
¼ tsp	ground ginger
⅓ cup	organic pomegranate juice
1 cup	hot filtered water
2 drops	liquid stevia

Mix all the ingredients together in a serving glass, and enjoy!

Makes 1½ cups.

Don't have time to make a hot beverage? Just remember to drink warm water between meals.

Pumpkin Pie Smoothie

If you've never tried a warm smoothie before, now is the time. This one is perfect for a cool, crisp morning because it contains warming spices that will keep you feeling cozy all day long. Pumpkin is filled with vitamins, minerals and essential fatty acids, and provides a good dose of fiber (5 grams per half cup), which will help your digestion run smoothly, remove toxins from the body and balance blood sugar.

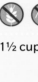

1½ cups	unsweetened almond milk or coconut beverage (page 127 or store-bought)
½ cup	pumpkin puree (see Tip)
½ cup	organic coconut milk
¼ cup	Hemp Hearts
2	medjool dates, pitted
1 tsp	pure vanilla extract
¼ tsp	ground ginger
⅛ tsp	ground cinnamon, plus more for serving
pinch	ground allspice
pinch	ground nutmeg
pinch	ground cloves

optional boosters

1 Tbsp	collagen powder
2 tsp	sunflower lecithin powder
pinch	pink rock or gray sea salt

1 In small saucepan over low heat, combine the almond milk and pumpkin puree. Heat gently, stirring occasionally until the mixture is very warm.

2 Meanwhile, place the rest of the ingredients, including any of the boosters if using, in a blender. Add the warmed pumpkin mixture and blend on high speed until smooth.

3 Serve with a pinch of cinnamon on top.

Makes 2½ cups.

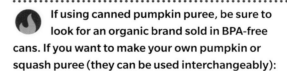

If using canned pumpkin puree, be sure to look for an organic brand sold in BPA-free cans. If you want to make your own pumpkin or squash puree (they can be used interchangeably):

1 Quarter an organic pumpkin or squash, discarding the stringy insides. Cut into chunks.

2 Place in a saucepan and cover with water. Bring to a boil and cook until the pumpkin chunks are tender.

3 Strain and let cool. Scoop out the flesh from the skin and puree in a blender until smooth.

Oh-So-Hardcore Detox Drink

Dandelion greens may seem scary, but once you juice them up, they become as tame as a circus lion. Dandelion is one of the most popular detox remedies for the kidneys, and turmeric is shown to protect the kidneys from damage and also cleanse the liver.

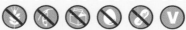

1 cup	fresh dandelion greens
½ head	cabbage, cut to fit the juicing tube
2	apples
1	organic lemon, peeled
2-inch piece fresh ginger	

optional boosters

8-inch piece fresh unpeeled burdock root	
½ tsp	roasted and ground dandelion root
½ tsp	ground turmeric

Using a juicer, process the dandelion greens, cabbage, apples, lemon and ginger, and the burdock if using. Stir in the ground dandelion root powder and/or turmeric if desired.

Makes 3 cups.

The Red Devil

The anthocyanins, phenols and flavanols in cherries are anti-inflammatory and help with muscle recovery. Studies show cherries can significantly reduce the risk of osteoarthritis, heart disease, cancer, metabolic syndrome and degenerative diseases.

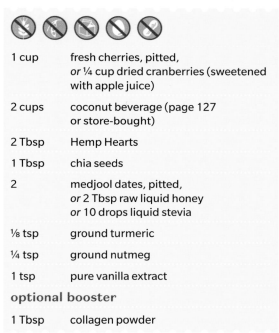

1 cup	fresh cherries, pitted, or ¼ cup dried cranberries (sweetened with apple juice)
2 cups	coconut beverage (page 127 or store-bought)
2 Tbsp	Hemp Hearts
1 Tbsp	chia seeds
2	medjool dates, pitted, or 2 Tbsp raw liquid honey or 10 drops liquid stevia
⅛ tsp	ground turmeric
¼ tsp	ground nutmeg
1 tsp	pure vanilla extract

optional booster

1 Tbsp	collagen powder

Place all the ingredients in a blender, including the collagen if using, and blend on high speed until smooth and silky.

Makes 3 cups.

If you use dried cranberries here, make sure you look for the ones that are juice sweetened and darker in color. Bright-red dried cranberries typically are loaded with added sugar.

Smooth Feeling

Apples contain calcium D-glucarate, a phytochemical that protects the body against cancer by increasing liver detoxification.

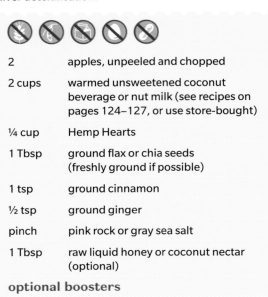

2	apples, unpeeled and chopped
2 cups	warmed unsweetened coconut beverage or nut milk (see recipes on pages 124–127, or use store-bought)
¼ cup	Hemp Hearts
1 Tbsp	ground flax or chia seeds (freshly ground if possible)
1 tsp	ground cinnamon
½ tsp	ground ginger
pinch	pink rock or gray sea salt
1 Tbsp	raw liquid honey or coconut nectar (optional)

optional boosters

¼ cup	unfiltered aloe vera juice
1 Tbsp	collagen powder

Place all the ingredients except the honey in a blender, including the aloe vera juice and/or collagen if using, and blend on high speed until smooth. Sweeten with honey if using.

Makes about 3 cups.

···

Aloe vera is a energetically "cool" food in traditional Chinese medicine. Aloe vera juice can reduce inflammation throughout the body and reduce constipation.

Tiger Spice Smoothie

This is a traditional Ayurvedic remedy for fall and winter exhaustion. Combining nuts, ginger, dates and cinnamon, with their warming effects, is said to raise *pitta* (the fire energy in the body). The high mineral content of these ingredients helps to soothe anxiety and aid in a peaceful sleep.

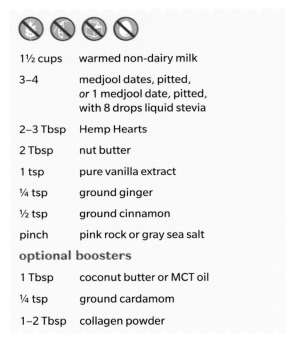

1½ cups	warmed non-dairy milk
3–4	medjool dates, pitted, *or* 1 medjool date, pitted, with 8 drops liquid stevia
2–3 Tbsp	Hemp Hearts
2 Tbsp	nut butter
1 tsp	pure vanilla extract
¼ tsp	ground ginger
½ tsp	ground cinnamon
pinch	pink rock or gray sea salt

optional boosters

1 Tbsp	coconut butter or MCT oil
¼ tsp	ground cardamom
1–2 Tbsp	collagen powder

Place all the ingredients in a blender, including any of the boosters if using, and blend on high speed until smooth.

Makes 3 cups.

···

Cinnamon is best when freshly ground, so try to buy whole cinnamon sticks and grind them as needed with a fine rasp grater or a sturdy spice or coffee grinder. You can also add a whole stick to soups and stews, where it can simmer with the broth.

Turmeric Spice Latte

This recipe is a wonderful way to take care of yourself and your family. My best friend Sarah swears by this drink to help her stay away from caffeine. It is very grounding and anti-inflammatory, so I think it will become one of your favorite beverages even after the Hot Detox is complete.

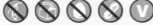

2 cups	warmed non-dairy milk
2	medjool dates, pitted, or 1 Tbsp coconut nectar
1 tsp	ground turmeric
1 tsp	freshly grated ginger or ½ tsp ground ginger
½ tsp	ground cinnamon

optional boosters

1 Tbsp	coconut butter (or coconut oil if coconut butter is unavailable)
¼ tsp	ground cardamom
2 threads	saffron

Place all the ingredients together in a blender, including any of the boosters if using, and blend on high speed until smooth. Serve warm.

Makes 2 cups.

Warm ACV and Honey Drink

Apple cider vinegar mixed with warm water and honey is a great start to your day. Acetic acid, the active ingredient in vinegar, reduces the hunger hormone ghrelin. It also improves digestion and helps you feel full faster and for a longer period of time. Activated charcoal is very detoxifying and may reduce diarrhea.

1 Tbsp	raw apple cider vinegar
1 tsp	raw liquid honey or 3–5 drops liquid stevia
1–1½ cups	warm filtered water (see Tip)

optional booster

½ tsp	activated charcoal

In a serving glass, combine vinegar, honey or stevia, and activated charcoal if using. Pour in warm water (see Tip) and stir well.

Makes 1 serving.

 For each serving, 1 cup of water will make a strong tonic, and 1½ cups will make a pleasant alternative to warm lemonade.

Drink this before meals to support digestion and regulate blood sugar.

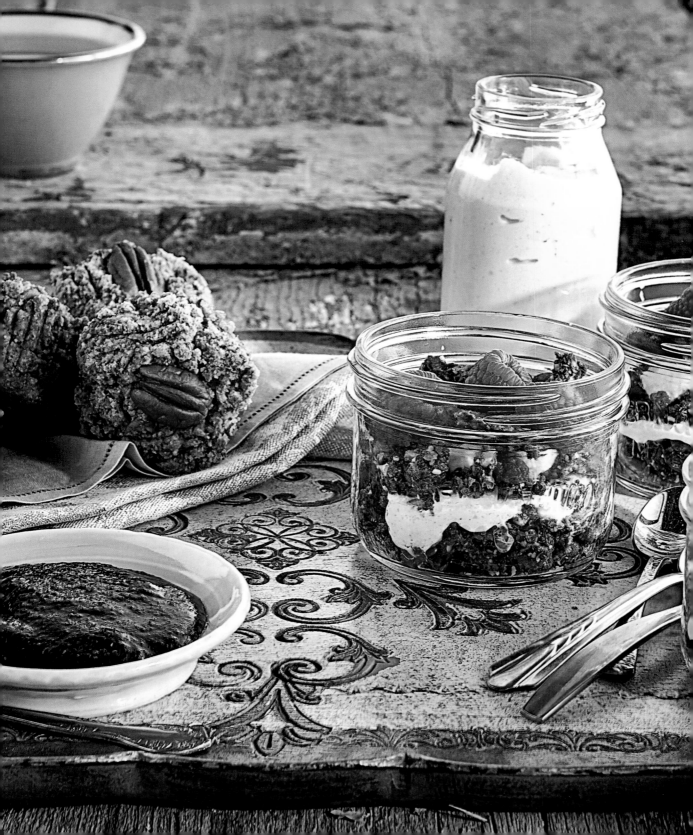

11

Meals to Begin the Day

Antioxidant Smoothie Bowl

Blueberries are loaded with many of the detoxifying antioxidants that are crucial for maintaining a healthy liver. A study published by the *World Journal of Gastroenterology* found that eating blueberries slowed the progression of liver diseases without the side effects commonly associated with conventional treatments. Choose wild blueberries whenever possible as they have twice the antioxidants of cultivated berries.

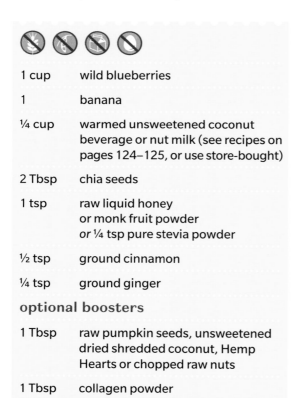

1 cup	wild blueberries
1	banana
¼ cup	warmed unsweetened coconut beverage or nut milk (see recipes on pages 124–125, or use store-bought)
2 Tbsp	chia seeds
1 tsp	raw liquid honey or monk fruit powder or ¼ tsp pure stevia powder
½ tsp	ground cinnamon
¼ tsp	ground ginger

optional boosters

1 Tbsp	raw pumpkin seeds, unsweetened dried shredded coconut, Hemp Hearts or chopped raw nuts
1 Tbsp	collagen powder
1 tsp	bee pollen or maca powder

Place all the ingredients in a high-speed blender, and blend until smooth. Top with boosters and fresh berries (if desired), and enjoy!

Makes 1 serving.

 Using frozen blueberries is fine. If you don't have time to defrost them, just warm up your non-dairy milk to take the chill off your smoothie bowl.

Monk fruit powder makes a great-tasting zero-calorie sweetener.

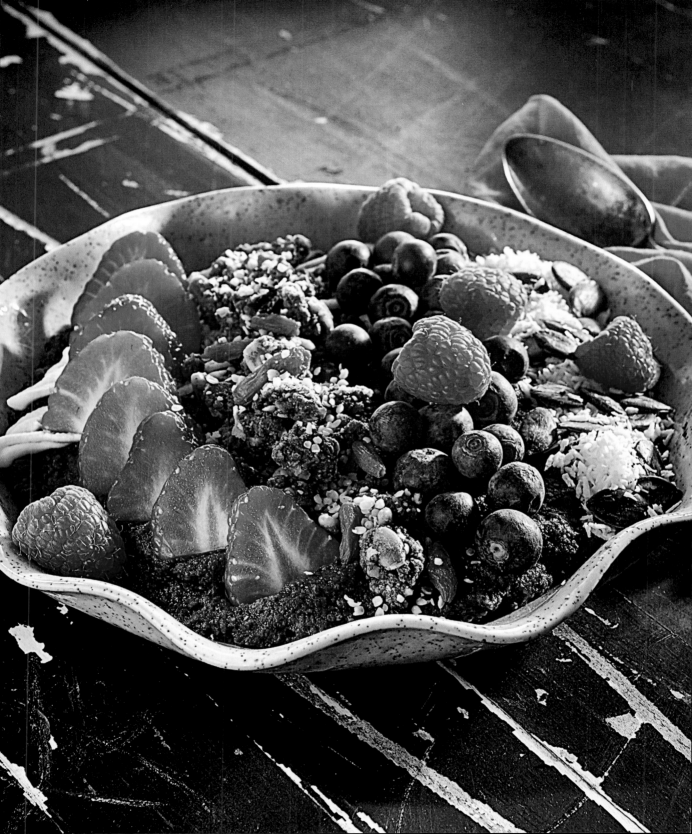

Apple Breakfast Bars

These tasty bars have a high amount of fiber, which helps to keep the bowel moving. And the polyphenols in apples regulate blood sugar levels, which are key in the prevention of cravings, overeating and even type 2 diabetes. Afternoon crashes will be a thing of the past! Be sure to enjoy lots of liquid along with these bars to help the fiber transit easily.

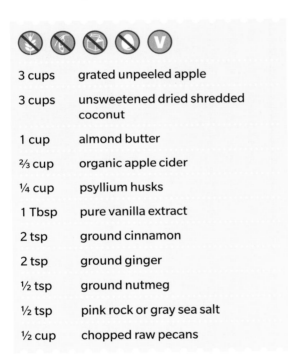

3 cups	grated unpeeled apple
3 cups	unsweetened dried shredded coconut
1 cup	almond butter
⅔ cup	organic apple cider
¼ cup	psyllium husks
1 Tbsp	pure vanilla extract
2 tsp	ground cinnamon
2 tsp	ground ginger
½ tsp	ground nutmeg
½ tsp	pink rock or gray sea salt
½ cup	chopped raw pecans

1　Preheat the oven to 350°F.

2　In a large bowl, mix all the ingredients except for the pecans until well combined.

3　Press into a parchment-lined 11-by-7-inch baking dish, and bake for 40 minutes.

4　Remove from the oven and immediately press pecans into the top. Serve warm.

Makes 12 bars. Will keep for up to 10 days in the fridge or 4 months in the freezer.

 Freeze the rest of the bars for those days of the Hot Detox that you don't feel like cooking breakfast or are pressed for time.

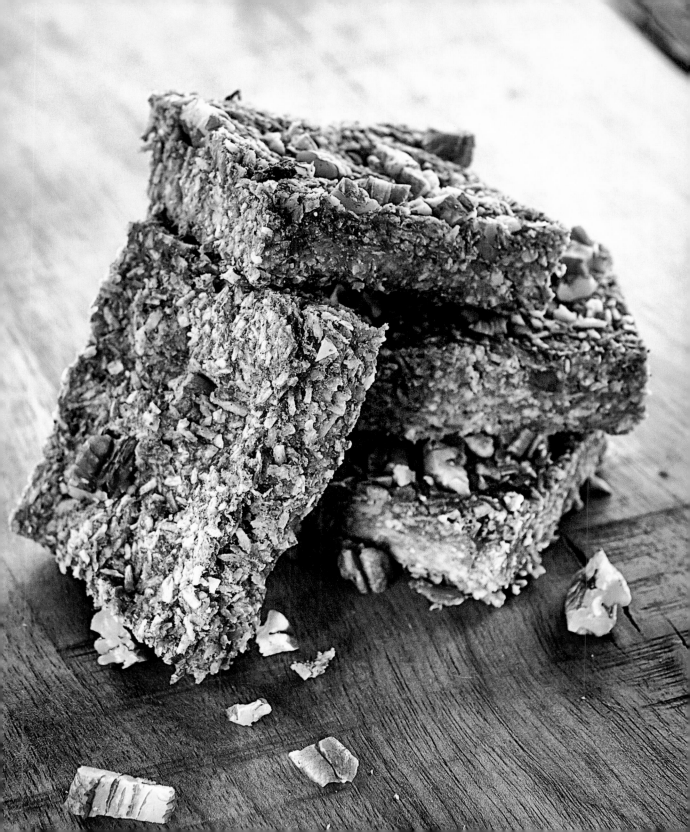

Banana Pecan Muffins

My sister, Lynn, is allergic to eggs, so muffins are usually off her menu. At one point she owned a bakery — muffins and cookies were a big part of her life. Then she learned about substituting eggs with ground chia seeds, and she went back into the kitchen to experiment. You'll agree that her results are incredibly tasty!

¼ cup	whole chia seeds (to make ⅓ cup ground chia seeds)
⅔ cup	filtered water
3	bananas, mashed
½ cup	raw pecan pieces
⅓ cup	coconut oil, melted
⅓ cup	coconut nectar
1 Tbsp	pure vanilla extract
¾ cup	coconut flour
½ tsp	baking soda
½ tsp	pink rock or gray sea salt
1 Tbsp	ground cinnamon
½ tsp	ground nutmeg
¼ tsp	ground turmeric
12	pecan halves for garnish

1 Preheat the oven to 350°F. Line a 12-cup muffin pan with baking cups (unbleached parchment paper or silicone).

2 Grind the chia seeds in a clean spice or coffee grinder. (If you don't have a grinder, use preground seeds.)

3 In a large bowl, mix the ground seeds and water. Let it sit for 2 to 3 minutes to gel.

4 Once the seeds gel, mix in the bananas, pecans, coconut oil, coconut nectar and vanilla.

5 In a small bowl, combine the coconut flour, baking soda, salt and spices.

6 Add the dry ingredients to the wet ingredients, and mix just until combined and there are no lumps.

7 Drop the batter into the lined muffin cups, and top each muffin with a pecan half. Bake for about 40 minutes.

Makes 12 muffins. Will keep for 3 days in an airtight container at room temperature or up to 3 months in the freezer.

Berry Chia Jam

Did you know that chia, the Aztec superseed, is a member of the mint family? It boasts exceptionally high amounts of soluble and insoluble fiber, which is necessary for maintaining a healthy digestive system (as long as you consume it with lots of water). The mucilaginous gel that coats the seeds helps the body sweep out wastes and toxins. This jam tastes as good as freezer jam, with a fraction of the sweetener.

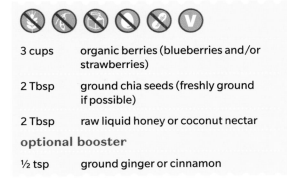

3 cups	organic berries (blueberries and/or strawberries)
2 Tbsp	ground chia seeds (freshly ground if possible)
2 Tbsp	raw liquid honey or coconut nectar

optional booster

| ½ tsp | ground ginger or cinnamon |

1 Add the berries, chia seeds and honey or coconut nectar to a food processor and process until smooth.

2 Transfer to a Mason jar, cover with the lid and refrigerate for a few hours to thicken.

Makes 2 cups. Will keep for up to 2 weeks in the fridge.

> This jam is so easy that I bet you won't go back to fussing with all that pectin and sugar! Make this recipe year-round using whatever berries you have on hand. It even works with frozen berries; just thaw them before blending.

Blueberry Seed Soak

Blueberries contain the building blocks for an antioxidant known as superoxide dismutase. SOD is important in disarming the most harmful of free radicals in our bodies — specifically the free radicals that like to break down the synovial fluid, which lubricates our joints. I love to use wild blueberries because they contain twice as many antioxidants as conventional blueberries.

½ cup	Hemp Hearts or raw sunflower seeds
¾ cup	wild blueberries, fresh or frozen (see Tip)
1 tsp	raw liquid honey or coconut nectar
½–¾ cup	warmed non-dairy milk (such as coconut beverage, hemp milk or cashew milk)

optional booster

| ¼ tsp | ground cinnamon or ginger |

Overnight version:

1 Mix the Hemp Hearts or sunflower seeds and blueberries in a glass or ceramic container, cover and let it sit on the counter overnight. (The seeds will soften up.)

2 In the morning, mix in the honey or coconut nectar, warm non-dairy milk and spices, if using.

Faster version:

1 To consume immediately, warm ¾ cup of non-dairy milk. Pour it over the blueberry mixture, and let sit long enough to defrost the berries and soften the seeds. Then add the honey or coconut nectar and spices, if using. Enjoy!

Makes 1 serving.

Carrot Cake Bars

Carrots have a phytonutrient called falcarinol that is being researched for its ability to fight colon cancer. Carrots also boast 4 grams of fiber per cup, making them a great bowel cleanser.

8	medjool dates, pitted, *or* 10 honey dates if medjool are unavailable
1 cup	filtered water, for soaking the dates
2 cups	raw hazelnuts or pecans
1 cup	raw sunflower seeds or Hemp Hearts
4 cups	grated carrots, divided
1 cup	diced apple
1 cup	chopped zucchini
½ tsp	pink rock or gray sea salt
¾ cup	whole flaxseeds (to make 1 cup ground flaxseeds)
1 cup	dried cranberries (sweetened with apple juice) or organic raisins
¼ cup	unsweetened dried shredded coconut
1 Tbsp	ground cinnamon
1 tsp	ground nutmeg
2 tsp	ground ginger
¼ tsp	ground cloves

1 Soak dates in water for 30 minutes.

2 Place the nuts and sunflower seeds or Hemp Hearts in a food processor, and process until finely chopped. Drain the dates and add them to the food processor along with 2 cups of the carrots and the apple, zucchini and salt. Process until you get a puree, about 1 minute. Transfer to a large mixing bowl.

3 Using a clean spice or coffee grinder, grind the flaxseeds finely. (If you don't have a grinder, use preground seeds.)

4 To the nut and carrot mixture, fold in the ground flax, the rest of the carrots, and the cranberries, coconut and spices. Stir until you have the consistency of cookie batter.

5 Preheat the oven or dehydrator to 150°F. On a parchment-lined rimmed baking sheet, spread batter evenly to form a ¼-inch-thick rectangle.

6 Dehydrate for 2 hours. Invert the pan onto a cutting board, and remove the parchment paper. Cut into 4-by-2-inch bars. Return bars to lined baking sheet and place pan back in the dehydrator or oven for about 4 more hours or until the bars are as firm as a moist cake.

Makes 18 bars.

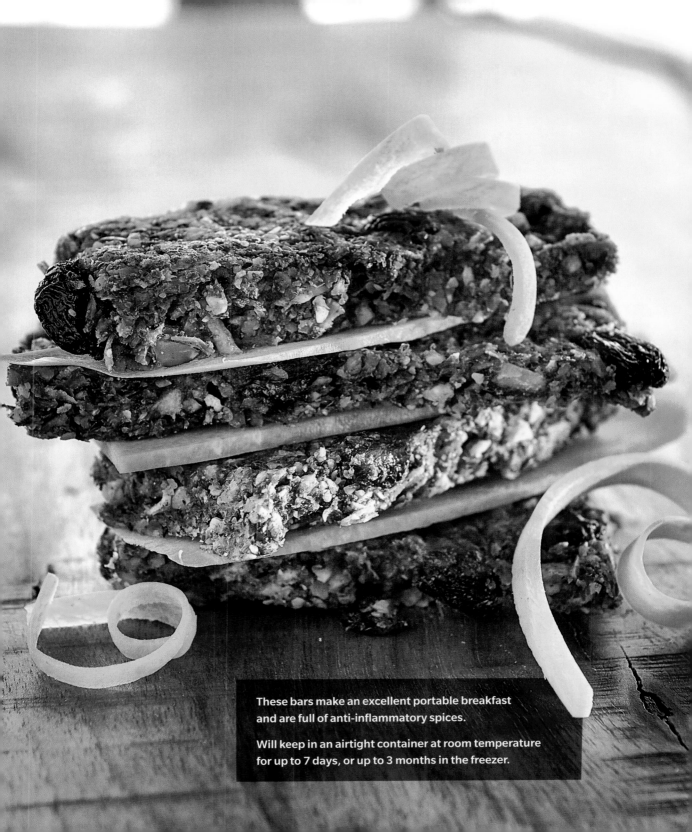

These bars make an excellent portable breakfast and are full of anti-inflammatory spices.

Will keep in an airtight container at room temperature for up to 7 days, or up to 3 months in the freezer.

Cran-Almond Muffins

Having this muffin for breakfast leaves me satisfied for hours, probably because of all the nut flour! A 28-month study involving 8,865 adults in Spain found that people who ate nuts at least two times per week were 31 percent less likely to gain weight than those who never (or almost never) ate nuts.

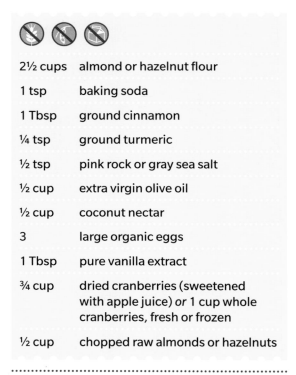

2½ cups	almond or hazelnut flour
1 tsp	baking soda
1 Tbsp	ground cinnamon
¼ tsp	ground turmeric
½ tsp	pink rock or gray sea salt
½ cup	extra virgin olive oil
½ cup	coconut nectar
3	large organic eggs
1 Tbsp	pure vanilla extract
¾ cup	dried cranberries (sweetened with apple juice) *or* 1 cup whole cranberries, fresh or frozen
½ cup	chopped raw almonds or hazelnuts

Fresh cranberries kill *H. pylori* bacteria responsible for ulcers.

1 Preheat the oven to 300°F. Line a 12-cup muffin pan with baking cups (unbleached parchment paper or silicone).

2 In a medium bowl, whisk together the nut flour, baking soda, cinnamon, turmeric and salt. Add the oil, coconut nectar, eggs and vanilla to the flour mixture, and stir until smooth. Using a spatula, gently fold in the cranberries just until evenly distributed throughout the batter.

3 Divide the batter between the muffin cups. Sprinkle with almonds or hazelnuts. Bake on the center rack for 35 minutes (or 40 minutes if using fresh cranberries), rotating the pan after 15 minutes. A toothpick inserted into the center of the muffin should come out clean.

4 Let the muffins cool in the muffin pan for 15 minutes, then transfer to a wire rack and let cool completely.

Makes 12 muffins. Will keep for up to 3 days in an airtight container at room temperature or 6 months in the freezer.

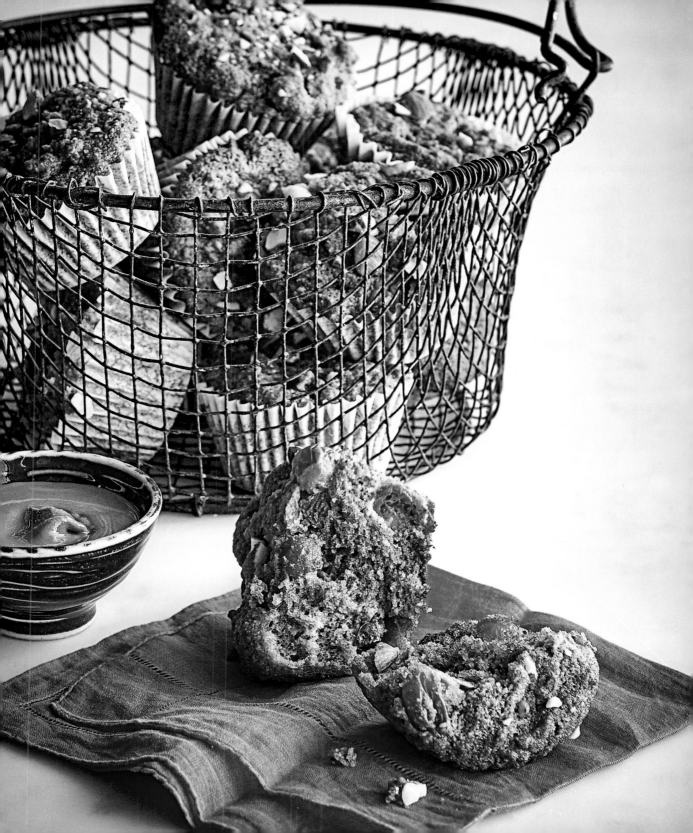

Coconut Cashew Yogurt

I can't tell you just how great it is to make your own dairy-free yogurt — it saves money and is so much healthier! Commercial dairy-free yogurts are often filled with thickeners and sweeteners. (Read the ingredients carefully if you do get store-bought, especially for this cleanse.)

This recipe is easier than you think. The preparation time is as short as for a smoothie; just let it sit and work its magic. Feel free to halve this recipe.

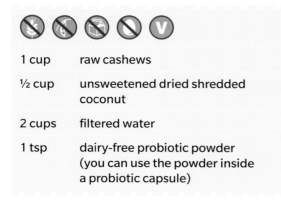

1 cup	raw cashews
½ cup	unsweetened dried shredded coconut
2 cups	filtered water
1 tsp	dairy-free probiotic powder (you can use the powder inside a probiotic capsule)

1 In a blender jar, mix the cashews and coconut in the water. Cover and refrigerate overnight (or 8 hours minimum) to soak.

2 Do not drain. Blend on high speed until smooth. Add the probiotic powder, and pulse until well mixed.

3 Transfer to a 1-quart (4 cups) Mason jar and cover with the lid. Leave space in the jar, as the yogurt will expand.

4 Let ferment on the countertop for 8 to 12 hours, until the mixture thickens and develops a slightly sour taste similar to yogurt. After the fermentation time is complete, refrigerate immediately to prevent it from fermenting too much. For Greek-style yogurt or a sour-cream consistency, during the middle of the fermenting time, transfer the mixture to a fine-mesh sieve lined with cheesecloth, placing a bowl beneath to catch liquid.

Makes 3 cups. Will keep for up to 4 days in the fridge.

For a fruity yogurt drink, add ½ cup of fresh or frozen and thawed berries or other fruit to the yogurt. Blend on high speed until smooth. Will keep covered for 3 days in the fridge.

Detox Flush Pudding

This pudding works like a broom to sweep the colon clean. Flax and chia are good sources of soluble fiber, which cleanses the colon and reduces cholesterol. Apples are rich in calcium D-glucarate, allowing the body to excrete used hormones (such as estrogen) before they can be reabsorbed. Warming spices will soothe your tummy.

5 cups	cubed unpeeled organic apples or pears
½ cup	filtered water
2 Tbsp	ground flaxseeds (freshly ground if possible)
1 Tbsp	minced fresh ginger or 1 tsp ground ginger
1 Tbsp	organic lemon juice
2 tsp	pure vanilla extract
1 tsp	ground cinnamon
pinch	pink rock or gray sea salt

optional boosters

2 Tbsp	Hemp Hearts
1 Tbsp	collagen powder
1–3 tsp	sunflower lecithin powder
1 tsp	dairy-free probiotic powder (you can use the powder inside a probiotic capsule)
1 tsp	raw liquid honey or coconut nectar
¼ tsp	ground turmeric

1 In a medium saucepan, bring the apples or pears and water to a boil, then cover, reduce the heat and simmer for 15 minutes. Using a whisk or fork, mash the apples in the pot.

2 Remove from the heat and stir in the remaining ingredients, including any of the boosters. Serve warm.

Makes 3 cups. Will keep for up to 4 days in the fridge. Can also be frozen.

 Apples contain approximately 3 to 5 grams of fiber, including pectin, which is very beneficial for cleansing the gallbladder.

Detox Frittata

Artichokes contain a substance that can increase the protective mucus that lines the stomach. That is, artichokes can keep the acids that break down our food from creating holes (ulcers) in the stomach lining. Artichokes, leeks, asparagus, arugula and herbs all help to cleanse the liver and bowel.

2 Tbsp	coconut oil, divided
2 cups	finely chopped leeks (white and green parts) or onions
1 ½ cups	asparagus, ends trimmed, cut into thirds
½ cup	olives, pitted and sliced
1 Tbsp	herbes de Provence
¼ tsp	pink rock or gray sea salt
2 cups	arugula or baby spinach
14 oz jar	water-packed artichoke hearts, drained
12	large organic eggs

to serve

½ cup	salsa

1 Preheat the oven to 350°F. Grease a 13-by-9-inch baking dish with 1 teaspoon of the coconut oil and set aside.

2 In a skillet over medium heat, melt the remaining coconut oil and sauté the leeks, asparagus, olives, herbes de Provence and salt for 5 minutes. Add the arugula or spinach and cook, stirring, until slightly wilted, about 2 minutes. Remove from the heat, add the artichoke hearts and mix well.

3 Spread the mixture evenly in the baking dish. Whisk the eggs in a large bowl, and pour over the vegetables.

4 Bake for 30 minutes or until eggs are set. Serve warm with a dollop of salsa.

Makes 8 servings.

 This is a great recipe to make ahead and enjoy on the busier days of the cleanse. I like to pair it up with **Messy Gingered Sweet Potatoes, shown opposite.**

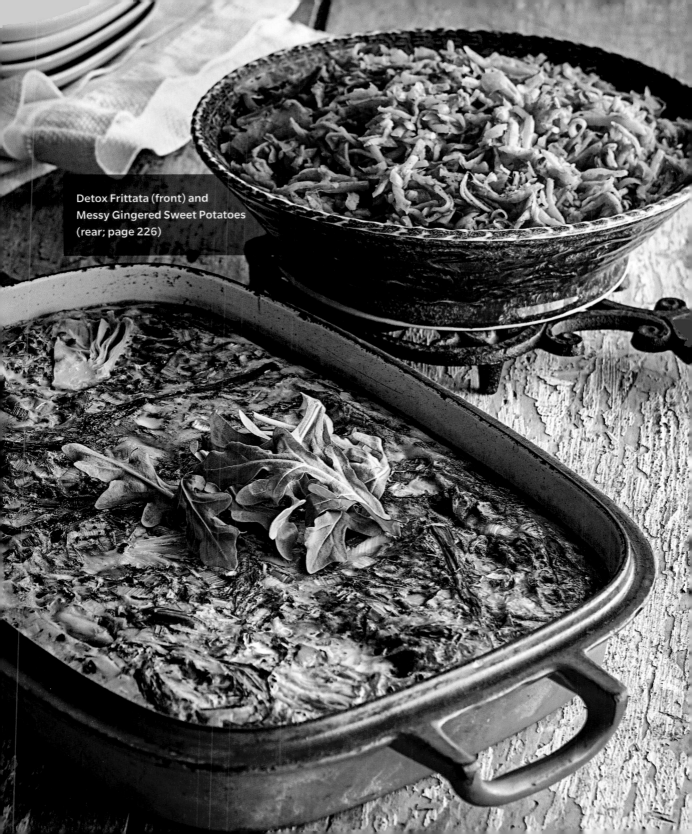

Detox Frittata (front) and Messy Gingered Sweet Potatoes (rear; page 226)

Detox Marmalade

I adore the taste of marmalade. Store-bought marmalade is normally packed with refined sugar, so try my version below, as it provides a higher concentration of citrus flavonoids. By eating the rind of organic citrus, you assist the liver to detox.

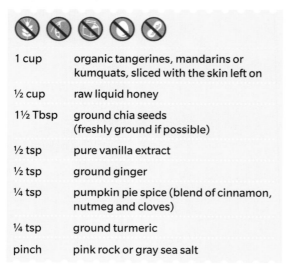

1 cup	organic tangerines, mandarins or kumquats, sliced with the skin left on
½ cup	raw liquid honey
1½ Tbsp	ground chia seeds (freshly ground if possible)
½ tsp	pure vanilla extract
½ tsp	ground ginger
¼ tsp	pumpkin pie spice (blend of cinnamon, nutmeg and cloves)
¼ tsp	ground turmeric
pinch	pink rock or gray sea salt

Place all the ingredients into a food processor or blender. Blend until it becomes jamlike (it should be a little chunky). Use immediately or transfer to a small Mason jar and store in the fridge.

Makes 1 cup. Will keep for up to 3 months in the fridge.

....

Flavonoids enhance the absorption of vitamin C, an important antioxidant that protects your body from toxins while they are being processed by the liver, especially during the intermediate step between Phase 1 and Phase 2.

Shamrock Butter

Spirulina is a microscopic blue–green algae that flourishes in fresh and salt water. It's rich in healing oils (including omega-3), detoxifying vitamins (B1, B2, B3, B6, B9 [folic acid], B12, C, D and E), and minerals such as potassium, calcium, chromium, iron, magnesium, manganese, selenium and zinc. You can take it in tablet form, but I like to mix the powder into raw-food recipes for extra nutrition and color.

¼ cup	nut or seed butter
1 tsp	Hawaiian spirulina powder
½ tsp	pure mint extract (about 10 drops)
⅛ tsp	stevia powder (1 packet) or 6 drops liquid stevia or 1 Tbsp raw liquid honey

optional booster

2 tsp	coconut oil

In a small bowl, stir together all the ingredients until well combined. If you're using stevia instead of honey, note that the optional coconut oil will make for a smoother texture.

Makes ¼ cup.

....

For a **Chai-Spice Butter**, replace the mint extract with a warming spice mix: ½ teaspoon each of ground cinnamon and ginger, ¼ teaspoon each of ground nutmeg and cardamom, and a pinch of pink rock or gray sea salt. This version is very soothing, with all the spices that ease digestion. Cardamom clears harmful bacteria in the body without destroying the beneficial bacteria of the gut.

Try one of these butters on a thinly sliced apple or toasted piece of Hot Detox Bread (page 168).

Extreme Ginger Bake

Ginger contains gingerol, an active anti-inflammatory that reduces pain. Its anti-spasmodic properties help settle the stomach, relieve gas and bloating, and support the enzymatic action of digestion. In this recipe, the fruit fiber helps to slowly release the sweetness to ensure satisfaction and balanced blood sugar.

8 cups	sliced unpeeled apples or pears
3 cups	organic berries or sliced unpeeled peaches
3 Tbsp	chopped fresh ginger
2 tsp	ground ginger
1 tsp	ground turmeric
1 tsp	ground nutmeg

topping

1 cup	raw pumpkin seeds
1 cup	unsweetened dried coconut flakes
1 cup	Hemp Hearts or raw sunflower seeds
½ cup	tahini
2 tsp	ground cinnamon
1 tsp	ground ginger
¼ tsp	pink rock or gray sea salt
½ cup	coconut nectar
½ cup	coconut oil

optional booster

½ cup	chopped raw hazelnuts

1 Preheat the oven to 300°F. In an ungreased 13-by-9-inch baking dish, mix together the fruit, ginger, turmeric and nutmeg.

2 In a large bowl, combine all the ingredients for the topping except for the coconut nectar and coconut oil. Add the hazelnuts if using, and the coconut nectar and coconut oil, and stir until just combined. Spread over the fruit.

3 Bake for 35 to 40 minutes. Serve warm.

Makes 12 servings. Keeps up to 5 days in the fridge.

 This divine recipe freezes well. Just heat from frozen in a 300°F oven until warmed through.

The Early Riser

My husband, Alan, came up with this great portable breakfast. The basil in this riser can help to protect you from bacteria, yeast and mold. This powerful plant contains several essential oils that have exhibited antimicrobial activity against a wide range of bacteria, such as listeria, staphylococcus and salmonella.

1½ cups	thinly sliced unpeeled winter squash or sweet potato, in half moons
1–2 cups	chopped baby spinach or Swiss chard, including stems (use 2 cups if not boosting with parsley)
12	large organic eggs
¼ cup	dairy- and nut-free basil pesto (such as Instant Pesto, page 257)
¼ tsp	pink rock or gray sea salt, more to taste

optional boosters

1 cup	chopped fresh parsley
1 cup	chopped green onions
¼ cup	chopped sun-dried tomatoes
¼ cup	sliced green or black olives
1 Tbsp	dulse flakes

1 Preheat the oven to 350°F. Line a 12-cup muffin pan or 12 ramekins with baking cups (unbleached parchment paper or silicone).

2 Layer the squash or sweet potato and spinach or chard equally into the cups or ramekins.

3 In a medium bowl, whisk together the eggs, pesto and salt.

4 Pour the mixture evenly over the squash and spinach. Top with any of the boosters, and a sprinkle of extra salt if desired.

5 Cook for 35 minutes or until eggs are set.

Makes 12 servings. Will keep for up to 4 days in the fridge and freezes well.

 I highly recommend adding all the optional ingredients for a truly gourmet dish. But if you're in a rush, the simple version will still impress anyone lucky enough to be served this. This recipe is great for shared meals and as a quick and convenient lunch to bring to work.

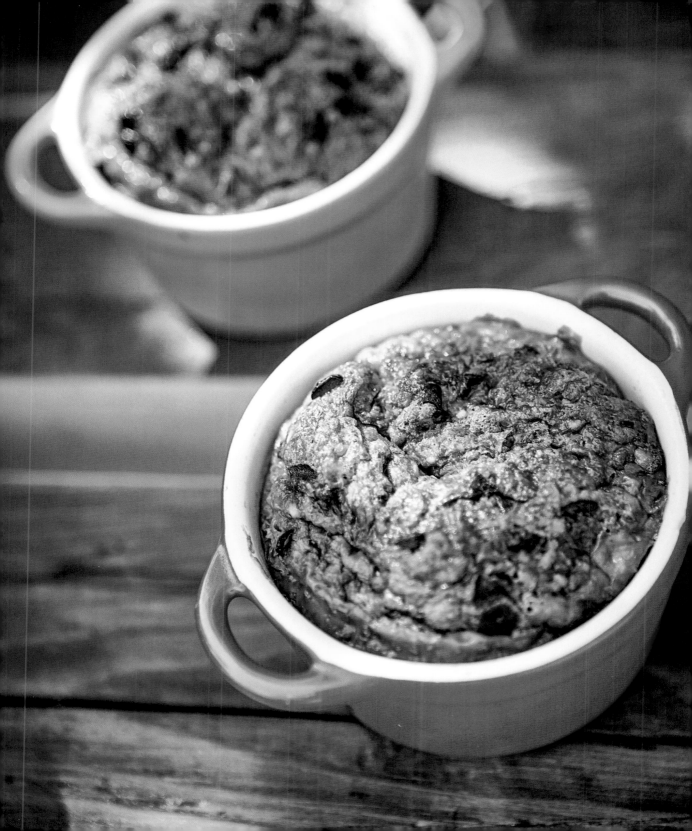

Faux-tmeal Breakfast

This is my sister's favorite detox breakfast. She eliminated her joint pain by following the Hot Detox's omnivore menu (dairy-, grain- and legume-free). Creating the perfect faux oatmeal gave her the comfort she craves and the healing she needs.

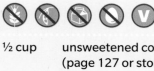

½ cup	unsweetened coconut beverage (page 127 or store-bought)
3 Tbsp	chia seeds
2 Tbsp	raw pecan or walnut pieces
1 Tbsp	dried currants or raisins
½ Tbsp	coconut oil
½ tsp	pure vanilla extract
½ tsp	ground cinnamon
pinch	pink rock or gray sea salt

optional booster

1 tsp	liquid honey or coconut nectar

1 Gently heat the coconut beverage until just warm.

2 In a bowl, mix together the rest of the ingredients.

3 Pour the coconut beverage over the mixture and let it gel for 5 to 10 minutes. Sweeten with honey or coconut nectar if using, before serving.

Makes 1 serving.

 Chia seeds are an excellent source of plant-based, cholesterol-free protein. Just one serving (28 grams/2 tablespoons) provides a remarkable 4.6 grams of easily absorbable protein.

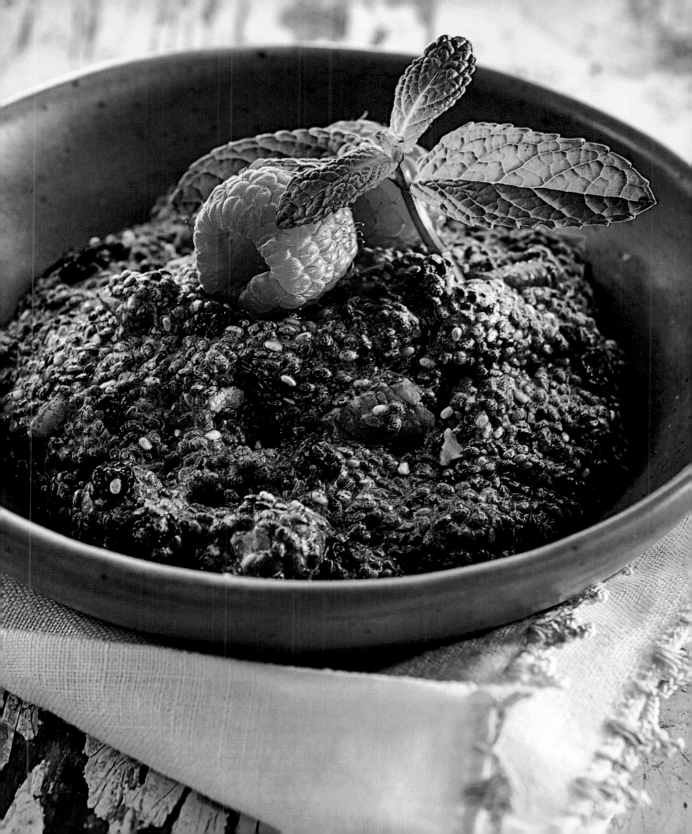

Hot Detox Bread

Sarah Britton of *My New Roots* (www.mynewroots.org) has come up with a brilliant loaf that contains oats. But because it's important to avoid grass grains for this detox, I instead use quinoa or buckwheat, and it works just as well. Look for rolled quinoa or rolled buckwheat in your local health-food store.

1½ cups	rolled quinoa flakes *or* 1¼ cups rolled buckwheat flakes
1 cup	raw sunflower seeds
½ cup	raw pumpkin seeds or almonds
½ cup	flaxseeds
¼ cup	psyllium husks (decrease to 3 Tbsp if using psyllium husk powder)
2 Tbsp	ground chia seeds (freshly ground if possible)
1 tsp	ground turmeric
1 tsp	ground ginger
1 tsp	pink rock or gray sea salt
3 Tbsp	coconut oil, melted, divided
1 Tbsp	coconut nectar
1½ cups	filtered water

1   Grease a 9-by-5-inch loaf pan with 1 tsp of the coconut oil.

2   In a large bowl, combine all the dry ingredients (everything except the last three ingredients), stirring well.

3   In a separate bowl, whisk together the remaining coconut oil, coconut nectar and water. Add this to the dry ingredients, and mix well (you should end up with a very thick dough).

4   Transfer dough to the loaf pan, and press very firmly to prevent a crumbly loaf.

5   Let sit on the counter for at least 2 hours or overnight, covered with a clean kitchen towel. The bread is ready to bake when it retains its shape but pulls away slightly from the edge of the pan.

6   Preheat the oven to 350°F.

7   Place the pan on the middle rack in the oven, and bake for 20 minutes.

8   Remove the bread from the pan and place it upside-down directly on the rack in the oven. Bake for another 25 minutes. The bread is done when it sounds hollow when tapped.

9   Let cool on a wire rack before slicing.

Makes one 9-by-5-inch loaf (12 slices). Will keep for up to 5 days in an airtight container in the fridge. Can also be sliced and frozen (with parchment between the slices) for up to 3 months.

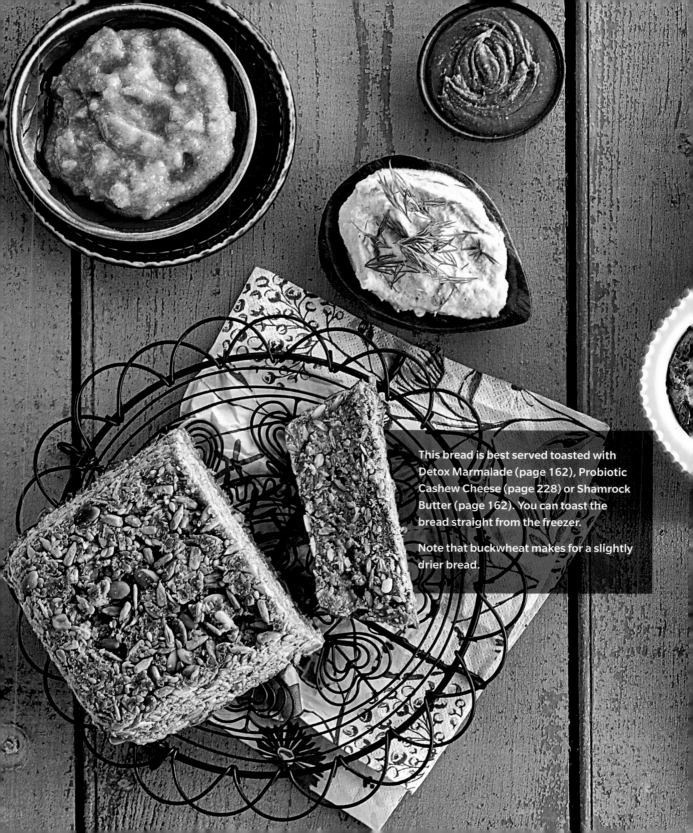

This bread is best served toasted with Detox Marmalade (page 162), Probiotic Cashew Cheese (page 228) or Shamrock Butter (page 162). You can toast the bread straight from the freezer.

Note that buckwheat makes for a slightly drier bread.

Hulk Flourless Pancakes

These pancakes are as healthy as a salad! They are bright green inside and packed with detoxifying B vitamins. Spirulina is optional, but note that it contains all the essential amino acids, which assist the liver with detoxification and is 55 to 70 percent protein — ounce for ounce, spirulina contains 12 times the digestible protein of beef. Coconut is naturally antifungal and helps to balance your digestive flora. These pancakes can be whipped together quickly and are a perfect high-protein weekend treat.

3	large organic eggs
⅓ cup	organic coconut milk
2 Tbsp	coconut nectar
1 Tbsp	pure vanilla extract
1 tsp	raw apple cider vinegar
1 cup	almond flour
1 tsp	ground cinnamon
½ tsp	baking soda
¼ tsp	pink rock or gray sea salt
2 cups	baby spinach
1 Tbsp	coconut oil (for coating the skillet)

optional booster

1 tsp	Hawaiian spirulina powder

blueberry sauce (optional)

2 cups	wild blueberries, fresh or frozen
2 Tbsp	coconut nectar

1 Place the eggs, coconut milk, coconut nectar, vanilla and vinegar in a blender (preferably a high-powered one). Then add the almond flour, cinnamon, baking soda and salt, and spirulina powder if using.

2 Blend on medium speed for 30 seconds, until well combined.

3 Use a spatula to scrape down the sides of the blender. Add the spinach, and blend on high speed until the spinach leaves are completely incorporated and the batter is smooth. Set aside.

4 Make the blueberry sauce, if desired. In a saucepan over medium heat, combine the blueberries and coconut nectar and cook, stirring frequently as the berries heat up and start to break down. Using the backside of a spoon, gently squash some of the blueberries. Cook for 4 to 5 minutes or until the sauce has become syruplike, with a few berries still intact. Remove from the heat and set aside.

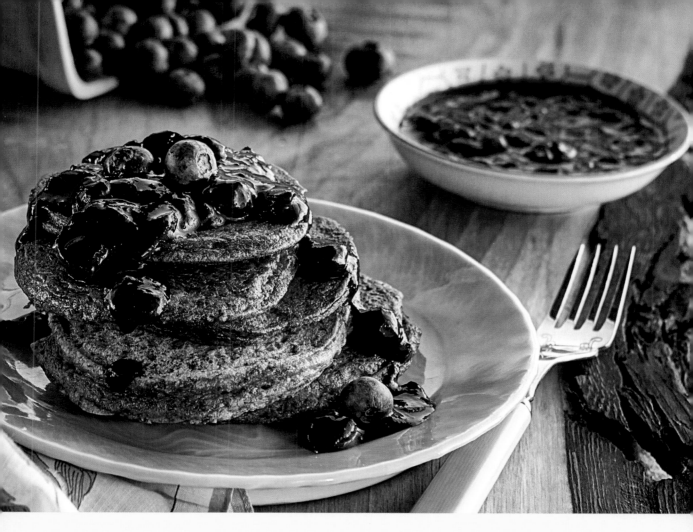

5 Heat a skillet or griddle on medium-high, and coat with coconut oil. Spoon the batter onto the skillet, keeping your pancakes approximately 3 inches in diameter. (They're much easier to flip when small.) Let cook for 2 to 3 minutes on one side, then flip and cook for an additional 1 to 2 minutes.

6 Serve immediately, with the blueberry sauce if you made it.

Makes 9 pancakes.

 If you want to make a savory pancake, leave out the coconut sweetener in the batter.

Joint-Healing Gell-O

It's been shown that in athletes, gelatin can lessen the inflammation that leads to joint pain and stiffness, and can repair small tears in cartilage. Gelatin is rich in an amino acid called glycine, which helps the liver clear toxins from your body. This recipe tastes so good that you may want to double it.

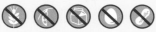

¼ cup   cold filtered water

1½ Tbsp   organic gelatin powder (from grass-fed or pasture-raised cows)

¼ cup   filtered water, just off the boil

1½ cups   organic fruit juice of choice

optional booster

1 cup   organic fresh fruit (such as strawberries and wild blueberries)

1 Have ready an 8-by-8-inch baking dish or several small ramekins.

2 Pour the cold water in a large mixing cup or quart-size Mason jar, and add the gelatin powder. Mix well until it thickens.

3 Add the boiling water and stir. Then add the juice and mix well.

4 If using fruit, place it in the baking dish or ramekins. Pour the gelatin mixture into the dish or ramekins, and if using fruit, stir lightly to coat. Cover and place in the fridge for at least 2 to 3 hours or overnight to set.

5 Bring gell-o to room temperature before unmolding and cutting into cubes or different shapes (you can use cookie cutters) and serving.

Makes 4 to 6 servings. Will keep for up to 5 days in the fridge.

 For extra detox nutrition, substitute carrot juice for half of the fruit juice.

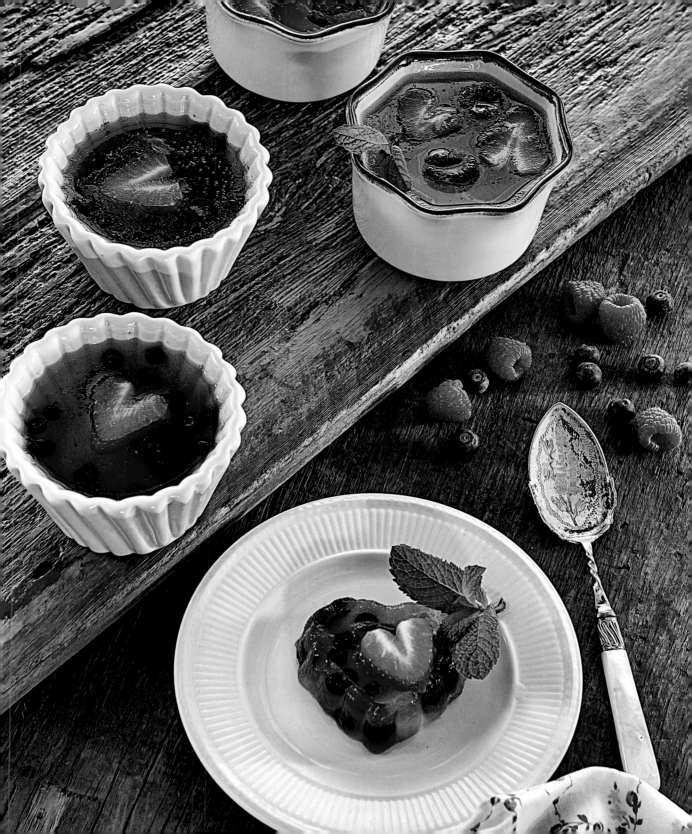

Vegan Lemon Gell-O

This vegan gell-o contains kudzu, a wonderful thickening agent. Combined with agar flakes, kudzu creates a perfect gell-o every time. Kudzu root contains a flavonoid called puerarin, which has been shown to help with headaches, high blood pressure or muscular tension; it also stabilizes blood sugar. Agar comes from seaweed that grows on the rocky areas in the tidal waters of Japan.

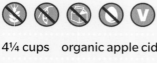

4¼ cups	organic apple cider, divided
½ cup	agar flakes
2 tsp	kudzu or arrowroot flour
¼ cup	organic lemon juice
¼ cup	coconut nectar
to serve	
¼ cup	raw slivered almonds or pumpkin seeds
1 cup	wild blueberries or sliced strawberries

1 Have ready an 8-by-8-inch baking dish or 10 small ramekins.

2 In a saucepan over medium heat, stir together 4 cups of the cider and the agar flakes, then simmer for 15 minutes. Meanwhile, in a small cup or bowl, dissolve the kudzu or arrowroot flour in the remaining ¼ cup cider.

3 Remove agar mixture from the heat, add the dissolved kudzu or arrowroot, and stir until clear. Add the lemon juice and coconut nectar, and stir well.

4 Pour into ramekins. Top with the almonds or pumpkin seeds and berries.

5 Place in the fridge for 1 hour to set.

Makes 10 servings. Will keep for up to 7 days in the fridge.

 Mix it with a liquid and agar becomes gelatinous and swells up, giving you a feeling of fullness; in this way, it's a great appetite suppressant. It also has a gentle laxative effect because it's so high in fiber. Agar is also rich in minerals.

Squeaky Clean Granola

My goal here was to create the cleanest granola that both my vegan and omnivore friends could eat. And it was a success! It's now a staple in my kitchen. (See page 177 for photo.)

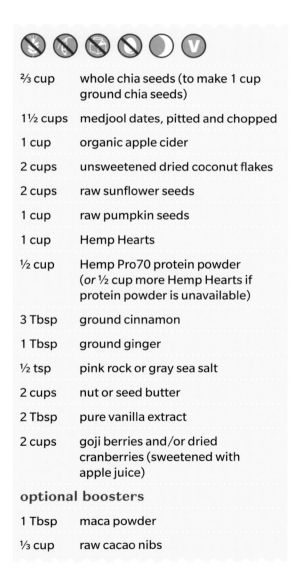

⅔ cup	whole chia seeds (to make 1 cup ground chia seeds)
1½ cups	medjool dates, pitted and chopped
1 cup	organic apple cider
2 cups	unsweetened dried coconut flakes
2 cups	raw sunflower seeds
1 cup	raw pumpkin seeds
1 cup	Hemp Hearts
½ cup	Hemp Pro70 protein powder (*or* ½ cup more Hemp Hearts if protein powder is unavailable)
3 Tbsp	ground cinnamon
1 Tbsp	ground ginger
½ tsp	pink rock or gray sea salt
2 cups	nut or seed butter
2 Tbsp	pure vanilla extract
2 cups	goji berries and/or dried cranberries (sweetened with apple juice)

optional boosters

1 Tbsp	maca powder
⅓ cup	raw cacao nibs

1 Using a clean spice or coffee grinder, grind the chia seeds. (If you don't have a grinder, use preground seeds.)

2 Add the ground chia seeds, dates and apple cider to a blender, and pulse until smooth.

3 In a bowl, mix together the rest of the ingredients except for the nut or seed butter, vanilla, goji and/or cranberries. Add the maca and/or cacao nibs if using.

4 In another bowl, combine the chia-date paste with the nut or seed butter and vanilla. Add the bowl of dry ingredients, and mix until well incorporated. The mixture will be quite sticky.

5 Preheat the oven or dehydrator to 150°F. Crumble the mixture evenly onto Teflex sheets (dehydrator sheets) or parchment-lined baking sheets, and bake for 8 hours or place in the dehydrator for 6 hours. If possible, stir the granola each hour to ensure even drying.

6 Combine the dried granola with the goji and/or cranberries.

Makes 14 cups. Will keep for up to 4 weeks in an airtight container at room temperature.

 Adding the fruit after the granola has been dehydrated preserves its anti-inflammatory benefits.

Pommy Paleo Pudding

This is one of my favorite superfood breakfasts because it can be made ahead and eaten on a busy day when you need the extra energy the most. Pomegranates, blueberries, apples, chia, Hemp Hearts and lecithin are all beneficial for bowel cleansing. Chia seeds are a rich source of soluble fiber, which helps the body sweep away wastes and toxins and minimizes your risk of developing constipation.

2 cups	wild blueberries, fresh or frozen
1 cup	filtered water, just off the boil if using frozen berries
1 cup	organic pomegranate or berry juice
1 cup	applesauce
½ cup	chia seeds
2 Tbsp	Hemp Hearts

optional boosters

2 tsp	sunflower lecithin powder
1 tsp	pure vanilla extract
½ tsp	ground ginger
½ tsp	ground cinnamon
5 drops	liquid stevia (if you like it sweeter)

to serve

1 cup	fresh pomegranate seeds (about ½ pomegranate), or other fresh fruit if pomegranate is unavailable
2 Tbsp	raw pumpkin seeds

1 Place the blueberries in a large bowl. If using frozen blueberries, pour boiling water over them, mixing gently to thaw; otherwise, add cold or room-temperature water.

2 Add the juice, applesauce, chia seeds and Hemp Hearts, and stir well.

3 Mix in any of the boosters if desired, and place in the refrigerator overnight to set.

4 In the morning, bring it to room temperature and serve topped with fresh fruit and pumpkin seeds.

Makes 4–6 servings. Will keep for up to 4 days in the fridge.

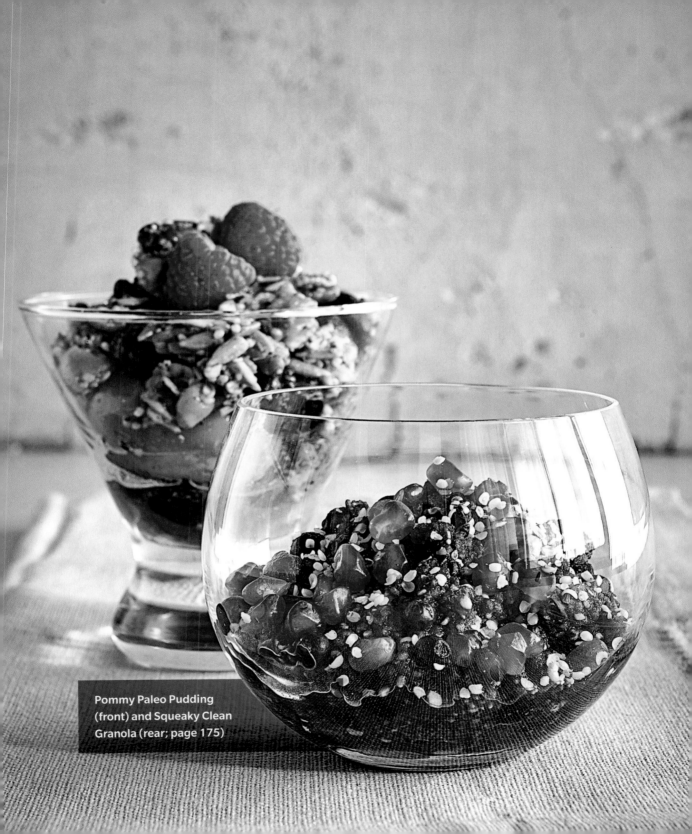

Pommy Paleo Pudding
(front) and Squeaky Clean
Granola (rear; page 175)

Paleo Pumpkin Bagels

This recipe was created by my sister, Lynn, and mom, Elaine, so everyone could enjoy a grab-and-go meal. These bagels are chewy and salty just like a classic bagel. They are amazing toasted with Probiotic Cashew Cheese (see page 228).

½ cup	whole chia seeds (to make ¾ cup ground chia seeds)
½ cup	full-fat organic coconut milk
2 cups	pumpkin puree (see Tip on page 142)
½ cup	coconut nectar
2 Tbsp	organic lemon juice
1 cup	coconut flour
2 tsp	garam masala or Julie's Curry Powder (page 269)
1 tsp	ground turmeric
2 tsp	baking soda
1 tsp	pink rock and gray sea salt

1 Grind the chia seeds in a clean spice or coffee grinder to make a flour. (If you don't have a grinder, use preground seeds.)

2 In a large bowl, whisk the coconut milk to a uniform consistency. (If you have a stand mixer, use the whisk attachment.) Add the ground chia and mix well. Add the pumpkin, coconut nectar and lemon juice, and mix well.

3 In a small bowl, sift together the dry ingredients—the coconut flour, spices, baking soda and salt. (If you have a stand mixer, switch to the dough hook.) Slowly add the dry ingredients to the wet and mix until a uniform dough forms. Divide into 12 even balls.

4 Preheat the oven to 350°F and line a baking sheet with parchment paper. Press down on each ball of dough to form a puck. Using a chopstick, pierce a whole in the center of each puck, then work the dough into a bagel shape and place on the baking sheet.

5 Bake for 30 to 40 minutes. Time can vary due to differences among oven temperatures so check carefully.

6 Let the bagels cool completely on pan before cutting.

Makes 12 small bagels. Will keep for up to 4 days in an airtight container at room temperature or up to 3 months in the freezer.

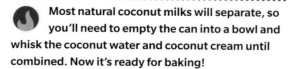 Most natural coconut milks will separate, so you'll need to empty the can into a bowl and whisk the coconut water and coconut cream until combined. Now it's ready for baking!

Pumpkin Spice Smoothie Bowl

Here's my formula for a superhealing recipe — think of every kind of tummy-soothing ingredient then mix it together and call it breakfast! This smoothie bowl blends easy-to-digest carbs, anti-inflammatory oils from the Hemp Hearts and chia, and protein. Two-thirds of the protein content of Hemp Hearts is what's called edestin, a protein easily digested and readily absorbed and utilized by the body.

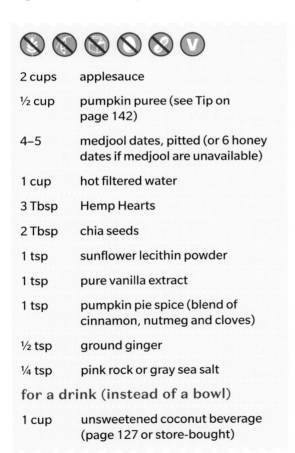

2 cups	applesauce
½ cup	pumpkin puree (see Tip on page 142)
4–5	medjool dates, pitted (or 6 honey dates if medjool are unavailable)
1 cup	hot filtered water
3 Tbsp	Hemp Hearts
2 Tbsp	chia seeds
1 tsp	sunflower lecithin powder
1 tsp	pure vanilla extract
1 tsp	pumpkin pie spice (blend of cinnamon, nutmeg and cloves)
½ tsp	ground ginger
¼ tsp	pink rock or gray sea salt

for a drink (instead of a bowl)

1 cup	unsweetened coconut beverage (page 127 or store-bought)

Combine all the ingredients in a blender or food processor; add the coconut beverage if making a smoothie drink instead of a bowl. Blend on high speed until smooth. Serve immediately.

Makes 4 cups. Any left over will keep for 3 days in the fridge. Warm in a saucepan before serving.

This recipe is hypoallergenic — that is, it has a low potential to trigger allergies, making it a great choice for people with soy and/or peanut allergies.

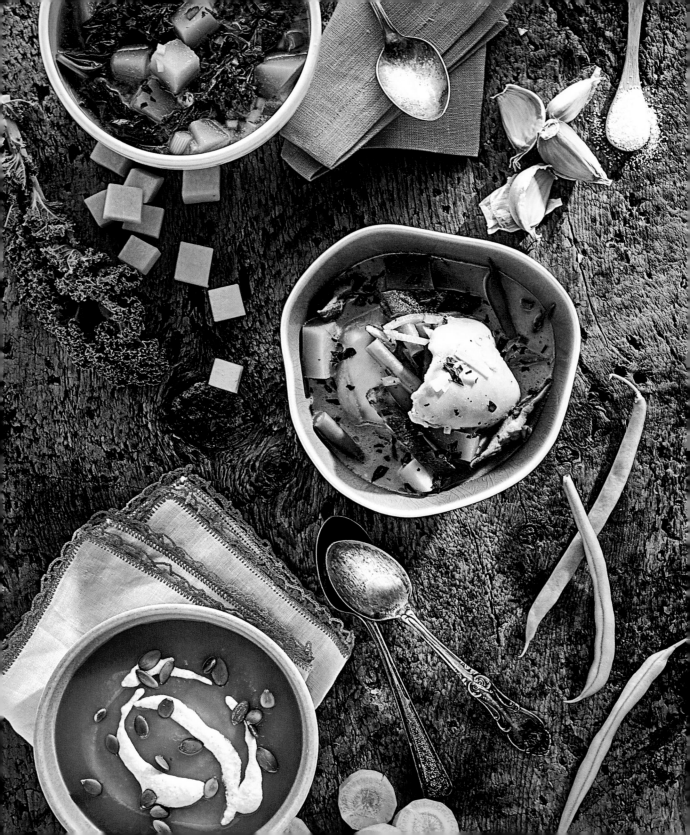

12

Soups and Sides

The Wonderful Healing Effects of Broth

Bone and seaweed broths have likely been popular as long as people have been cooking over fire. It's wonderful to see these healing recipes make such a big comeback. My recipe for Rich Bone Broth is at the core of this cleanse. Take the time to make it at the start of the Hot Detox, and use it in all the recipes. It freezes well, so don't be scared to make a double batch. (You can have both the large slow cooker and large stockpot going!)

Reasons to Cook Bone Broth

- **It rebuilds your gut lining.** Bone broth is full of gelatin and collagen, both of which can soothe the intestines and heal leaky gut syndrome. Antibiotics, Aspirin and other non-steroidal anti-inflammatory drugs, refined sugar and flour, caffeine, alcohol and fried food can damage our intestines. The matrix of minerals and special proteins in bone broth can reverse dietary damage and repair the gut lining.
- **It reduces inflammation.** As ancient healing wisdom goes, "Eat what ails you." Broth made from bones and joints contains nutrients that help strengthen your own skeletal system. Glucosamine and chondroitin help repair bones and joints and may reduce inflammation throughout the whole body.
- **It ups your mineral intake.** The minerals in bone broths include calcium, iron, magnesium, potassium, zinc and selenium. Our food supply contains less minerals than it did before. Minerals are critical for everything from our bones and joints to our mood.
- **It nourishes your immune system.** Chicken soup is a popular remedy for colds and flus that really works! (See my recipe for Golden Chicken Bone Broth, page 186.) The amino acid cysteine thins mucus, making it easier for the body to get rid of it.

- **It maintains healthy skin.** Your skin contains a matrix of collagen that breaks down after the age of 21, leading to wrinkles. Eating collagen will fight wrinkles! Bone broth also contains the amino acids glycine and proline, which your skin will appreciate.
- **It heals your brain.** There is mounting evidence that brain inflammation is linked to conditions such as ADHD, depression and dementia. Many people report that a diet rich in bone broth has meant that their moods and their memory improve, and that they feel calmer and more able to cope with daily stress.

Tips for Bone Broth Success

- Buy bones from organic or grass-fed animals, sourced from your local health-food store, butcher or farmers' market. Ask the vendor to cut up the bones to expose the marrow to yield maximum surface area.
- Consider saving your leftover meat bones and keeping them in the freezer until you have enough to make a broth on a weekend. Use an unbreakable container. Make sure to label it so you can track the date you put them in, and use them within 6 months.
- Do NOT skip the apple cider vinegar, as it draws the minerals out of the bones and adds a nice flavor. If you're sensitive to cider vinegar, use lemon juice instead.
- Bone broth should simmer over a low heat (the stove or slow cooker/Crock-Pot) for 12 to 48 hours. Do be careful with this: make sure you have enough fluid in the pot before you go to bed to prevent burning the pot — or starting a house fire! If you're thinking of buying a slow cooker, get the largest capacity you can find. It will give you peace of mind.

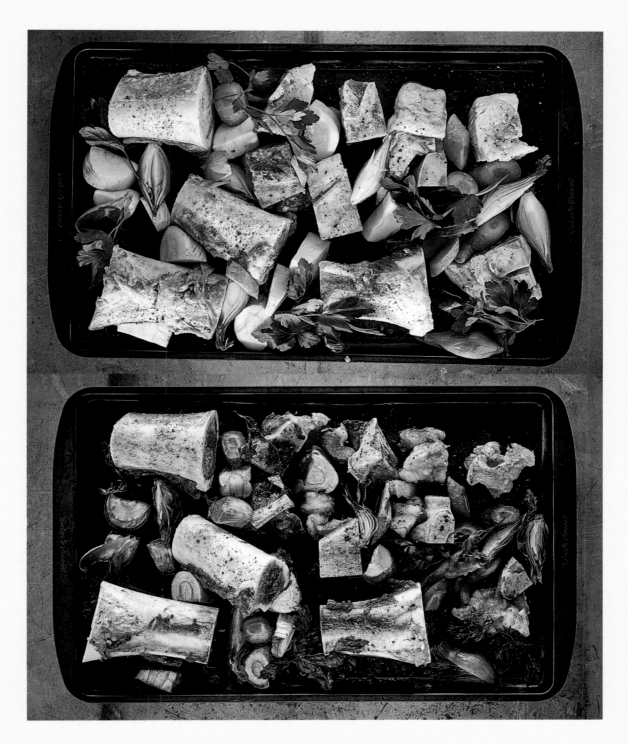

Rich Bone Broth

Remember, roasting the bones before they simmer adds a ton of flavor. If you don't own a big enough pot, just halve the recipe.

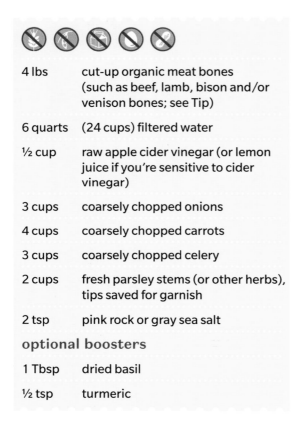

4 lbs	cut-up organic meat bones (such as beef, lamb, bison and/or venison bones; see Tip)
6 quarts	(24 cups) filtered water
½ cup	raw apple cider vinegar (or lemon juice if you're sensitive to cider vinegar)
3 cups	coarsely chopped onions
4 cups	coarsely chopped carrots
3 cups	coarsely chopped celery
2 cups	fresh parsley stems (or other herbs), tips saved for garnish
2 tsp	pink rock or gray sea salt

optional boosters

1 Tbsp	dried basil
½ tsp	turmeric

1 Preheat the oven to 350°F. Place the bones on a large baking sheet or roasting pan, and brown in the oven for 45 minutes.

2 Remove from the oven and cool slightly. Using a small knife, remove the marrow and meaty bits from the bones and store in a Mason jar. (Use in pâté or gravy.)

3 Place the bones into a stockpot or slow cooker, and add the water, vinegar, vegetables, parsley stems and salt.

4 Bring to a boil, skimming off the scum/foam that rises to the top. Do not keep it at a high boil for too long or you may risk making your broth high in glutamate. Reduce the heat, cover and simmer for at least 12 hours and as long as 48 hours. The longer you cook the broth, the more rich and flavorful it will be.

5 Strain the broth into a large bowl (discard solids). Set aside what you'll be using immediately, then pour into Mason jars. Seal and let cool until they are just warm to the touch, then refrigerate. A layer of fat will form at the top, which will preserve the broth and keep microbes out. If you're going to freeze the broth, leave room in the jars for the broth to expand. (Loosen the seal before freezing to avoid breaking the glass.)

Makes 8 cups. Will keep for 4 days in the fridge or up to 12 months in the freezer.

 When buying bones, ask your butcher to cut the bones so that the marrow is exposed.

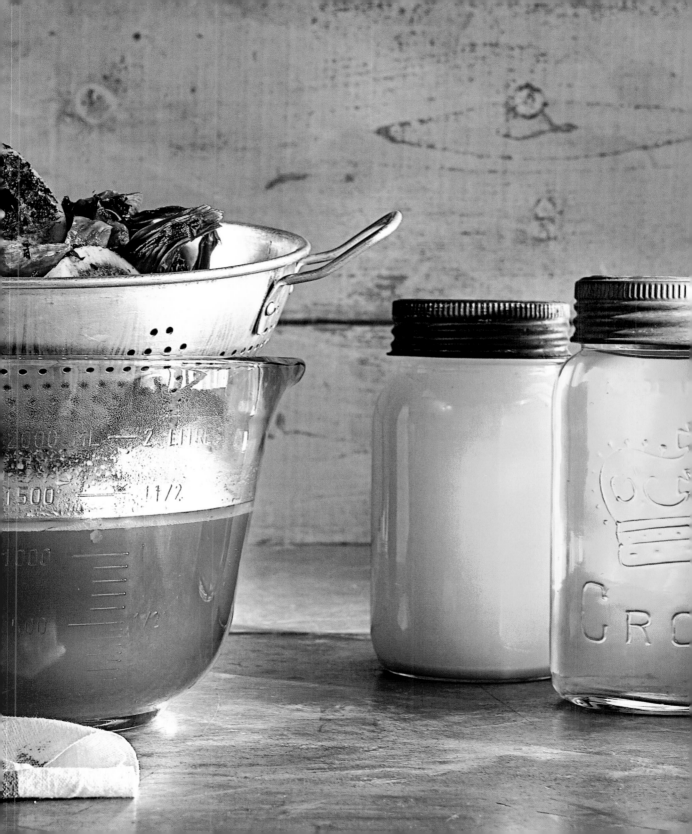

Golden Chicken Bone Broth

This broth is easy to make and brimming with detox nutrients. Turmeric adds a lovely golden hue and helps accelerate detoxification.

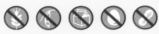

1 lb	raw and/or leftover organic chicken bones (from 1 average-size chicken carcass)
3 quarts (12 cups) filtered water	
2 cups	chopped carrot or winter squash
2 cups	chopped celery
2 cups	fresh parsley, cilantro or basil stems
1½ cups	sliced onions
¼ cup	raw apple cider vinegar
½ tsp	ground turmeric
1 tsp	pink rock or gray sea salt

optional booster

½ tsp	ground ginger

1 If using chicken backs and necks, you can leave the meat on the bones, but otherwise strip the bones of any meat, setting it aside to use in a soup later on. Put all the ingredients into a large pot, including the ground ginger if using, and bring to a boil, stirring occasionally. Alternatively, you can cook this in a slow cooker on low for 12 to 24 hours.

2 Reduce the heat, cover and simmer for a minimum of 4 hours, but ideally for 12 hours or more. (If using backs and necks, cook for an hour before removing the meat from the bones for later use; return the bones to the broth and continue simmering.)

3 Strain the broth through a stainless-steel colander or strainer. Set aside what you'll be using immediately, and transfer the rest to Mason jars. Let cool completely, then seal. If you're going to freeze the broth, leave room in the containers for the broth to expand. (Loosen the seal prior to freezing to avoid breaking the glass.)

Makes 8 cups. Will keep for 4 days in the fridge or up to 12 months in the freezer.

 After you eat a roast chicken, throw all the bones in the freezer and make the broth on the weekend. Save your vegetable trimmings (such as celery leaves and onion and carrot ends) to use in broth instead of fresh vegetables. With these two tips, you are virtually making broth for free!

Vegan Broth

The main benefit of bone broth is it provides so many easy-to-absorb minerals. If you choose to avoid all animal products on this cleanse, then seaweed will help you get enough minerals. In my opinion, dulse tastes the best of all the seaweed products, and it's often harvested from areas of the eastern coast of Canada and the United States where toxins are low.

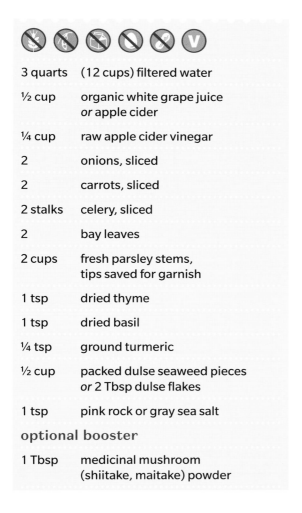

3 quarts	(12 cups) filtered water
½ cup	organic white grape juice *or* apple cider
¼ cup	raw apple cider vinegar
2	onions, sliced
2	carrots, sliced
2 stalks	celery, sliced
2	bay leaves
2 cups	fresh parsley stems, tips saved for garnish
1 tsp	dried thyme
1 tsp	dried basil
¼ tsp	ground turmeric
½ cup	packed dulse seaweed pieces *or* 2 Tbsp dulse flakes
1 tsp	pink rock or gray sea salt

optional booster

1 Tbsp	medicinal mushroom (shiitake, maitake) powder

1 In a large pot over high heat, bring all the ingredients to a boil. Reduce the heat, and simmer for 1 hour. Alternatively, you can cook this in a slow cooker on low for 6 hours.

2 Strain the broth through a stainless-steel colander or strainer. Set aside what you'll be using immediately, and transfer the rest to Mason jars. Let cool completely, then seal. If you're going to freeze the broth, leave room in the jars for the broth to expand. (Loosen the seal prior to freezing to avoid breaking the glass.)

Makes about 10 cups. Will keep for 4 days in the fridge or up to 12 months in the freezer.

Asian Onion Soup

Move over, gooey French onion soup — this version is packed with healing nutrients and flavor! Shiitake mushrooms are effective in protecting liver cells from toxins. Considering that the liver is your major detox organ, it's a great idea to give it the help it needs by including shiitakes in your diet. Fennel seed is a wonderful carminative spice; in other words, it's commonly used to reduce intestinal gas and aid digestion.

8 cups	bone or vegan broth (see pages 184–187 for broth recipes), divided
4 cups	thinly sliced onions
6 cloves	garlic, sliced
1 inch	fresh ginger, sliced
1 tsp	ground cinnamon
½ tsp	pink rock or gray sea salt
6	whole cloves
3	whole star anise
1 tsp	fennel seeds
6	fresh shiitake or cremini mushrooms, sliced
1 tsp	organic lemon juice
1 Tbsp	coconut aminos
1 Tbsp	coconut nectar

1 In a soup pot over medium heat, bring ½ cup of the broth to a boil.

2 Add the onion, garlic, ginger, cinnamon and salt, and gently simmer.

3 Meanwhile, using kitchen twine, tie up the cloves, star anise and fennel seed in a little cheesecloth package.

4 When the onions are soft (this takes about 3 minutes), add the remaining 7½ cups broth, along with the spice bag. Bring to a boil, then cover, reduce the heat to medium-low and simmer for 20 minutes.

5 Remove the spice bag from the broth. Add the mushrooms. Bring to a boil, then reduce the heat and simmer for another 10 minutes.

6 Remove the pan from the heat and stir in the lemon juice, coconut aminos and coconut nectar.

Makes 6 servings.

 Whole star anise is for beauty and flavor. Discard before eating.

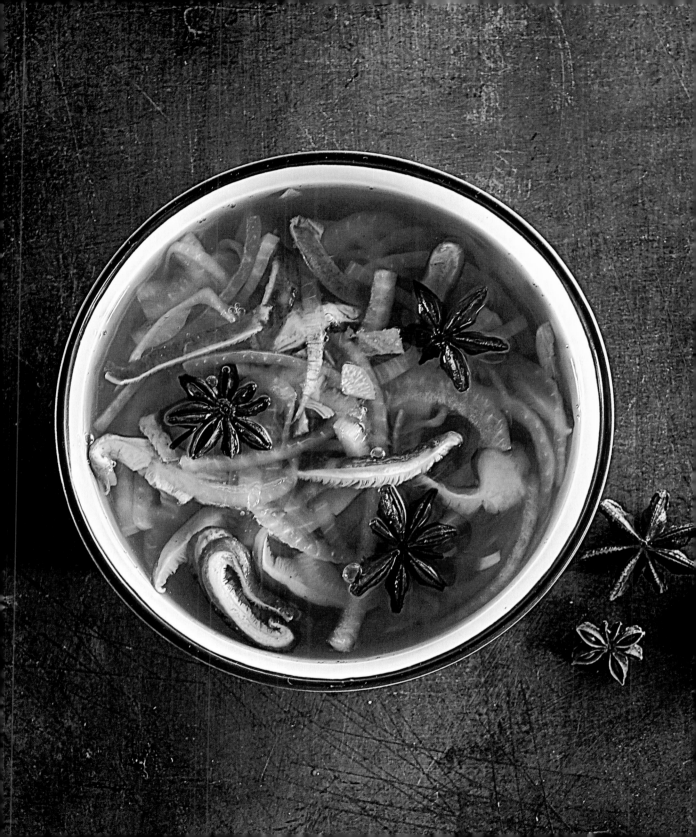

Lynn's Quick Borscht

My sister's tasty beet soup increases the body's nitric oxide, a powerful vasodilator (something that dilates your blood vessels). A study found that cyclists who consumed 2 cups of beet juice 2½ hours before a 2½-mile race experienced a 2.8 percent improvement in their time trials. The cyclists showed up to an 11 percent improvement in power output with no increase in the rate of oxygen being used. That could make the difference between winning the race and not making the podium.

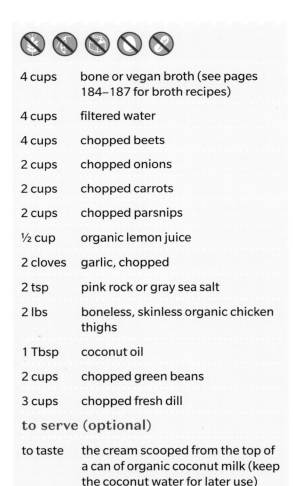

4 cups	bone or vegan broth (see pages 184–187 for broth recipes)
4 cups	filtered water
4 cups	chopped beets
2 cups	chopped onions
2 cups	chopped carrots
2 cups	chopped parsnips
½ cup	organic lemon juice
2 cloves	garlic, chopped
2 tsp	pink rock or gray sea salt
2 lbs	boneless, skinless organic chicken thighs
1 Tbsp	coconut oil
2 cups	chopped green beans
3 cups	chopped fresh dill

to serve (optional)

to taste	the cream scooped from the top of a can of organic coconut milk (keep the coconut water for later use)

1 In a large soup pot, combine the broth, water, beets, onions, carrots, parsnips, lemon juice, garlic and salt. Bring to a boil, then cover and simmer for 20 to 30 minutes or until all the vegetables are very soft.

2 Meanwhile, in a skillet over medium heat, sauté the chicken in the coconut oil until cooked through. Remove the chicken from the skillet, and chop into cubes.

3 Add the cooked chicken and green beans to the soup, and cook on low heat for another 10 minutes.

4 Remove from the heat, and stir in the dill. Serve with a dollop of coconut cream if desired.

Makes 12 servings. Keeps in the fridge for 4 days or in the freezer for 6 months.

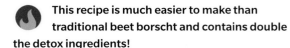

This recipe is much easier to make than traditional beet borscht and contains double the detox ingredients!

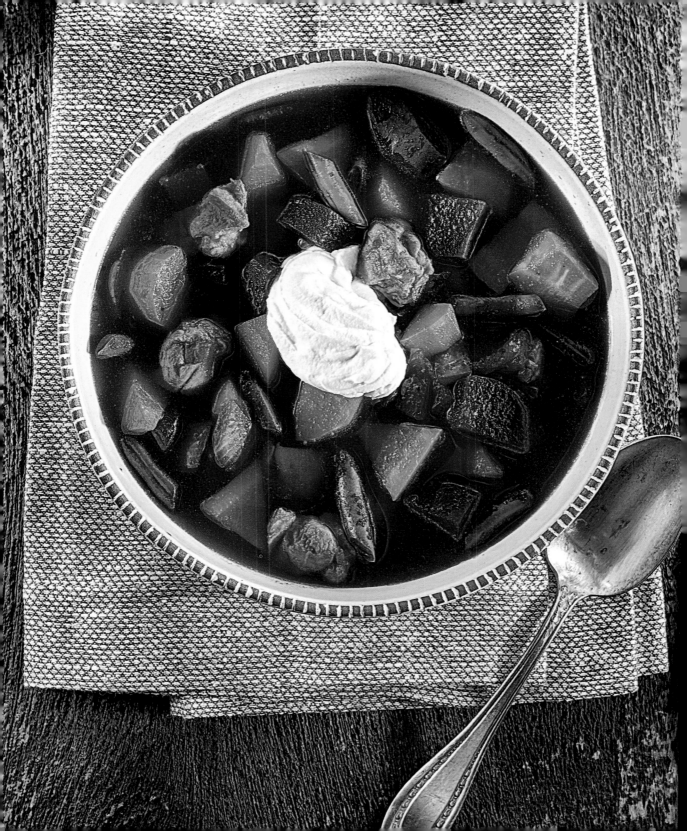

Broccoli Lentil Soup

Broccoli is high in a chemical called sulforaphane, which increases the amount of detox enzymes. These enzymes neutralize the harmful toxins we breathe in every day, toxins that can cause respiratory distress, especially in people who have asthma and other similar conditions.

2 Tbsp	coconut oil
1½ cups	chopped onions
2 tsp	minced garlic
2 cups	chopped green beans
1 cup	chopped carrots
1 cup	chopped celery
1 Tbsp	dried basil
1 tsp	dried thyme
½ tsp	dried oregano
½ tsp	pink rock or gray sea salt
3 cups	chopped broccoli (1 large head)
¾ cup	dried green lentils, rinsed well
6 cups	bone or vegan broth (see pages 184–187 for broth recipes)

optional booster

1 Tbsp	Julie's Curry Powder (page 269)

to serve

¼ cup	chopped green onions

1 Heat the coconut oil in a large soup pot over medium heat. Add the onions and sauté for 3 minutes.

2 Add the garlic, green beans, carrots, celery, dried herbs and salt, and curry powder if using, and cook for a few more minutes until the vegetables are nicely coated in spices.

3 Add the broccoli, lentils and broth, and bring to a boil. Reduce the heat, cover and simmer for 1 hour.

4 Using an immersion blender, puree until smooth. Garnish with chopped green onions if desired.

Makes 6 servings.

A soup doesn't need to contain dairy to be creamy and delicious. You can puree almost any soup with an immersion blender (or regular blender) for a creamy effect. But you can also save time here by skipping this step for a chunkier broccoli soup.

Butternut Squash Puree or Soup

Both traditional Chinese medicine and Ayurveda suggest quashing your sweet cravings by adding more naturally sweet, highly nutritious orange foods. Butternut squash is a great example, with deep-orange-colored flesh and a sweet flavor. It's filled with alpha- and beta-carotene, powerful antioxidant and anti-inflammatory agents.

1	large butternut squash (about 6 cups)
1 Tbsp	coconut oil
to taste	pink rock or gray sea salt
1 tsp	organic lemon zest
1 tsp	organic lemon juice (use 1 Tbsp if using sweetener)
1 Tbsp	coconut butter (or extra coconut oil), softened
⅛ tsp	ground cinnamon

optional boosters

1 tsp	coconut nectar
1 tsp	pure vanilla extract

to make a soup

1 cup	bone or vegan broth (see pages 184–187 for broth recipes)
1½ cups	organic coconut milk

1 Preheat the oven to 350°F.

2 Halve the squash lengthwise, and remove the seeds and stringy matter. Rub the insides and cut surface with coconut oil, and season with salt.

3 Place cut side up in a roasting pan, and bake for 1 hour or until fork-tender.

4 Remove the squash from the oven. Scoop out the flesh and place in a food processor.

5 Add the lemon zest, lemon juice and coconut butter, and coconut nectar and vanilla if using. Puree until smooth.

6 Add the cinnamon, and more salt to taste, and pulse a few times to mix well. Serve as a puree.

7 To make this into a soup, place the puree in a saucepan. Stir in broth and coconut milk, and heat until simmering.

Makes 4 cups puree or 10 cups soup. Keeps in the fridge for up to 1 week.

 This should be your go-to recipe when you have an upset tummy. It's easy to digest and will keep up your strength.

Spotlight: The Hot Detox Spices

Now that you understand the basics of the Hot Detox, it's time to decide if you want to turn up the heat and accelerate this program. How far do you want to take this cleanse? You can stick with the soothing menu I suggest, or take it to the next level just by adding extra culinary spices. Spices such as cinnamon, ginger, turmeric, cardamom and coriander boast not only rich colors and fragrances but also strong therapeutic effects. Indeed, there is a world of healing treasures hidden in your spice cupboard. The Hot Detox is the perfect time to dip into your stash of warming spices to bolster your body's immunity. Let's explore some of my favorites.

Cinnamon (*Cinnamomum verum*)

A member of the *Lauraceae* family. Cinnamon is a delicious warming spice that, according to traditional Chinese medicine, helps to reduce dampness in the body by increasing circulation. It is antiseptic, an excellent digestive tonic, and known to act like insulin (the hormone that regulates blood sugar). By stimulating insulin receptors on the muscle and fat cells, cinnamon helps to usher sugar out of the blood and into the cells. As a result, the simple addition of 1 gram of cinnamon (about ¼ teaspoon) to the daily diet of people with type 2 diabetes has been shown to improve blood sugar levels, as well as blood fats, and to reduce their risk factor for cardiovascular disease.

Adding cinnamon to the diet can also help reduce muscle soreness after exercise. Cinnamon contains a range of compounds that help reduce the damage of oxidation and inflammation — both of which are elevated after an intense workout. Recent studies show that less than 1 teaspoon per day of cinnamon or ginger can significantly reduce this type of muscle soreness.

Look for Ceylon cinnamon from Sri Lanka — it's considered to be the best quality.

Ginger (*Zingiber officinale*)

A member of the *Zingiberaceae* family. Like cinnamon, ginger improves circulation in all parts of the body. This fragrant root has been used to soothe an upset stomach for centuries. Scientists have found that ginger suppresses the release of vasopressin, a hormone thought to be responsible for the feeling of motion sickness.

You can also use ginger to stop nausea and vomiting during pregnancy; in recent studies, ginger was shown to be just as effective at this as pharmaceutical drugs. Further, it can boost the immune systems of both mother and baby. Ginger also has a cleansing effect on the digestive tract, and reduces the stress put on the liver during pregnancy.

Ginger has the ability to heal painful inflammation by inhibiting the effects of arachidonic acid, a fatty acid responsible for triggering inflammation, which ultimately leads to pain. Moreover, choosing ginger over anti-inflammatory drugs gives the liver a break from working to clear a drug from your system.

If you buy organic ginger, there is no need to peel it, which will save you time and deliver greater flavor.

Turmeric (*Curcuma longa*)

Like ginger, a member of the *Zingiberaceae* family. Turmeric, known for its intense yellow–orange color, is a deeply warming spice that has powerful antioxidant and anti-inflammatory properties. It has played an important role in many traditional cultures for thousands of years and is highly valued in the practice of Ayurveda.

Turmeric improves circulation by reducing elevated blood levels of fibrinogen, a plasma protein that plays a key role in the process of blood clotting. Elevated levels of this protein are known to be a major risk factor for heart attack and stroke. Turmeric also inhibits platelet aggregation, which can reduce the risk of blood clots.

Curcumin, the active ingredient in turmeric, works by stimulating the liver and gallbladder to produce bile. Curcumin also reduces symptoms of bloating and gas in people suffering from indigestion.

Turmeric is best known for its amazing ability to reduce inflammation. Curcumin can protect and heal almost every organ in the body! It's an antioxidant — preventing oxidation in the organs and thereby reducing the low-grade inflammation that comes with chronic disease.

Turmeric is a root that looks a lot like ginger but is much more difficult to grind yourself. If you buy your turmeric already ground, make sure you buy small quantities of good-quality powder, and use it up before you buy more.

Cardamom (Elettaria cardamomum)

Another member of the *Zingiberaceae* family. Cardamom, also known as the "queen of spices," is the small seed pod of the perennial cardamom plant. The seeds have a pleasant aroma with a warm, slightly sweet and pungent taste. Cardamom is widely used in South Asian cooking and is an essential ingredient in garam masala.

Cardamom helps to reduce symptoms of gastrointestinal disorders such as constipation and diarrhea. It can have a positive effect on blood pressure — a 3-gram serving has been shown to significantly decrease diastolic pressure, without side effects. Cardamom also has a strong antimicrobial effect on the microorganisms that cause dental cavities and bad breath.

You only need a little to give your recipes a sweet, aromatic vanilla undertone.

Coriander (Coriandrum sativum)

Belongs to the *Apiaceae* family. Coriander is the seed of the coriander herb (also known as cilantro). The seeds have a sweet, nutty taste that is very different from the leaves of the plant, and are packed with volatile oils that provide powerful antioxidant protection.

Studies show that people who suffer from the abdominal pain, cramping and bloating of irritable bowel syndrome see improvements after taking coriander seeds, as the spice possesses antispasmodic properties that help to relax the overactive muscles of the digestive tract. This relaxing effect also works on the arteries of the cardiovascular system, helping to lower blood pressure.

Coriander has a positive impact on blood lipids. Adding coriander seeds to the diet can help reduce your blood levels of cholesterol and triglycerides. The seeds help to increase the amount of bile that the liver produces, and assist in the breakdown and excretion of cholesterol.

Pure Red Chili Powder and Cayenne (Capsicum annuum)

Pure red chili powder can be made from various peppers such as ancho, and can vary in heat; cayenne is dependably fiery. These two are worthy of special mention as they add an intense heat to any dish they contain. Chilies can be beneficial for people with a "cold" constitution in Ayurveda (see page 14) and who can handle hot spices. (They should be tested with care, and avoided if you have a sensitivity to nightshades.) However, these spices are not recommended for those with excess *pitta* (i.e., a "hot" constitution; see page 14) as they can increase excess internal heat.

Fast Carrot Soup

This soup is traditionally prepared in India for people with digestive troubles. Carrots contain a phytonutrient called falcarinol, currently being researched for its ability to fight intestinal cancer. The vanilla, ginger and cinnamon make this soup so comforting, you will want to make it again and again.

4 cups	thinly sliced carrots
3 cups	bone or vegan broth (see pages 184–187 for broth recipes)
⅓ cup	Hemp Hearts
3 Tbsp	organic lemon juice
2 tsp	freshly grated ginger *or* 1 tsp ground ginger
1 tsp	pure vanilla extract
¼ tsp	ground cinnamon
¼ tsp	ground cumin
½ tsp	ground turmeric
1 tsp	pink rock or gray sea salt

optional booster

½ cup	cooked lentils (for the extra protein), plus 1 cup extra broth

to serve (optional)

2 Tbsp	onion flakes
2 Tbsp	raw pumpkin seeds
¼ cup	Coconut Cashew Yogurt (page 158) *or* organic coconut milk

1. In a soup pot, bring the carrots and broth to a boil. Reduce the heat, cover and simmer for 10 minutes.

2. Add the rest of the soup ingredients, including the lentils if using, and mix to combine. Transfer to a blender (you may need to do this in 2 batches) and blend on high speed until smooth. Be careful to hold down the blender lid as the hot soup will expand and the lid could pop off.

3. If desired, serve topped with the onion flakes, pumpkin seeds and/or coconut yogurt or coconut milk.

Makes 6 cups. Keeps up to 5 days in the fridge. Freezes well.

Fresh ginger is more potent than dried powder. Chop up some ginger and add it to a stir-fry, or grate some into your mint tea. You can even add chunks of ginger to your bath! Soaking in a hot ginger bath will relax the muscles, raise the body temperature and induce sweating — all of which help to fight off colds and flus.

Quick Cauliflower Soup

This is an excellent mild recipe for when you are convalescing. This soup provides lots of detox nutrients, including omega-3, vitamins B1, B2, B3, B5, B6 and B9, choline and magnesium, and a lot of fiber as well.

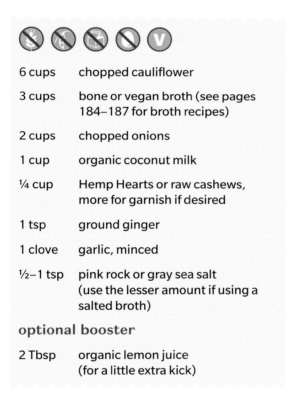

6 cups	chopped cauliflower
3 cups	bone or vegan broth (see pages 184–187 for broth recipes)
2 cups	chopped onions
1 cup	organic coconut milk
¼ cup	Hemp Hearts or raw cashews, more for garnish if desired
1 tsp	ground ginger
1 clove	garlic, minced
½–1 tsp	pink rock or gray sea salt (use the lesser amount if using a salted broth)

optional booster

2 Tbsp	organic lemon juice (for a little extra kick)

1. Place the cauliflower, broth and onions in a large soup pot. Bring to a boil, then reduce the heat and simmer until the cauliflower is soft, about 8 minutes.

2. Transfer to a blender, and add all the remaining ingredients, including the lemon juice if using. Blend on high speed until very smooth. Be careful to hold down the blender lid as the hot soup will expand and the lid could pop off.

3. Serve garnished with extra Hemp Hearts if desired.

Makes 8 cups. Keeps up to 5 days in the fridge. Freezes well.

Comforting Chicken Soup

This chicken soup is food for both body and soul. It provides electrolyte minerals, which your body uses to carry electrical signals from cell to cell.

2 Tbsp	extra virgin olive oil
2 cups	finely chopped onions
5 cloves	garlic, 3 cloves sliced and 2 cloves minced, divided
2-inch	piece of fresh ginger, minced
2 cups	chopped leeks (white and green parts)
2 cups	chopped fresh shiitake mushrooms
2 cups	sliced carrots, in ¼-inch rounds
2 cups	diced unpeeled sweet potatoes
1 cup	sliced celery
8	boneless, skinless organic chicken thighs, cut into cubes
8 cups	chicken broth (see page 186 for Golden Chicken Bone Broth)
2	bay leaves
½ tsp	pink rock or gray sea salt
4 cups	chopped kale
1 cup	chopped snow peas or green beans
½ cup	each chopped fresh parsley and basil
1 Tbsp	each chopped fresh oregano, thyme and rosemary

1   Heat the olive oil in a soup pot over medium heat. Add the onions, sliced garlic, ginger and leeks. Cook until softened, about 3 minutes.

2   Add the shiitake, carrots, sweet potatoes, celery, chicken, broth, bay leaves and salt. Increase the temperature to high, bring to a boil and then reduce the heat and simmer for about 25 minutes or until the vegetables soften but don't become mushy.

3   Stir in the kale, snow peas or green beans, the fresh herbs and the minced garlic. Simmer for another few minutes to meld the flavors and soften the kale. (Adding these ingredients at the end means that the veggies stay bright green and the garlic provides maximum immune benefit.)

Makes 12 servings. Will keep for up to 3 days in the fridge and 3 months in the freezer.

 It's important to use real chicken or turkey broth that has been made with the bones (see page 186). Poultry bones contain nutrients such as B vitamins (in the marrow), calcium, magnesium and zinc, which can assist your immune cells to better fight off viruses and build collagen.

Use fresh herbs whenever possible; their flavor and levels of essential oils are at their peak. If fresh herbs are unavailable, substitute 1 tsp each dried.

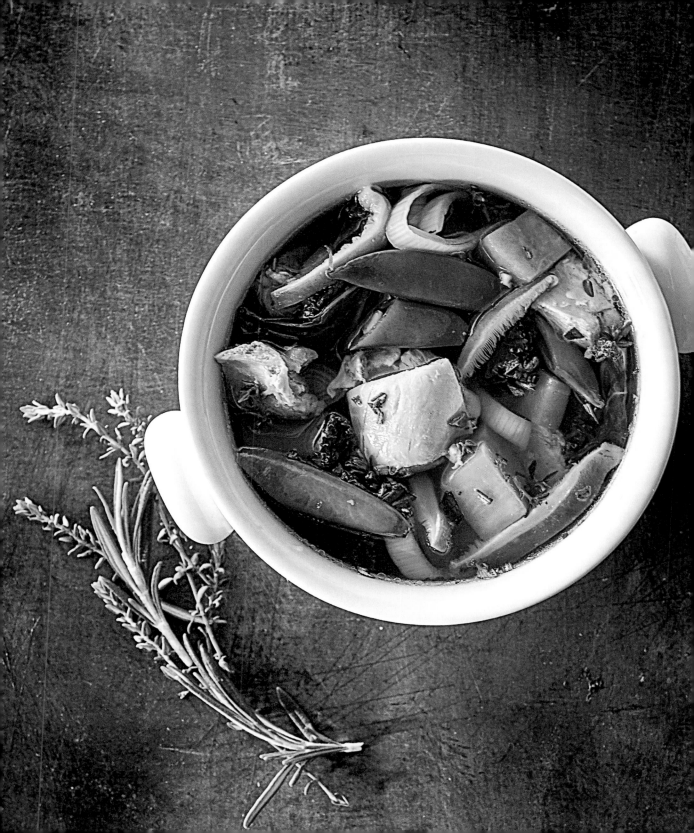

Dijon Chicken or Lentil Soup

This delicate, simple dish tastes superb and may become a family favorite! Be sure to use a Dijon mustard that doesn't contain sugar. Mustard seeds contain selenium, a nutrient that can lessen the severity of asthma and rheumatoid arthritis.

6 cups	chicken broth *or* 7 cups vegan broth (see pages 186 and 187)
¼ cup	Dijon mustard
1 Tbsp	Italian seasoning (basil, oregano, rosemary, sage, savory and thyme)
8	large boneless, skinless organic chicken thighs *or* 1½ cups dried split red lentils *or* split yellow mung beans, rinsed well
3 cups	cubed turnips, parsnips or celeriac
3 cups	cubed peeled butternut squash *or* unpeeled sweet potatoes
2 cups	green beans (or any green vegetable), cut into 2-inch pieces
1 cup	finely chopped onions
1 cup	organic coconut milk
½ tsp	pink rock or gray sea salt (reduce to ¼ tsp if using a salted broth)

optional boosters

2 cups	sliced fresh shiitake mushrooms, stems removed

to serve

2 cups	chopped fresh parsley

1 In a large pot, bring the broth, mustard and Italian seasoning to a boil. Add the chicken, lentils or mung beans; turnips, parsnips or celeriac; and squash or sweet potatoes. If desired, add the shiitakes. Reduce the heat and simmer for 20 minutes for the chicken soup version, 25 minutes for the vegetarian version.

2 Add green beans, onions, coconut milk and salt, and simmer for 4 minutes.

3 Serve hot. For the chicken soup, place a chicken piece in each soup bowl, and divide the vegetables around it. Spoon over the broth.

Makes 8 servings. Chicken soup keeps up to 3 days in the fridge and lentil soup up to 5 days.

The soup can be frozen and reheated, and the quick cooking times in the recipe mean the vegetables will still hold up well. However, if you suffer from digestive stress, increase the cooking time to ensure that the root vegetables are cooked until tender. You should be able to easily stick a fork through the squash.

Gentle Healing Dal

Want to do the Hot Detox for just 10 dollars a day? Lean into this recipe and save a bundle. This soup is from the yogic tradition and eaten regularly on a cleanse to correct "digestive fire" (*agni*). The spices can eliminate negative microbes that are influencing your mood and immune system.

5 cups	bone or vegan broth (see pages 184–187 for broth recipes) or filtered water
1 cup	dried split yellow mung beans or split red lentils, rinsed well
1 tsp	ground turmeric
½ tsp	pink rock or gray sea salt, or to taste
1 Tbsp	coconut oil
1 tsp	cumin seeds
1 cup	chopped onions
3 cloves	garlic, chopped
2 tsp	ground coriander
2 tsp	Julie's Curry Powder (page 269)
3 Tbsp	organic lemon juice
10 oz pkg	frozen spinach, thawed, *or* 4 cups chopped fresh baby spinach
1 cup	organic coconut milk

to serve

to taste	fresh cilantro

1 Bring the broth or water to a boil in a soup pot, and add the mung beans or lentils, turmeric and salt. Lower the heat to medium, cover and simmer for 35 minutes. (After 20 minutes of cooking, skim off the foam with a spoon, then cover again.)

2 While the beans or lentils are cooking, heat the coconut oil in a skillet over medium heat, and add the cumin seeds. As they start to pop, add the onions and sauté until translucent. Add the garlic, coriander and curry powder and cook, stirring, for 2 minutes.

3 When the beans or lentils are cooked, stir in the onion mixture, lemon juice, spinach and coconut milk. Cook for 3 to 4 minutes or until heated through. Garnish with cilantro and serve.

Makes 6 servings.

 As with other spices, it's best to buy coriander in seed form and grind as needed. Coriander is often sold ground, but it's likely that the oils will have dissipated and lost their healing potential.

The Hot Detox Soup Mix

This is a fabulous detox meal that is ready to go whenever you need something instantly. Make up a few jars of this soup mix before you start the cleanse.

½ cup	dried green split peas or split mung beans
½ cup	dried split red lentils
½ cup	quinoa or kasha (toasted buckwheat groats)
2 Tbsp	unsweetened dried shredded coconut
2 Tbsp	onion flakes
2 Tbsp	dried parsley or cilantro
2 Tbsp	dried basil
1 Tbsp	Julie's Curry Powder (page 269)
2 tsp	pink rock or gray sea salt
½ tsp	garlic powder

optional boosters

1 cup	freeze-dried carrots or peas
1 cup	crumbled kale chips
1 tsp	vanilla bean powder

to cook

7 cups	bone or vegan broth (see pages 184–187 for broth recipes) or non-dairy milk
14 oz can	organic coconut milk
2 Tbsp	organic lemon juice

to serve

to taste	fresh sprouts

1 Using a canning funnel, layer all the soup mix ingredients attractively in a wide-mouthed half-quart (2 cup) Mason jar, including any or all of the boosters, and tightly seal the lid.

2 To make soup with the soup mix, add the contents of the jar to a medium saucepan with the broth or non-dairy milk. Bring to a boil, then simmer for 45 minutes. Add the coconut milk and lemon juice, and stir well. Garnish with fresh sprouts.

Makes 2 cups of soup mix, which makes 10 cups of soup.

 This soup tastes good made with just water, for those times when you don't have broth.

A jar of this is a wonderful gift for a friend feeling under the weather.

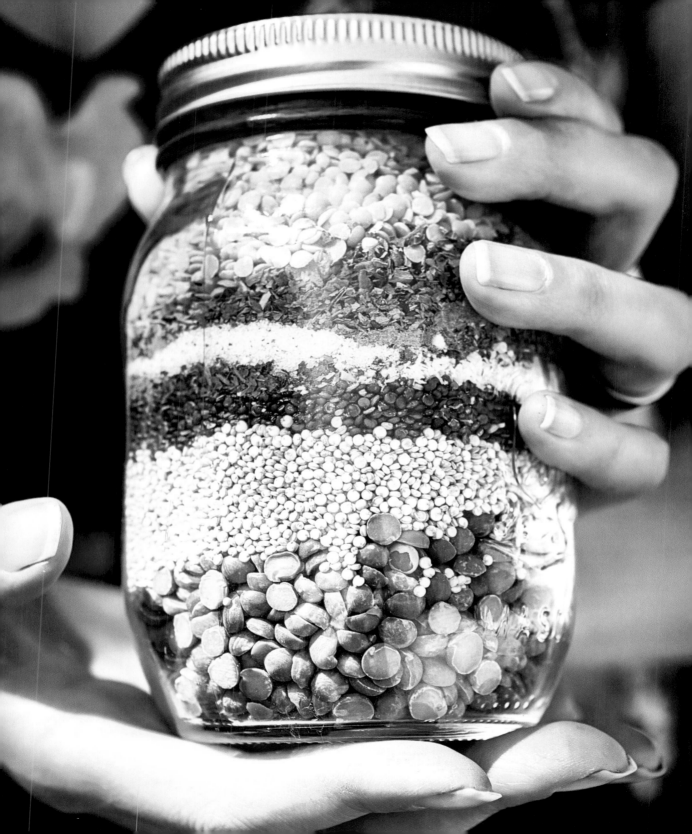

Kale Squash Soup

My sister makes our family this soup when we're in the mood for something fast, easy and tasty. It's creamy and delicious, full of fiber and vitamin A, and the perfect meal for a cold day.

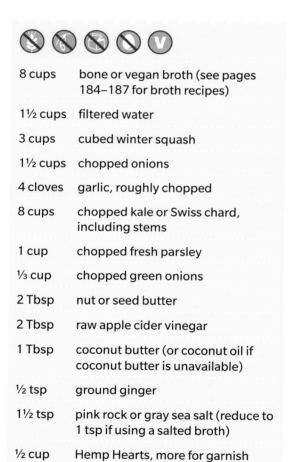

8 cups	bone or vegan broth (see pages 184–187 for broth recipes)
1½ cups	filtered water
3 cups	cubed winter squash
1½ cups	chopped onions
4 cloves	garlic, roughly chopped
8 cups	chopped kale or Swiss chard, including stems
1 cup	chopped fresh parsley
⅓ cup	chopped green onions
2 Tbsp	nut or seed butter
2 Tbsp	raw apple cider vinegar
1 Tbsp	coconut butter (or coconut oil if coconut butter is unavailable)
½ tsp	ground ginger
1½ tsp	pink rock or gray sea salt (reduce to 1 tsp if using a salted broth)
½ cup	Hemp Hearts, more for garnish

1 Bring the broth and water to a boil in a large soup pot.

2 Add the squash, onions and garlic, and reduce the heat to medium. Cover and cook until the squash is soft, about 20 minutes.

3 Add the kale or Swiss chard, and simmer until it has wilted, about 5 minutes.

4 Remove from the heat and add the remaining ingredients except for the Hemp Hearts.

5 Using an immersion blender (or blender), puree until smooth. Add the Hemp Hearts, and then blend to desired consistency. Garnish with extra Hemp Hearts if desired.

Makes 8 servings. Keeps up to 1 week in the fridge. Freezes well.

 This is a perfect soup for Phase 2 of the Hot Detox program, when you need the maximum amount of easy-to-digest nutrition.

Salad Soup

Traditional Chinese medicine considers leafy vegetables to be "cold," energetically speaking. People with tummy troubles often find lettuce difficult to digest. By cooking down the lettuce with delicious ingredients, you'll find you get all the nutrition without the bloat.

2 cups	thinly sliced leeks (white and green parts), in rounds (or green onions if leeks are unavailable)
1½ cups	thinly sliced fresh shiitake or oyster mushrooms
1 Tbsp	organic lemon juice
1 Tbsp	herbes de Provence or Italian seasoning
½ –1 tsp	pink rock or gray sea salt (use the lesser amount if using a salted broth)
6 cups	bone or vegan broth (see pages 184–187 for broth recipes)
5 cups	sliced romaine lettuce, in thin ribbons, or watercress, separated
2 cups	peas (frozen is fine)
1 Tbsp	tahini

optional boosters

1 cup	sliced water chestnuts or the center core of a pineapple sliced into coins (when sliced, the texture of pineapple core is the same as water chestnut)

to serve

1 cup	chopped fresh parsley or cilantro
¼ cup	Hemp Hearts or other seeds

1 To a soup pot, add the leeks, mushrooms, water chestnuts or pineapple if using, lemon juice, dried herbs and salt, along with the broth. Bring to a boil, then reduce the heat and simmer for 10 minutes.

2 Add the lettuce or watercress, peas and tahini, and cook for 2 more minutes. Serve garnished with fresh herbs and Hemp Hearts or other seeds.

Makes 8 cups. Keeps up to 5 days in the fridge. (Do not freeze.)

 The shiitake mushrooms here are highly recommended. A 2010 study found they were effective in protecting liver cells from toxins.

Beet Kvass

Drink this each morning to improve digestion. Beets contain phytonutrients called betalains that support liver detoxification through the important Phase 2 of the detox process. You can also enjoy the beets, which taste pickled and make a nice garnish for steamed greens.

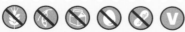

2 cups	cubed beets (see Tip)
2 Tbsp	sauerkraut juice or raw apple cider vinegar
½ Tbsp	pink rock or gray sea salt
2 cups	filtered water

optional booster

1–2 Tbsp	grated fresh ginger

1 Place the beets in a 1-quart (4-cup) Mason jar.

2 Add the sauerkraut juice or vinegar, along with the salt, and fill the rest of the jar with water.

3 Cover with a towel or cheesecloth, and leave on the counter at room temperature for 1 day to ferment.

4 Transfer the jar to the fridge, and consume the liquid as desired in 2-ounce (¼ cup) amounts each time. Enjoy the beets as well.

Makes 2 cups liquid and 2 cups fermented beets. Keeps for 6 months in the fridge.

 Wash and peel the beets if you cannot find them certified organic.

Ginger Kimchi

This recipe is from my dear friend Marni Wasserman (www.marniwasserman.com), the culinary nutritionist who cohosts the *Ultimate Health Podcast*. We both agree that kimchi is better when made with ginger instead of chili pepper.

8 cups	napa cabbage, washed, cored and chopped into ½- to 1-inch pieces (approx. ½ head)
1- to 2-inch piece fresh ginger	
½	medium onion
½ head	garlic
¼ cup	pink rock or gray sea salt
1 cup	sliced carrots
2 Tbsp	coconut aminos

1 Place a layer of cabbage in a 1-gallon (4-quart) Mason jar (or use four 4-cup jars). Sprinkle some of the salt over the cabbage. Repeat layers until all cabbage is used. Let the cabbage and salt to sit at room temperature for 6 hours. Rinse the salt off the cabbage under running water, drain well, and place in a large bowl.

2 Peel and finely chop the ginger and onion. Peel the garlic, but leave the cloves whole.

3 Mix the ginger, onions, garlic, carrots and aminos with the cabbage. Place the mixture back into the jar. Cover the jar with cheesecloth.

4 Let ferment at room temperature for 2 days. Cover with the lid and place in the refrigerator to ferment for another week or until the desired taste has developed.

Makes 4 cups. Keeps for 6 months in the fridge.

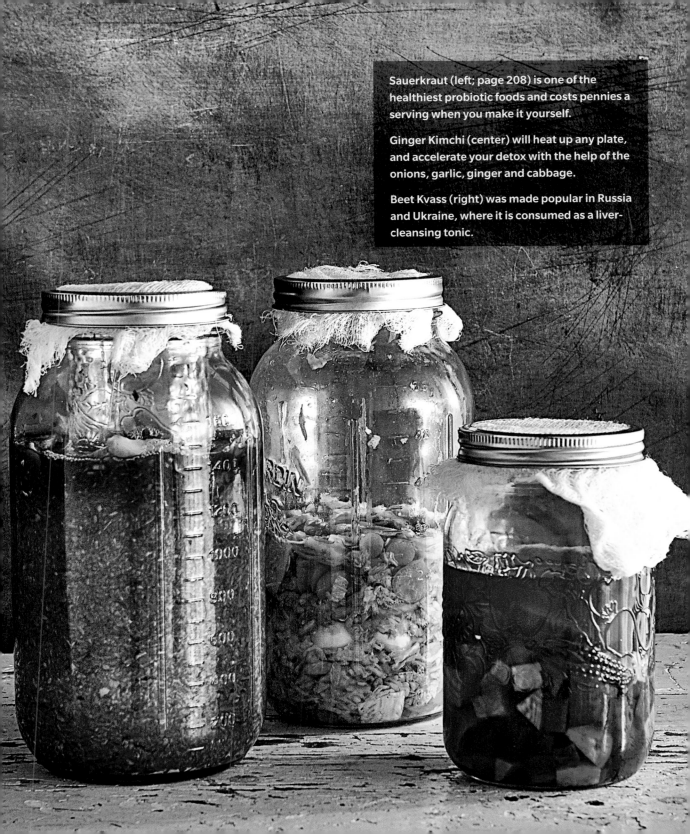

Sauerkraut (left; page 208) is one of the healthiest probiotic foods and costs pennies a serving when you make it yourself.

Ginger Kimchi (center) will heat up any plate, and accelerate your detox with the help of the onions, garlic, ginger and cabbage.

Beet Kvass (right) was made popular in Russia and Ukraine, where it is consumed as a liver-cleansing tonic.

Pretty Purple Sauerkraut

Here is another recipe from my dear friend Marni Wasserman (www.marniwasserman.com). Sauerkraut is sour because of lacto-fermentation, a process in which probiotic bacteria break down the cabbage.

A serving of sauerkraut gives you a powerful dose of these healthy probiotics, which aid digestion, and research has found raw sauerkraut prevents cancer cells from forming. It contains sulfur-containing compounds known as glucosinolates, which help the liver eliminate excess estrogen and xenoestrogen. I use purple cabbage because it also contains anthocyanins, a powerful antioxidant.

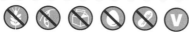

| 5 lbs | purple cabbage (about 1 large head) |
| 3 Tbsp | pickling salt |

optional boosters

2 tsp	dill or cumin seeds
2 tsp	whole coriander seeds
2	whole cloves or ⅛ tsp ground cloves
1 tsp	ground ginger
2	bay leaves, crumbled
4 cloves	garlic, halved

1 Discard any damaged outer leaves of the cabbage. Quarter the cabbage and remove the hard core. Finely slice the cabbage by hand or with a food processor.

2 Sterilize four 4-cup widemouthed Mason jars in boiling water. Meanwhile, combine cabbage, salt and any boosters in a large bowl and mix until evenly coated (this helps to leach any juice from the cabbage faster).

3 Divide the cabbage evenly among the jars, tamping firmly with a wooden utensil to remove any hidden air pockets and to bruise the cabbage, making it release juice.

4 Cover each jar with a coffee filter secured by a rubber band. Let it sit for 2 hours. Every 30 minutes, tamp down the cabbage to help draw out the juices and submerge the cabbage in the brine.

 It's very important that the cabbage stays submerged in the brine as it ferments so mold doesn't form. After the fermentation is complete, store the jars in the fridge.

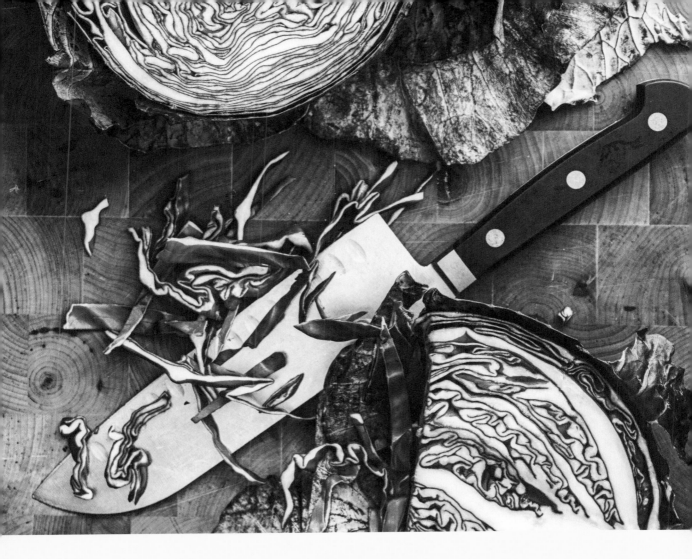

5 After 2 hours, if you still don't have enough natural brine, dissolve 1 teaspoon pickling salt in 1 cup of filtered water, and pour over the cabbage. When it's fully submerged, replace the coffee filter with a small saucer that fits just inside the top of the jar so it rests directly on the submerged cabbage. Add a weight, such as a water-filled ½-cup Mason jar, to keep the saucer under the brine.

6 Cover the jars with a clean dishcloth to keep out dust and insects. Place the jars out of the way, at room temperature, for 3 to 4 weeks. Check them daily to skim off any scum that may build up on the top, and cover with more brine if necessary. Replace the dishcloth with a clean one each time you remove scum buildup.

Makes 4 quarts (16 cups).

Coco Quinoa

Quinoa is gluten-free and easier to digest than common grass grains such as wheat and rye. Combining quinoa with coconut and spices ensures that it is brimming with detox nutrients.

1 cup	quinoa
½ tsp	pink rock or gray sea salt (reduce to ¼ tsp if using broth instead of water)
1 cup	bone or vegan broth (see pages 184–187 for broth recipes) or filtered water
1 cup	organic coconut milk

optional boosters

1 cup	peas (frozen are fine)
2 tsp	Julie's Curry Powder (page 269)

to serve

½ cup	unsweetened dried shredded coconut, lightly toasted
1 cup	chopped fresh cilantro or parsley

1 Combine the quinoa, salt, broth or water, and coconut milk in a medium saucepan. Bring to a boil, then reduce the heat to low, cover and simmer for 15 minutes. If using peas, add at the 10-minute mark and let them steam on top of the quinoa for the last 5 minutes of the cooking time.

2 Remove the pan from the heat and let stand without lifting the lid for 5 minutes or until ready to serve.

3 Add the curry powder if using. Fluff the quinoa with a fork, transfer to a serving bowl and garnish with the coconut and fresh herbs.

Makes 6 servings.

Garlic Cauliflower Mash

This tasty dish, very similar to mashed potato, will really help you bust carb cravings during the cleanse. Once chopped, cauliflower contains a compound called sulforaphane, which acts as an antibacterial agent against *Helicobacter pylori*. This bacteria can be present in the stomach, and not only can it cause gastric ulcers, it's linked to stomach cancer.

4 cups	cauliflower florets (about 1 small head)
2 cups	chopped parsnips or extra cauliflower
2 cups	filtered water
¼ cup	extra virgin olive oil
¼ cup	organic coconut milk
2 tsp	organic lemon juice
2–3 cloves	garlic, chopped (depending on how garlicky you like it!)
1 tsp	pink rock or gray sea salt

1 Combine the cauliflower, parsnips and water in a medium saucepan. Bring to a boil. Reduce the heat and simmer until the vegetables are very tender.

2 Drain the vegetables, then transfer to a blender or food processor. Add all the remaining ingredients and blend on high speed until very smooth.

Makes 4 cups.

Cauliflower Crust Pizza

Cauliflower is a good source of the B vitamins, vitamin C and fiber, all of which are important for detoxification.

3 cups	cauliflower florets (about ½ head)
1 clove	garlic, chopped
¼ cup	filtered water
2	large organic eggs
1 tsp	dried basil
4 Tbsp	almond flour
½ tsp	dried oregano or thyme
¼ tsp	pink rock or gray sea salt
2 Tbsp	dairy- and nut-free basil pesto (such as Instant Pesto, page 257)
½ cup	sliced red bell pepper
½ cup	fresh sprouts (e.g., arugula, basil, broccoli, pea, sunflower)
2	water-packed (in a jar) artichoke hearts, quartered
8	olives, sliced

1 In a food processor, pulse the cauliflower until it becomes crumblike. Place the cauliflower crumbs, garlic and water in a saucepan. Cover and cook on medium heat for 6 minutes or until cauliflower is tender. Avoid stirring, which will make it mushy.

2 Meanwhile, preheat the oven to 375°F. Line 2 baking sheets with parchment paper.

3 Drain the cauliflower in a sieve, then transfer to a clean kitchen towel and firmly squeeze out as much water as possible. Transfer to a bowl, and add the eggs, almond flour, dried herbs and salt.

4 Form 2 circles of "dough" on the baking sheets. Using a spatula, press down the dough so it forms a layer about ½ inch thick. Keep the crusts compact. There should be no parchment showing through the dough.

5 Bake for about 17 minutes or until dry and pliable. Gently transfer to a wire rack to cool, removing the parchment paper so the bottom does not become soggy.

6 Top with pesto, artichokes, red peppers, olives and sprouts.

Makes 2 pizzas.

Cauliflower is the perfect vegetable for veggie haters because it tastes quite similar to potato.

Baba's Sautéed Cabbage

This fast and inexpensive side dish was a staple in my grandma's home. Cabbage and other members of the cruciferous vegetable family contain glucosinolates, which help the liver produce toxin-removing enzymes. The purple pigment in purple cabbage is anthocyanins, which protect cells from being damaged by free radicals. They also protect you against allergies, diabetes and certain cancers.

2 cups	sliced onions
1½ Tbsp	coconut oil
8 cups	sliced purple cabbage (approx. half a cabbage; use green cabbage if purple is unavailable)
½–¾ tsp	pink rock or gray sea salt
1 Tbsp	cumin seeds

1 In a very large skillet or sauté pan over medium heat, sauté the onions in the coconut oil until translucent.

2 Stir in the cabbage 1 cup at a time, adding a bit of salt and cumin each time and stirring to evenly distribute.

3 Cover and reduce the heat to medium-low. Cook until the cabbage is tender. Do not overcook. If the cabbage is still wet near the end of the cooking time, leave it uncovered to let the excess moisture evaporate.

Makes 6 servings.

 Don't omit the cumin seeds; they help to reduce any gas that may occur from eating cabbage.

Tea-Time Eggs

The protein-bound sulfur found in egg yolks is needed for cytochrome P450 detoxification, the Phase 1 pathway in the liver. The dark tea creates a beautiful pattern on the eggs, reminiscent of spiderwebs. The scent of spices from the tea permeates the eggs, leaving a trace of sweet and spicy flavor. These spices also happen to be anti-inflammatory.

 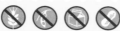

6	large organic eggs
3 teabags	chai tea
1 tsp	pink rock or gray sea salt

1 Lower the eggs carefully into a pot of boiling water, and boil for 8 minutes.

2 Drain the eggs. When cool enough to touch, hold each egg in your palm and crack the shell very gently all over with the back of a spoon but leave the shell intact (do not peel).

3 Add the teabags, salt and eggs to a saucepan, adding enough water to cover the eggs. Bring to a boil, cover and simmer for 10 minutes.

4 Remove from the heat, and let the eggs to cool in the liquid. Transfer the pan to the fridge to steep overnight.

5 In the morning, carefully peel the eggs, and enjoy.

Makes 6 eggs.

Eggs are high in selenium, which is used to create one of our body's most powerful antioxidants: superoxide dismutase (SOD). A study published in the *Journal of Neurotoxicology* reports that selenium effectively reduces toxic mercury buildup.

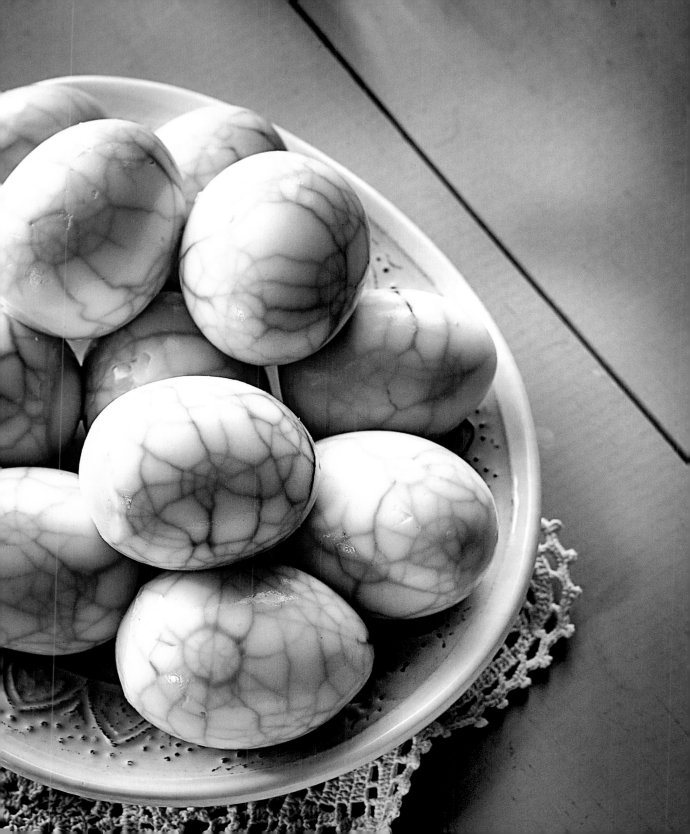

Fasolakia Lemonata (Lemon Green Beans)

This is my favorite way to make green beans. If you like Greek food, you will crave this dish long after the detox is over. The garlic activates enzymes in the liver to help with overall digestion and the flushing out of toxins.

4 cups	green beans, washed and trimmed
2 Tbsp	finely chopped fresh dill
2 Tbsp	organic lemon juice (if marinating overnight, you'll need 2 Tbsp more for serving)
2 Tbsp	extra virgin olive oil
1	green onion, thinly sliced
1 tsp	minced garlic
½ tsp	pink rock or gray sea salt

optional boosters

¼ cup	chopped red bell pepper
2 Tbsp	Hemp Hearts
½ tsp	organic lemon zest

1 In a large pot, bring salted filtered water to a boil. Add the green beans and cook for 4 to 5 minutes, then drain and run cold water over them to stop the cooking. Drain again.

2 Place the green beans in a bowl, and add the rest of the ingredients and any of the boosters if using.

3 Toss together until well coated. Serve immediately or marinate in the refrigerator overnight. If you let it marinate overnight, don't forget to add the extra lemon juice before serving.

Makes 4 servings.

 Dill has been shown to activate the enzyme glutathione-S-transferase. This enzyme helps the antioxidant glutathione reduce free radicals, which cause aging.

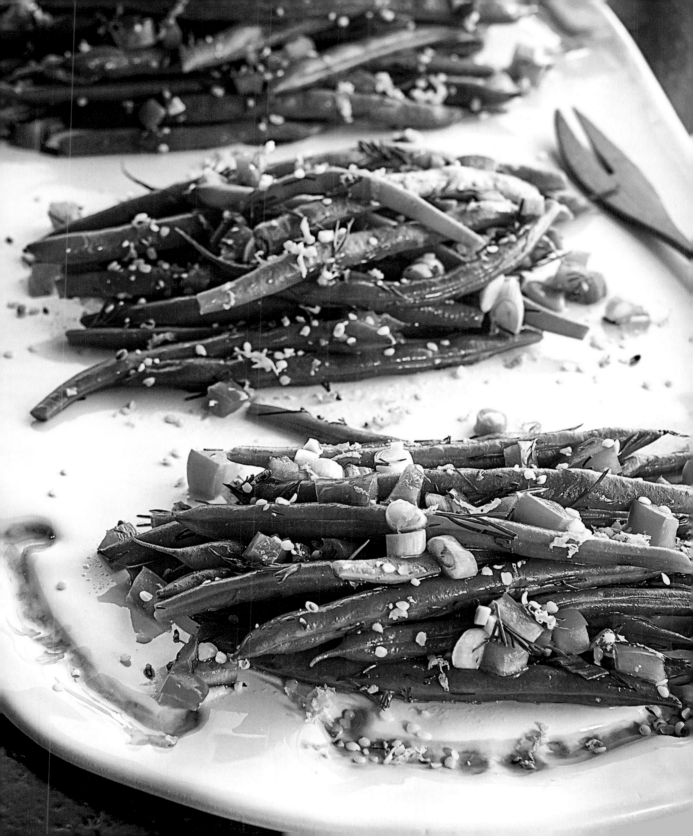

Garlic Dandelion Greens

Dandelion greens are excellent for you! Though many people know of the benefits of eating these nutrient-dense weeds, they shy away from the bitter taste. The younger the leaf, the less bitter it is, but there is no denying that dandelions have a strong flavor. If you are especially daring, drink the water used to steam the dandelion as a tea.

4 cups	chopped fresh dandelion greens
½ cup	filtered water
1 Tbsp	coconut oil
6 cloves	garlic, sliced
½ tsp	pink rock or gray sea salt

1 Wash the dandelion greens well by submerging them in a bowl of water. Drain the water and repeat until there is no sign of grit. Lightly shake the water from the greens.

2 In a skillet over medium heat, cook the dandelion greens with the ½ cup water just until wilted. Drain off the liquid (or save it to drink).

3 In a separate skillet, melt the coconut oil over low heat. Cook the garlic for about 5 minutes or until softened and transparent.

4 Pour the coconut oil/garlic mixture over the wilted dandelion, season with salt and toss to combine. Serve immediately.

Makes 1 large serving or 2 side servings.

 Fortunately, dandelion's strong taste can be mitigated. Like rapini, dandelion is particularly tasty with coconut oil and garlic. The trick is to cook the garlic over a low heat so that it slowly softens, becoming a sweet accent to the bitter green.

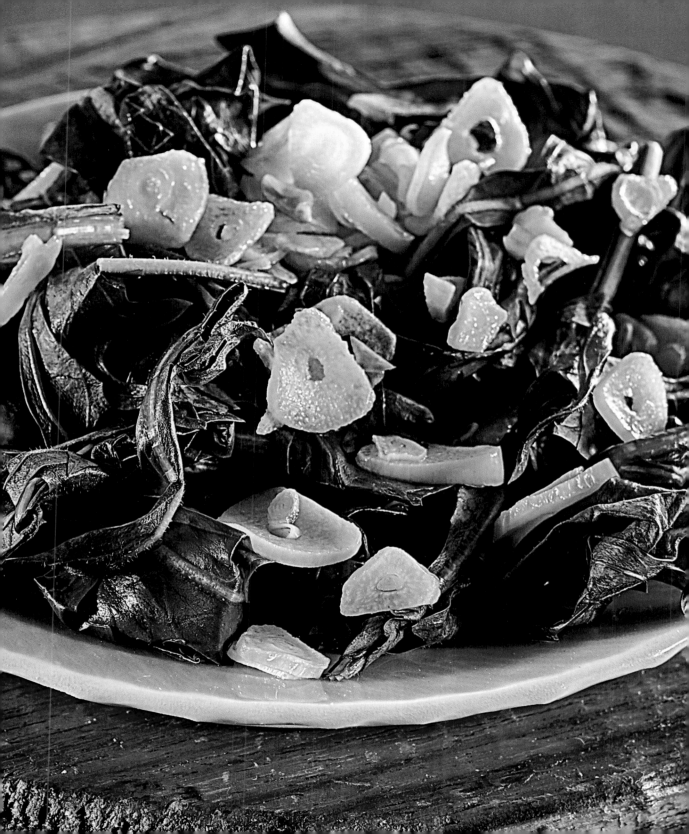

Garlic Roasted Asparagus

Succulent and tender asparagus is one of the most detoxifying items in the produce aisle. Eat it raw when you're feeling bloated — it's a natural diuretic. Asparagus is high in both anti-inflammatory and antioxidant nutrients. It contains vitamins C and E; beta-carotene; the minerals zinc, manganese, chromium and selenium; and the amino acid asparagine, which helps insulin transport glucose into cells to be used as fuel.

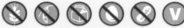

2 lbs	fresh asparagus, ends trimmed, rinsed and patted dry
3 Tbsp	coconut oil
1–2	cloves garlic, minced
½ tsp	pink rock or gray sea salt, more to taste
1 Tbsp	organic lemon juice, more to taste

optional booster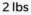

2 tsp	freshly grated organic lemon zest

1 Preheat the oven to 350°F. In a large glass baking dish, toss the asparagus with the coconut oil, garlic and salt.

2 Bake until the asparagus is tender-crisp, about 20 minutes. Stir gently at the 10-minute mark and 15-minute mark.

3 Remove the baking dish from the oven and toss the cooked asparagus with the lemon juice. Adjust the salt or lemon, if necessary. Serve warm or at room temperature.

Makes 8 servings.

 This recipe tastes amazing the next day and takes little time to make. Enjoy it often!

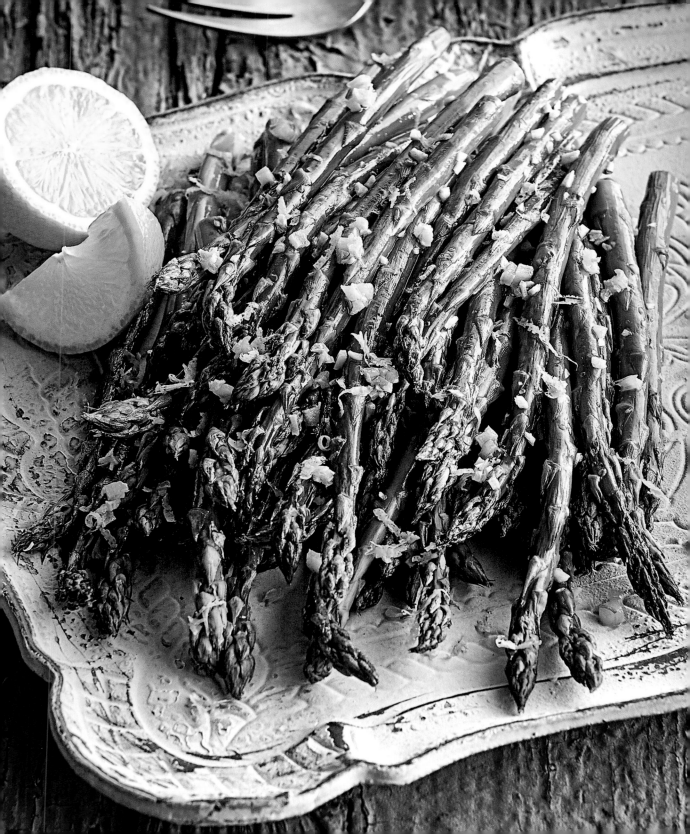

Garlic Steamed Artichokes

Though commonly thought of as a vegetable, artichokes (also called globe artichokes) are actually a flower bud. A relative of the famous milk thistle, artichokes stimulate bile flow, which helps to carry toxins out of your body. Artichokes have been used as an indigestion remedy in Europe for more than a century. One artichoke contains about 25 percent of our daily fiber needs and 16 essential nutrients, including vitamin C, potassium, folic acid, calcium and magnesium.

     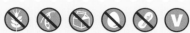

4	fresh artichokes
pinch	pink rock or gray sea salt
2 Tbsp	organic lemon juice
2–3	cloves garlic
1 recipe	Heart-Healthy Dipping Sauce (see page 223)

1 Cut off some of the stem, and the tips of the artichoke leaves.

2 In a large pot, bring filtered water (enough to cover the artichokes) to a boil, and add the salt. Add the artichokes, lemon juice and garlic.

3 Simmer for 15 minutes or until tender (older artichokes may take longer to cook). Prepare the dipping sauce while the artichokes cook.

4 To test for doneness, pull off a leaf; it should come off easily. Drain well, discarding the garlic, and dry the artichokes by squeezing gently in a clean kitchen towel.

5 Enjoy pulling off the leaves one at a time and dipping them in the sauce. Remove the "chokes" (the hairy center) and discard. Marinate the hearts in the rest of the sauce or add to your next salad.

Makes 4 servings.

 Classically, artichokes are served with melted butter. Try my Heart-Healthy Dipping Sauce (page 223) instead and be happily surprised that you don't actually miss the saturated fat.

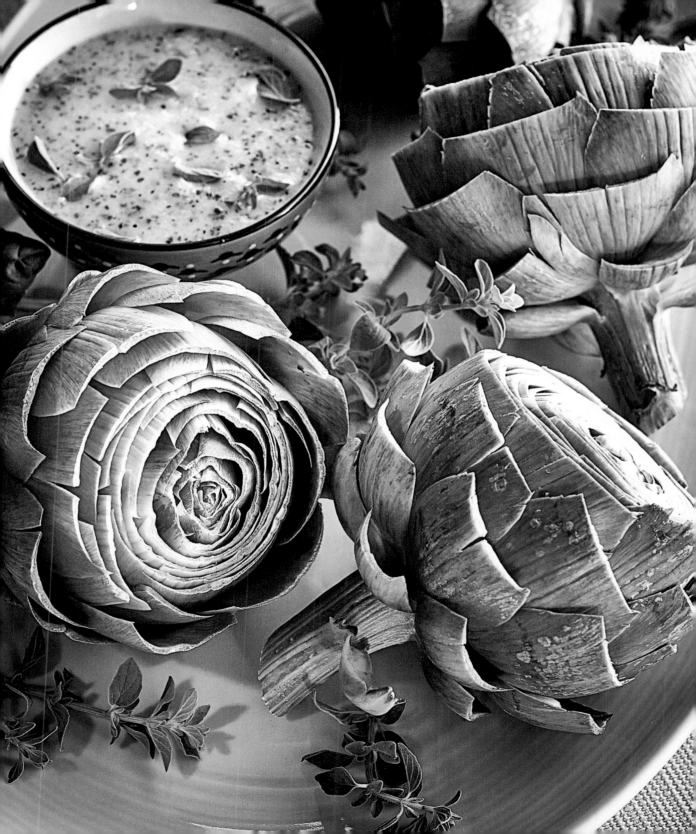

The Green Goddess

Choosing almond butter for this recipe will provide an awesome 95 percent of your daily recommended intake of magnesium, a key detox nutrient. The high potassium helps with the functioning of your adrenal glands, which regulate the balance of sodium and potassium in the blood. Adrenals secrete a hormone called aldosterone, which signals to the kidneys to release potassium in the urine while reabsorbing sodium. High-sodium diets, which are often a result of eating salt that is devoid of potassium, can lead to electrolyte imbalances, as well as hyperstimulation of the adrenal glands.

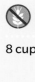 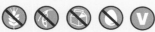

8 cups	baby spinach, chopped Swiss chard or beet greens, including stems *or* 6 cups chopped kale or collards

dressing

½ cup	nut or seed butter
¼ cup	filtered water
2 Tbsp	raw apple cider vinegar or organic lemon juice
1 Tbsp	raw liquid honey or coconut nectar
½ tsp	ground turmeric
½ tsp	pink rock or gray sea salt (omit if using a booster)

optional boosters

1 Tbsp	coconut aminos
1 tsp	umeboshi paste

1. Combine all the dressing ingredients in a small bowl or Mason jar, including the coconut aminos and/or umeboshi if using, and mix well.

2. Place the washed greens in a stainless-steel steamer basket set over boiling water (make sure the water doesn't come up to the bottom of the basket). Cover the pot. Steam for 2 minutes for spinach, 3 minutes for chard or beet greens, and 5 minutes for kale or collards. Transfer the steamed greens to a large bowl and let them cool slightly.

3. Pour half the dressing over the greens, and enjoy while still warm.

Makes 4 servings plus an additional ½ cup dressing. Dressing will keep for up to 1 week in the fridge.

 Rich and creamy almond butter is a delectable way to nourish your adrenals and makes steamed greens come alive!

Roasted Garlic

Garlic has strong antimicrobial properties but can be a bit harsh on the stomach if eaten raw. Roasting garlic makes it sweeter and easier to digest. This recipe is a lovely addition to roast chicken or fish dishes.

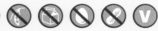

4 heads	garlic
½ tsp	pink rock or gray sea salt
1 Tbsp	toasted sesame oil or coconut oil

1 Preheat the oven to 375°F.

2 Leaving the heads of garlic whole, cut off the tops to expose the cloves. Season with the salt, and drizzle with the sesame or coconut oil.

3 Place the whole heads of garlic in a baking dish and cover with parchment paper. Bake in the oven for 1 hour or until each clove is softened and golden brown.

4 Serve immediately, or let cool and squeeze out each of the garlic cloves from the papery shells and store (see below).

Makes 12 servings. Will keep for up to 3 weeks in the fridge.

Optional: Puree roasted garlic cloves. Store in a Mason jar and refrigerate. Alternatively, fill the compartments of an ice cube tray with pureed garlic and freeze, then transfer frozen cubes to a resealable bag. Will keep in the fridge for 3 weeks; can also be frozen for up to 1 year.

 Garlic is loaded with sulfur, a mineral that helps rid the body of toxins. A deficiency of sulfur reduces the production of glutathione, a key molecule that helps to remove heavy metals from the body.

Heart-Healthy Dipping Sauce

This sauce is so tasty that you can use it to flavor any steamed greens, not just artichokes.

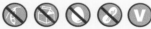

⅓ cup	extra virgin olive oil
1 clove	garlic, minced
2 Tbsp	raw apple cider vinegar
2 Tbsp	organic apple cider
1 tsp	raw liquid honey or coconut nectar
1 tsp	Dijon mustard
1 tsp	dried basil
½ tsp	dried oregano
¼ tsp	pink rock or gray sea salt

Add all the ingredients to a blender, and blend on high speed until emulsified.

Makes ½ cup.

If you find your broth or soup needs a little extra zip, just add a few tablespoons of this sauce or any of the detox salad dressings in the next chapter. It's a flavor bomb!

Hot Detox Flax Wraps

This wrap is perfect as a replacement for sandwich bread. I love it with every filling imaginable. Try sprouts and a pickled vegetable (ideally fermented) with your choice of protein. You may eventually want to double the recipe, especially if you own a larger dehydrator, once you realize you can't live without these!

Flaxseeds are an unparalleled source of lignans, which balance the hormones. They are also an excellent source of omega-3 essential fatty acids and a good source of vitamins and minerals, including selenium, that support detox.

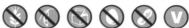

1½ cups	whole flaxseeds (to make 2 cups ground flaxseeds)
1½ cups	filtered water
2 Tbsp	coconut oil
2 Tbsp	organic lemon juice
1 Tbsp	dried parsley or cilantro *or* ¼ cup chopped fresh
1 Tbsp	onion flakes *or* ¼ cup chopped fresh onion
2 tsp	Italian seasoning (basil, oregano, rosemary, sage, savory and thyme)
½ tsp	ground turmeric
¼ tsp	ground ginger
½ tsp	pink rock or gray sea salt
2 cups	grated carrots (use a food processor)

1 Using a clean spice or coffee grinder, grind the flaxseeds. (If you don't have a grinder, use preground seeds.) Transfer ground flaxseeds to a bowl, add the water and mix well. Set aside.

2 In a food processor, combine all of the ingredients except the grated carrots. Add the flax mixture. Process until smooth, occasionally stopping to scrape down the sides of the work bowl. At the end, add the grated carrots and pulse just a few times so the carrots maintain their texture.

3 Preheat the oven to 150°F or dehydrator to 125°F. Line a few baking sheets or dehydrator trays with parchment paper. With moistened hands, spread ½ cup of the mixture as evenly as possible in a circular motion until it's as thin as a tortilla (⅛ of an inch). Repeat with the rest of the mixture. You should end up with 6 wraps.

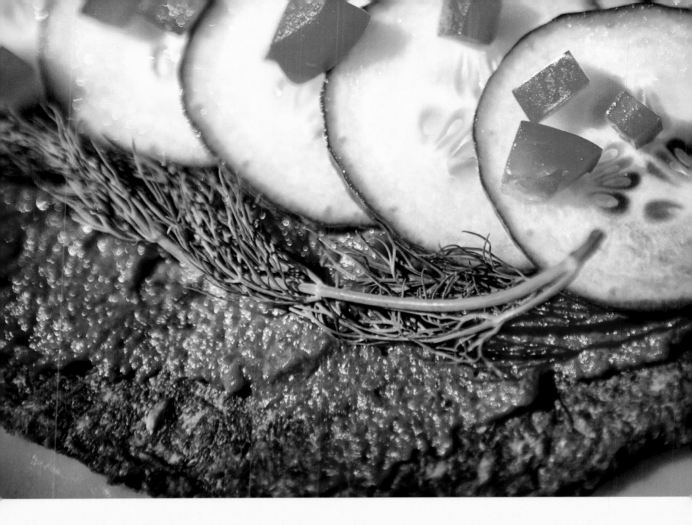

4 Bake in the oven for 5 to 7 hours or dehydrate for 5 to 8 hours, flipping the wraps halfway through to ensure even drying. Avoid doing this overnight. If you go too long without checking, the wraps may lose their pliability and resemble a cracker. There is a big variation in cooking times because every oven is different.

5 Remove from the oven and let the wraps cool for 20 minutes, then place in a resealable bag so they stay moist and soft.

Makes 6 wraps. Will keep for 1 week in a sealed bag in the fridge or up to 4 months in the freezer.

Freshly grind whole flaxseed whenever possible to ensure the highest amount of omega-3 nutrition. Golden flaxseed is prettier than brown flaxseed for this recipe.

Messy Gingered Sweet Potatoes

Are you missing hash browns? These golden jewels made with sweet potatoes are great with eggs for a tasty weekend brunch. The coconut oil will increase the absorption of the beta-carotene, which becomes vitamin A in the liver and protects the lungs, skin and digestive tract. The ginger and cinnamon give a nice tropical twist and warm up the dish beautifully. (See page 161 for photo.)

2 Tbsp	coconut oil
½ cup	finely chopped onions
2 Tbsp	freshly grated ginger
4 cups	grated unpeeled sweet potatoes
2 Tbsp	organic lemon juice
1 tsp	ground cinnamon
¼–½ tsp	pink rock or gray sea salt

1 Place the coconut oil in a large pan over medium heat, and sauté the onions and ginger until soft, about 5 minutes.

2 Add the grated sweet potatoes and lemon juice. Reduce the heat to low and sauté for 10 minutes, stirring constantly, until the sweet potatoes start to soften.

3 Season with the cinnamon and salt to taste. Cook for another 2 to 3 minutes. Remove from the heat and serve warm.

Makes 6 servings.

To add a protein punch to this recipe, add two eggs to the grated sweet potatoes and omit the lemon juice. Recipe will resemble latkes.

Olive Tapenade

This robust dip is superb served with roasted vegetables over an arugula salad. Olives are a good source of vitamin E, iron, copper and fiber. They are also high in monounsaturated fat, which acts as an anti-inflammatory.

2 cups	olives, pitted (kalamata is a great choice)
⅓ cup	extra virgin olive oil
6 cloves	roasted garlic or 2 Tbsp Roasted Garlic Puree (page 223)
½ cup	chopped fresh parsley or cilantro
1 Tbsp	organic lemon zest
2–4 Tbsp	organic lemon juice

1 In a food processor, process the olives, olive oil and garlic until smooth. Add the parsley or cilantro and lemon zest and pulse until well combined.

2 If serving the dip immediately, add 2 tablespoons of lemon juice. If serving the next day, add 4 tablespoons of lemon juice, as lemon juice mellows overnight. Pulse until combined. Transfer to a serving bowl or container.

Makes 2 cups. Will keep for up to 3 weeks in an airtight container in the fridge.

You may be tempted to skip the lemon zest, but not only does it add a ton of extra flavor, it contains important flavonoids that will deepen your detox.

Detox Olive Crackers

If you crave chips, the salty olives in this recipe will be a lifesaver. This cracker is worth the effort, so take the time to make this at least once near the beginning of the cleanse.

¾ cup	whole flaxseeds (to make 1 cup ground) or ⅔ cup whole chia seeds (to make 1 cup ground)
½ cup	filtered water, for soaking the seeds
2 cups	grated carrots (use food processor)
2 cups	grated beets (use food processor)
2 cups	Hemp Hearts and/or raw sunflower seeds
1 cup	tightly packed baby spinach
1 cup	tightly packed fresh parsley or cilantro leaves
1 cup	black olives, pitted
1 cup	chopped red onions
1 clove	garlic, sliced
2 tsp	ground turmeric
1 ½ tsp	pink rock or gray sea salt

optional boosters

1 Tbsp	chopped fresh rosemary or thyme
1 Tbsp	Julie's Curry Powder (page 269)

Save 2 hours of drying time by substituting pulp from the Anti-inflammatory Powerhouse juice (page 130) for the grated carrots and beets.

1 Using a clean spice or coffee grinder, grind the whole flax- or chia seeds. (If you don't have a grinder, use preground seeds.)

2 In a bowl, soak the flax- or chia seeds in the water for 20 minutes.

3 In a food processor, add the soaked flax- or chia seeds, grated beets, Hemp Hearts and/or sunflower seeds, spinach, parsley or cilantro, olives, onions, garlic, turmeric and salt, and desired herbs and/or curry powder if using, and process until well combined. Transfer to a bowl, then fold in the grated carrots.

4 Preheat the oven to 200°F or the dehydrator to 145°F. Line 2 baking sheets with parchment paper. Spread the mixture evenly over the parchment, smoothing it out to a ¼-inch thickness.

5 Bake or dehydrate for 5 hours. Invert the baking sheet onto a cutting board, and remove the parchment from the crackers. Using a pair a scissors, cut and separate into 2-by-2-inch squares. Return the crackers to the baking sheet, and bake or dehydrate for another 2 to 3 hours. If the crackers are still pliable, turn off the oven and leave them in overnight or continue to dehydrate for another hour or two.

Makes 48 crackers.

Probiotic Cashew Cheese

When I first created this recipe, I was so excited that I made it over and over again to share with friends. They all loved the texture and flavor. And they had no idea how easy it was to make! This is a delightful way to ingest the probiotic bacteria you need, in a tasty format. Did you know that a single course of antibiotics can alter the gut microbiome for up to a year? This cheese will help speed recovery and improve your digestion.

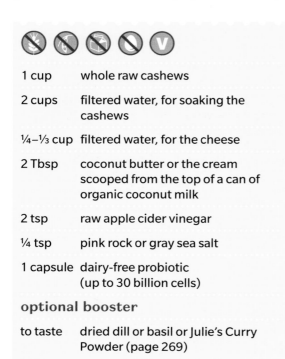

1 cup   whole raw cashews

2 cups   filtered water, for soaking the cashews

¼–⅓ cup   filtered water, for the cheese

2 Tbsp   coconut butter or the cream scooped from the top of a can of organic coconut milk

2 tsp   raw apple cider vinegar

¼ tsp   pink rock or gray sea salt

1 capsule   dairy-free probiotic (up to 30 billion cells)

optional booster

to taste   dried dill or basil or Julie's Curry Powder (page 269)

1 In a bowl, combine the cashews and water and set aside overnight to soak.

2 Rinse the soaked cashews in cold water and drain, then transfer to a blender or food processor. Add ¼ cup water, coconut butter or cream, vinegar and salt, and puree until very smooth. Add some more water if the mixture looks a bit dry.

3 Open the probiotic capsule and add the powder to the cashew puree. Pulse until well combined.

4 Transfer the mixture to a Mason jar (scalded in boiling water or sanitized in the dishwasher). Cover the jar with a thin clean cloth, and secure with a rubber band. Place in a dark, dry spot such as your kitchen cupboard, and let it ferment for 12 hours.

5 If desired, stir in herbs or spices. Enjoy it as a spreadable cheese.

Makes ¾ cup. Will keep for up to 1 week in the fridge.

Want to make a fancy cheese ball for a party? Line a fine-mesh sieve with cheesecloth. Sprinkle your chosen herbs or spices (dill, basil, curry) right onto the cheesecloth, and transfer the cheese mixture from the food processor onto the cloth. Gather up the cloth and tie a knot at the top, making sure the cheese forms a ball. Place in a dark, dry place such as your kitchen cupboard, and let it ferment for 12 hours.

Spiced Sweet Potato Mash

Sweet potatoes are rich in manganese, which facilitates the metabolism, regulates blood sugar levels and promotes the optimal functioning of the thyroid. They are also a good source of potassium, which functions as an energy-boosting electrolyte, reducing the risk of high blood pressure and stroke.

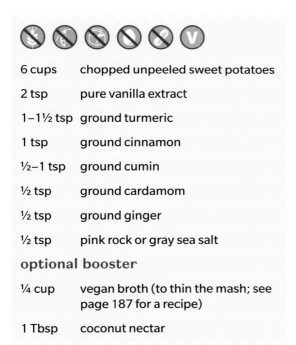

6 cups	chopped unpeeled sweet potatoes
2 tsp	pure vanilla extract
1–1½ tsp	ground turmeric
1 tsp	ground cinnamon
½–1 tsp	ground cumin
½ tsp	ground cardamom
½ tsp	ground ginger
½ tsp	pink rock or gray sea salt

optional booster

¼ cup	vegan broth (to thin the mash; see page 187 for a recipe)
1 Tbsp	coconut nectar

1 Preheat the oven to 375°F. Line a baking sheet with parchment paper.

2 Arrange the sweet potatoes in a single layer on the baking sheet and roast in the oven for about an hour. (Alternatively, boil them in 4 cups of filtered water until tender, about 12 minutes, then drain well.)

3 When the sweet potatoes are tender, transfer to a food processor with the remaining ingredients, and pulse until you reach the desired texture. Alternatively, mash using a potato masher.

4 If the sweet potato mash is too thick, thin with broth to reach desired consistency.

Makes 10 servings. Keeps up to 5 days in the fridge or 6 months in the freezer.

 If time permits, I prefer roasting over boiling for this recipe as it creates a nicer flavor. To make this into a tasty soup, thin with more broth.

Roasted Leeks with Olives and Garlic

Leeks contain the bioactive form of folate called 5-methyltetrahydrofolate (5-MTHF), which is helpful for people who struggle with methylation, a critical detox pathway in the liver that helps eliminate excess estrogen. Olives are rich in the polyphenol phytonutrient hydroxytyrosol, which is being researched for cancer prevention. The spices protect the olive oil from potentially being damaged by being heated, but if you are concerned, substitute coconut oil.

4	medium leeks
¼ cup	extra virgin olive oil or coconut oil, melted
2	large cloves garlic, coarsely chopped
½ tsp	pink rock or gray sea salt
½ cup	kalamata olives, pitted and halved

optional boosters

1 Tbsp	chopped fresh oregano *or* 1 tsp dried
1 cup	finely diced red bell pepper

to serve

1	organic lemon, quartered

1 Preheat the oven to 350°F.

2 Remove the green leaves of the leeks where they begin to fan out and reserve for when you make soup or broth.

Cut the 4 leeks in half so that you have 8 pieces. Halve each piece lengthwise (to make 16 pieces). Rinse well.

3 Using the back of a chef's knife, lightly pound the cut side of the leek to open up the layers.

4 Place the leeks in a roasting pan, cut side up, and coat evenly with oil. Sprinkle with garlic, and the oregano if using, and a generous amount of salt. Bake for 25 to 30 minutes.

5 Sprinkle the baked leeks with the olives and the red pepper if using. Place in oven about 6 inches from the broiler and broil for 5 minutes or until the leeks begin to lightly brown at the edges.

6 Serve hot or at room temperature with wedges of lemon.

Makes 8 servings. Will keep for up to 3 days in the fridge.

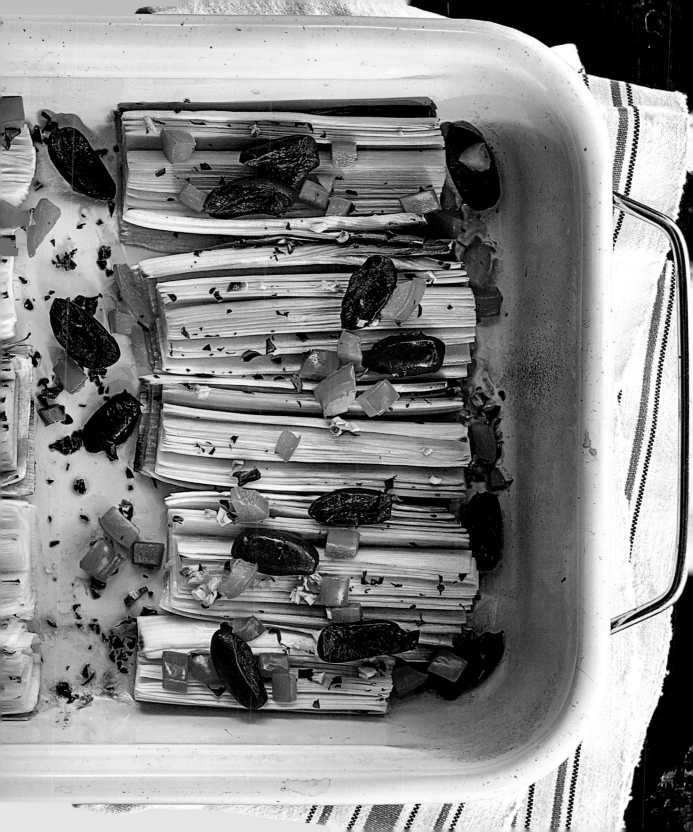

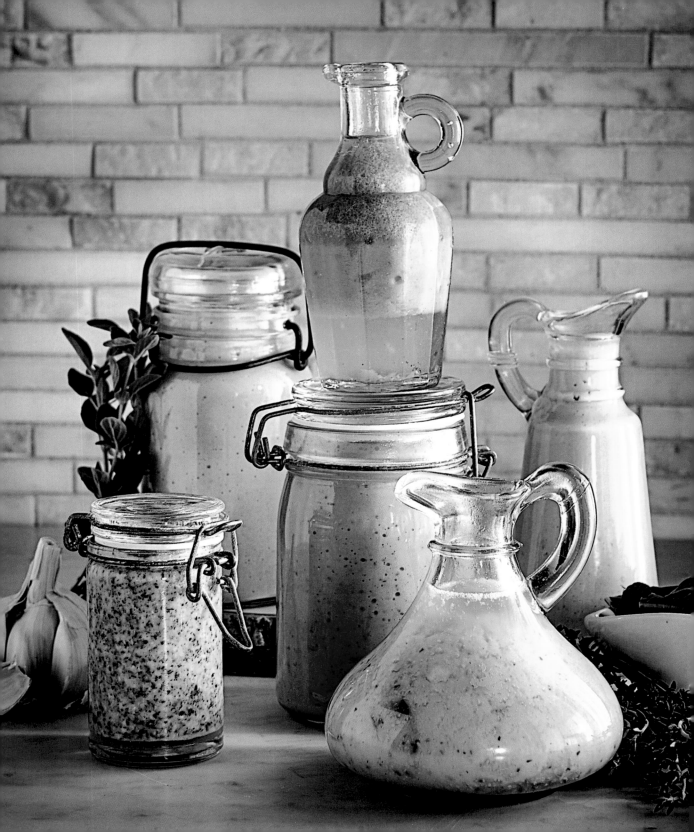

Salads, Dips and Dressings

Asian Salad Bowl

Pumpkin seeds, sesame seeds and turkey or black beans — this salad is packed with protein. Protein helps stabilize blood sugar, which helps prevent adrenal strain. The amino acid tyrosine is especially important for the adrenal glands as it supports the synthesis of adrenaline (aka epinephrine). Most varieties of seaweed provide all the essential minerals your body needs to support enzyme activity, repair tissues and balance hormones.

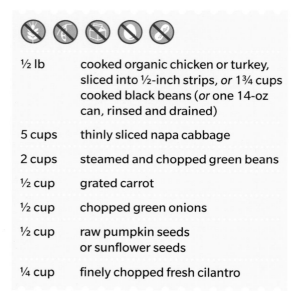

½ lb	cooked organic chicken or turkey, sliced into ½-inch strips, *or* 1¾ cups cooked black beans (*or* one 14-oz can, rinsed and drained)
5 cups	thinly sliced napa cabbage
2 cups	steamed and chopped green beans
½ cup	grated carrot
½ cup	chopped green onions
½ cup	raw pumpkin seeds or sunflower seeds
¼ cup	finely chopped fresh cilantro

dressing

3 Tbsp	raw sesame oil *or* extra virgin olive oil
⅓ cup	dulse flakes
¼ cup	raw apple cider vinegar
3 Tbsp	raw liquid honey or coconut nectar
2 Tbsp	coconut aminos
½ tsp	pink rock or gray sea salt

to serve

2 Tbsp	raw sesame seeds

1 In a bowl, mix together all the salad ingredients.

2 Combine the dressing ingredients in a small bowl or Mason jar. Pour over the salad and toss gently. Sprinkle with sesame seeds and serve.

Makes 4 servings.

Sea vegetables are especially rich in iodine, which is key for supporting thyroid function. With a balanced thyroid, your adrenals function at their best — these glands are connected.

This recipe is cooling, so enjoy if you need a break from hot recipes.

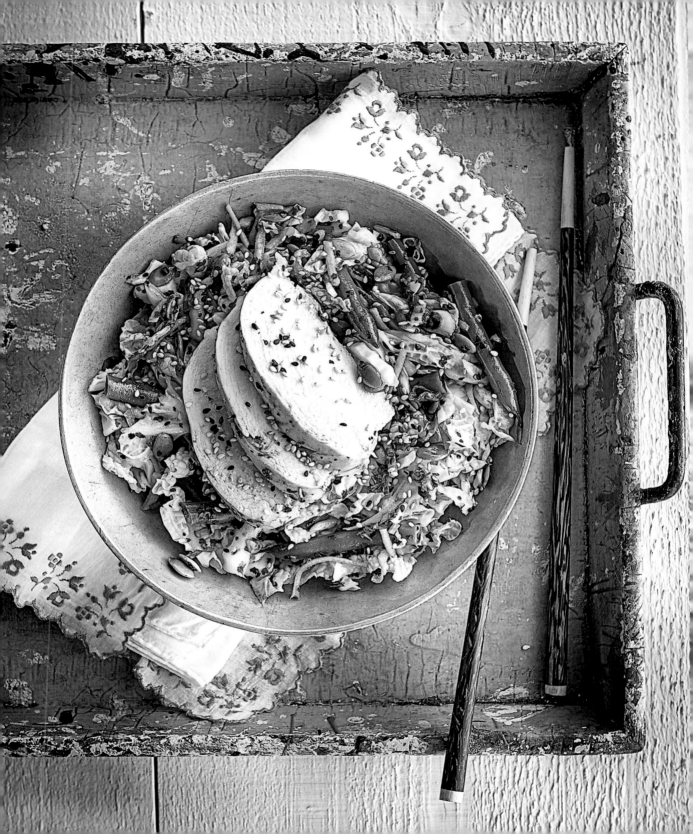

Beet Bop Salad

Beets are one of the best plant sources of betalains, which are potent anti-inflammatory phytochemicals that decrease the risk of heart disease and conditions associated with chronic inflammation. Pea sprouts are high in beta-carotene and vitamin A. Retinol, which is an active form of vitamin A, plays a pivotal role in the development of immune cells, which fight off the foreign invaders that cause inflammation.

   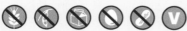

4 cups	grated raw beets
2 cups	pea shoots
2	pears, cored and chopped
½ cup	raw pumpkin seeds
1 Tbsp	poppy seeds

dressing

¼ cup	organic lemon juice
¼ cup	extra virgin olive oil
1 Tbsp	freshly grated ginger
½ tsp	pink rock or gray sea salt

1 In a large bowl, combine all the salad ingredients.

2 In a small bowl, mix together all the dressing ingredients. Pour the dressing over the salad, toss and serve.

Makes 4 servings or 8 side salads. Keep refrigerated and use within 4 days.

 Why so much salad? Because this one tastes better on the second day and makes a perfect snack or side salad.

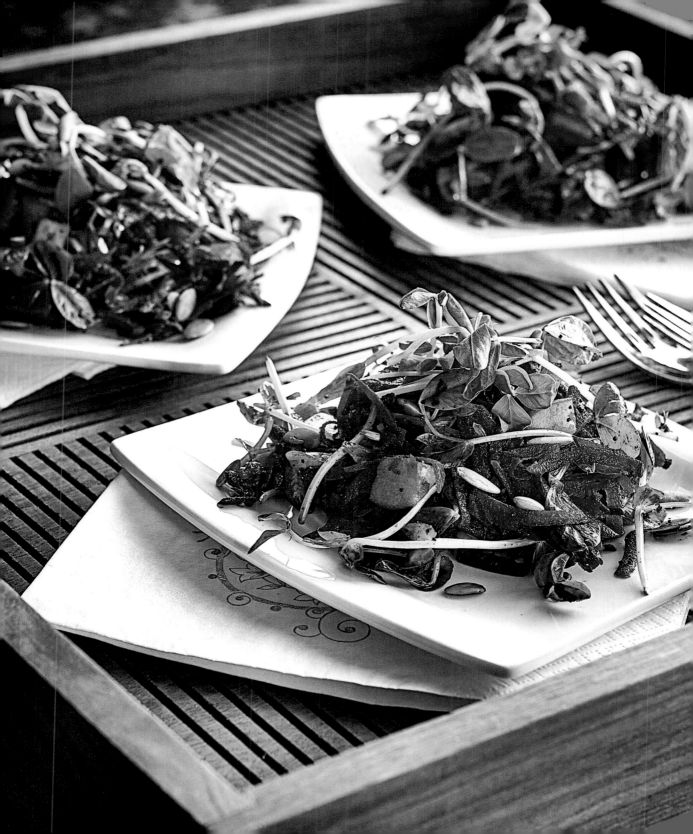

Fennel Ginger Salad

The hazelnuts (and hemp seeds in the mayo, if using) provide a good amount of vitamin E in one meal, which is wonderful for nourishing your adrenal glands. Adrenals are among the organs that store vitamin E, an important nutrient that fights stress. Vitamin E also restores glutathione levels in the liver, which is important for detoxification.

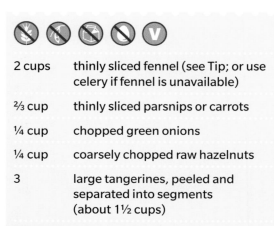

2 cups	thinly sliced fennel (see Tip; or use celery if fennel is unavailable)
⅔ cup	thinly sliced parsnips or carrots
¼ cup	chopped green onions
¼ cup	coarsely chopped raw hazelnuts
3	large tangerines, peeled and separated into segments (about 1½ cups)

dressing

¼ cup	chopped pickled ginger
¼ cup	Hemp Mayo (page 260) or Vegenaise
2 Tbsp	raw apple cider vinegar
½ tsp	pink rock or gray sea salt *or* 1 tsp umeboshi paste

1 Using a mandoline or food processor, slice the fennel and parsnips or carrots, and place in a large bowl.

2 Add the green onions, hazelnuts and tangerine sections. Mix to combine.

3 In a small bowl, whisk together all the dressing ingredients.

4 Pour over the salad. Toss gently, and serve immediately.

Makes 8 servings.

Fennel fronds make a fantastic garnish for this salad, so keep them out of the compost bin!

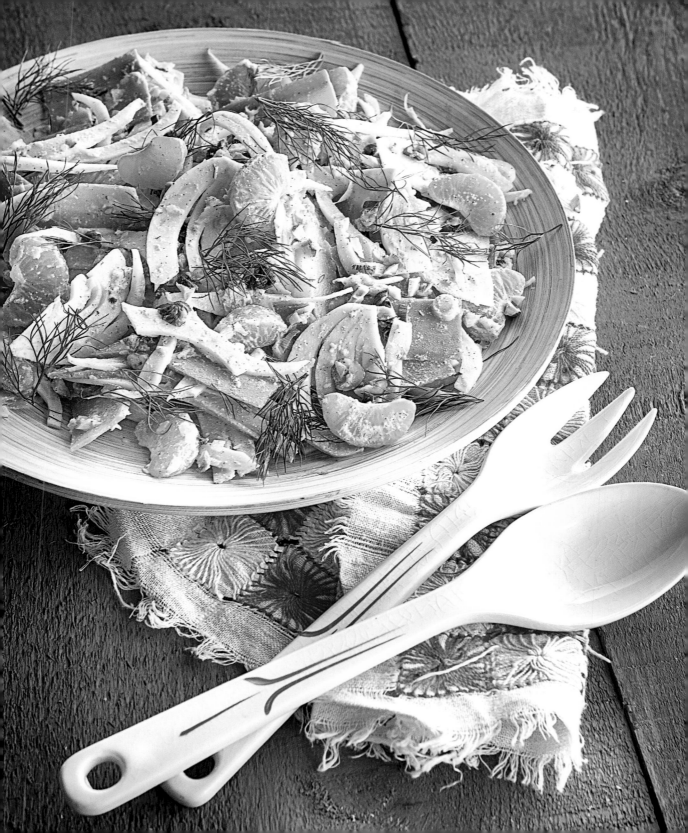

JFC Coleslaw (or Stir-Fry)

This is a great replacement for conventional coleslaw and is sure to be a crowd favorite. The sulfur compounds in cabbage help the liver break down excess hormones and neutralize the effects of damaging toxic compounds (found in household cleaners and cigarette smoke — secondhand too) and endocrine disruptors.

  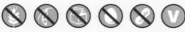

6 cups	shredded purple cabbage
2 cups	grated carrots
½ cup	Hemp Hearts or raw sunflower seeds
½ tsp	pink rock or gray sea salt

optional boosters

½ cup	finely chopped green onions
½ cup	dried currants *or* 2 Tbsp raw liquid honey
1 tsp	ground cinnamon
½ tsp	ground turmeric

dressing

½ cup	Hemp Mayo (page 260) *or* Sunny Anti-inflammatory Dressing (page 261)
3 Tbsp	extra virgin olive oil
3 Tbsp	raw apple cider vinegar

1 In a large bowl, combine the cabbage, carrots, Hemp Hearts or sunflower seeds, and salt, as well as any of the optional boosters.

2 In a small bowl, whisk together the dressing ingredients. Add the dressing to the salad, and toss until evenly coated.

3 If you want to make a stir-fry, omit the honey and the Hemp Mayo or Anti-inflammatory Dressing, and halve the cinnamon, if using. Sauté the dressed salad on medium heat for 5 to 7 minutes, stirring occasionally.

Makes 9 cups of coleslaw or 5 cups of stir-fry. Coleslaw keeps up to 5 days in the fridge; stir-fry keeps up to 3 days.

 Consider the stir-fry option if you have irritable bowel syndrome or inflammatory bowel disease (IBS/IBD) or an underactive thyroid and are intolerant of raw vegetables.

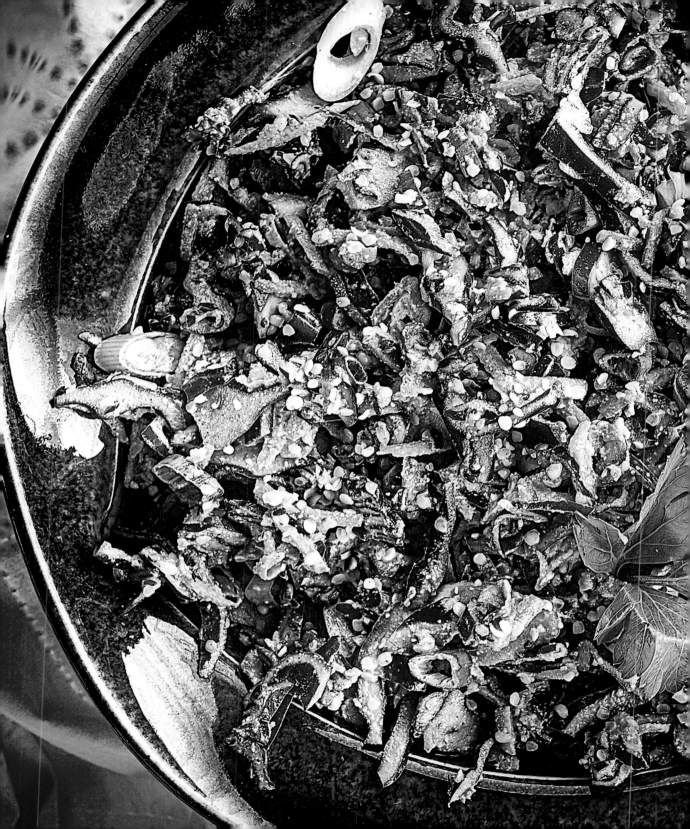

Pressed Radish Salad

I used to hate radishes until I discovered that they are only as good as the farmer who grows them! Commercial radishes can be woody in the center, but buy them fresh and they are incredibly sweet and juicy with just a touch of spice, as refreshing and crunchy as spicy apple.

Radishes contain a special compound — called phospholipid hydroperoxide glutathione peroxidase (PHGPx) — that acts as an antioxidant in the Phase 2 liver detoxification pathway. This pathway disarms harmful chemicals such as pain relievers, nicotine, insecticides and other cancer-causing substances. Between the detoxifying benefits and their great taste, fresh organic radishes are a must-try if you think you don't like them.

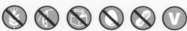

2 cups	thinly sliced red radishes
½ cup	thinly sliced apple

dressing

¼ cup	raw apple cider vinegar
1 Tbsp	coconut aminos
2 tsp	toasted sesame oil

to serve

¼ cup	chopped fresh basil
1 Tbsp	gomashio or pink rock or gray sea salt, to taste

1 In a large bowl, combine the radishes and apples. In another bowl, whisk together the dressing ingredients. Pour the dressing over the apple and radishes and toss well.

2 Place another bowl on top of the mixture and weigh it down with a jug of water or other heavy object to help squeeze out the juices.

3 Let it sit for 25 minutes. Holding the bowls together, drain off the liquid (there should be ¼ to ⅓ cup).

4 Serve the salad topped with the basil and gomashio or salt. You can also serve this on top of baby spinach — for each serving of 2 cups spinach, use ½ cup of this salad.

Makes 4 servings.

 By pressing veggies with some vinegar and salt (or in this case, coconut aminos), you're making a fresh pickle. The process has a similar effect to cooking, by making vegetables more digestible, yet preserves the active enzymes in the plants.

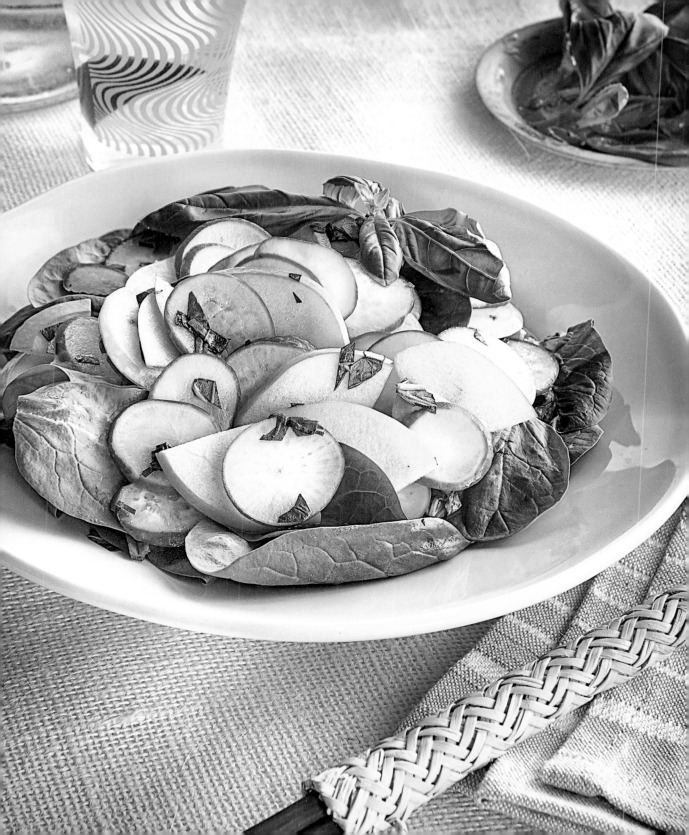

Roasted Squash and Dried Cherry Salad

Prepare to fall in love with arugula! Arugula tastes peppery and contains the bioactive compounds indole-3-carbinol and isothiocyanates, which detox the liver and suppress inflammation. Squash makes this sweet salad cleansing to the digestive system.

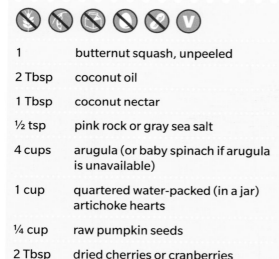

1	butternut squash, unpeeled
2 Tbsp	coconut oil
1 Tbsp	coconut nectar
½ tsp	pink rock or gray sea salt
4 cups	arugula (or baby spinach if arugula is unavailable)
1 cup	quartered water-packed (in a jar) artichoke hearts
¼ cup	raw pumpkin seeds
2 Tbsp	dried cherries or cranberries (sweetened with apple juice)

dressing

¾ cup	organic apple cider
2 Tbsp	raw apple cider vinegar
2 cloves	garlic, minced
2 tsp	Dijon mustard
¼ tsp	ground turmeric
3 Tbsp	extra virgin olive oil

1 Position racks in the upper and lower thirds of the oven. Preheat to 350°F. Line 2 large baking sheets with parchment paper.

2 Cut the squash in half, and discard the seeds and stringy matter. Cut into ½-inch-thick slices. In a bowl, toss together squash, coconut oil, coconut nectar and salt until well coated. Spread out evenly on the baking sheets, and roast until just tender and edges are starting to brown, about 40 minutes.

3 For the dressing, combine the apple cider, vinegar and garlic in a small saucepan and bring to a boil. Continue boiling until the mixture is reduced to ¼ cup, about 10 minutes. Remove the pan from the heat, and whisk in the Dijon, turmeric and olive oil.

4 Divide the arugula evenly among serving plates. Top with the warm squash. Drizzle with the dressing, and top with artichokes, pumpkin seeds and dried cherries or cranberries.

Makes 4 servings, with extra roasted squash (which will keep in the fridge for up to 3 days).

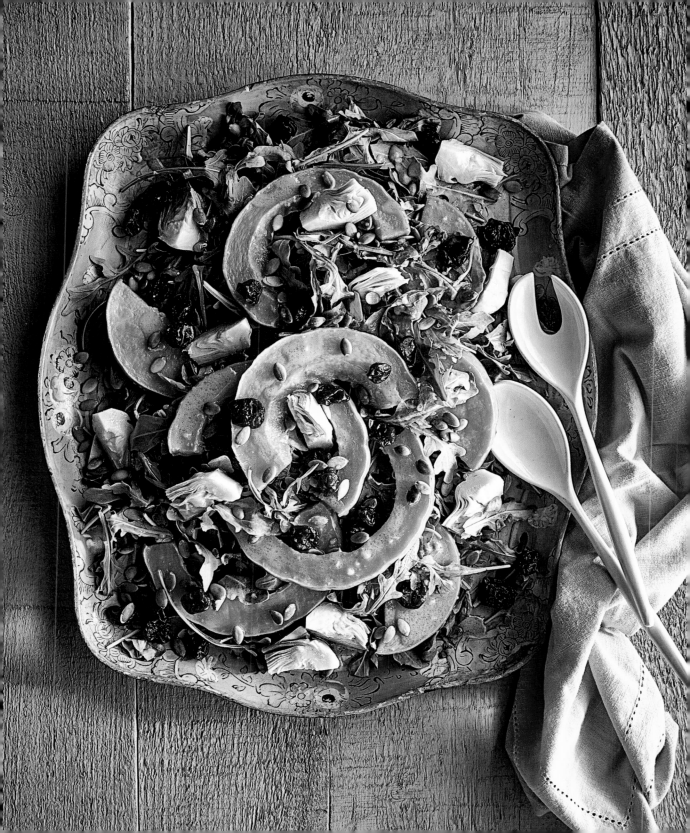

Salmon Niçoise Salad

The artichokes, green beans and spinach all provide vitamin B to help your liver detox pathways. The salmon and eggs provide omega-3 fats, which are required for many functions in the body including detoxification.

3 or 4	large organic eggs
1 cup	green beans
1 Tbsp	coconut oil
2 fillets	salmon, without skin (about ½ lb each)
¼ tsp	pink rock or gray sea salt
1 Tbsp	Italian seasoning (basil, oregano, rosemary and thyme)
4	water-packed (in a jar) artichoke hearts
¼ cup	thinly sliced red onion or chopped green onions
6 cups	baby spinach or other greens
½ cup	kalamata or green olives, pitted
½ cup	sliced radishes
1 cup	fresh sprouts

dressing

¼ cup	extra virgin olive oil
2 Tbsp	organic lemon juice
1 Tbsp	Dijon mustard
¼ tsp	pink rock or gray sea salt

1 Carefully place the eggs into a pot of boiling filtered water and boil for 10 minutes, then remove the eggs and let them cool.

2 Have ready a bowl of ice water. Add the green beans to a fresh pot of boiling filtered water. Cover and cook, stirring occasionally, until tender, 4 to 6 minutes. Using a slotted spoon, transfer the cooked beans to the ice water to stop the cooking. Rinse under cool water, drain and set aside.

3 In a deep skillet, warm the coconut oil over medium heat. Season the salmon on both sides with the salt and Italian seasoning. Cook the salmon in the skillet for 3 minutes per side. Transfer to a plate, and let cool. Slice each fillet in half, lengthwise, using a sharp knife.

4 Quarter the artichokes, and peel and quarter the boiled eggs.

5 In a small bowl, whisk together all of the dressing ingredients.

6 On a large platter or 4 serving plates, arrange the spinach, salmon, green beans, eggs, artichokes, onions, radishes and olives. Serve with the dressing and sprouts on the side.

Makes 4 servings.

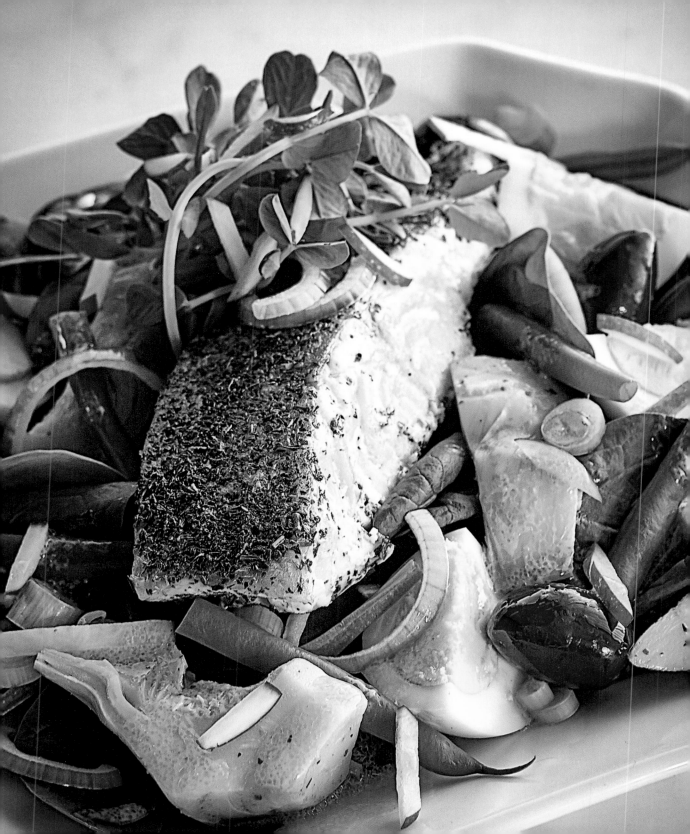

Sweet Potato and Asparagus Salad

Sweet potatoes are rich in beta-carotene, which is a natural anti-inflammatory nutrient your body loves! Asparagus is high in the B vitamin thiamine, a fundamental component of proper brain and liver function.

3 cups	chopped unpeeled sweet potatoes, in 1-inch cubes
½ tsp	pink rock or gray sea salt, for cooking the sweet potatoes, more for seasoning salad
2 cups	fresh asparagus, ends trimmed, cut into 3-inch pieces
2 Tbsp	extra virgin olive oil
1 cup	thinly sliced onions
½ tsp	ground turmeric
½ tsp	mustard seeds
½ tsp	cumin seeds
1 Tbsp	garam masala or Julie's Curry Powder (page 269)
3 Tbsp	fresh cilantro leaves
1 to 2 Tbsp organic lemon juice	

to serve

1 Tbsp	organic lemon zest

1 Fill a pot with cold filtered water, add the salt and bring to a boil. Reduce the heat to medium-high and cook the potatoes for 10 minutes or until just barely tender.

2 Add the asparagus, and blanch for 1 minute. Strain the vegetables, rinse with cold water and spread out to dry on a clean kitchen towel.

3 In a large skillet, sauté the onions in the oil for 3 minutes or until transparent.

4 Add the turmeric, mustard seeds, cumin and garam masala or curry powder. Cook until fragrant, then add the sweet potatoes and the asparagus and gently toss until evenly coated.

5 Cook for 2 minutes to heat through, then stir in the cilantro and lemon juice. Season well with sea salt and garnish with lemon zest.

Makes 4 servings.

Asparagus contains two classes of antioxidants called phenolics and flavonoids. These powerful antioxidants have the ability to scavenge free radicals in the body.

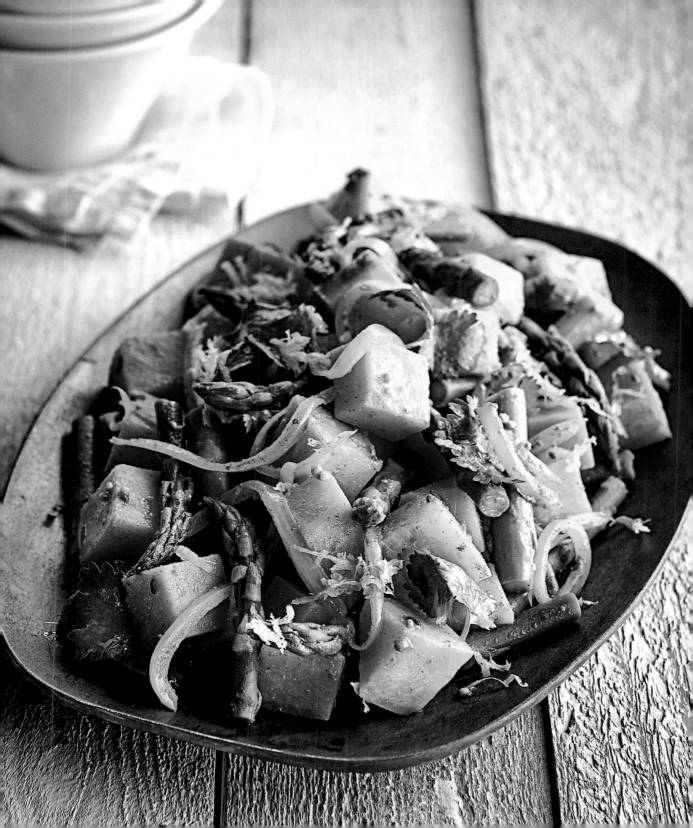

Quick Lentil Salad

Have you ever wanted to nourish yourself fast, but the idea of cooking from scratch is just daunting? Every once in a while, my husband, Alan, and I make a meal from canned goods, usually when we're traveling and the only other option is fast food. It's always best to use fresh ingredients of course, but this is one of our favorite dishes when we're in a pinch.

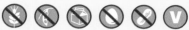

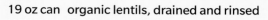

In a large bowl, combine all the ingredients, including any or all of the boosters, and mix well. Serve on steamed greens.

Makes 4 cups. Will keep for up to 3 days in the fridge.

19 oz can	organic lentils, drained and rinsed
14 oz can	black olives, drained and quartered
14 oz jar	water-packed artichoke hearts, drained and quartered
10 oz can	sliced organic mushrooms, drained
¼ cup	Hemp Hearts
2 Tbsp	dairy- and nut-free basil pesto (such as Instant Pesto, page 257)
2–4 Tbsp	organic lemon juice

optional boosters

1 Tbsp	Italian seasoning (basil, oregano, rosemary, sage, savory and thyme) *or* 3 Tbsp fresh herbs of choice
1 Tbsp	minced fresh ginger
1 clove	garlic, minced

 Use cans that aren't lined with BPA. If you want to cook the lentils from scratch, check out my first book, *Meals That Heal Inflammation*.

If you're eating this salad after it's been stored in the fridge, refresh it with some more lemon juice.

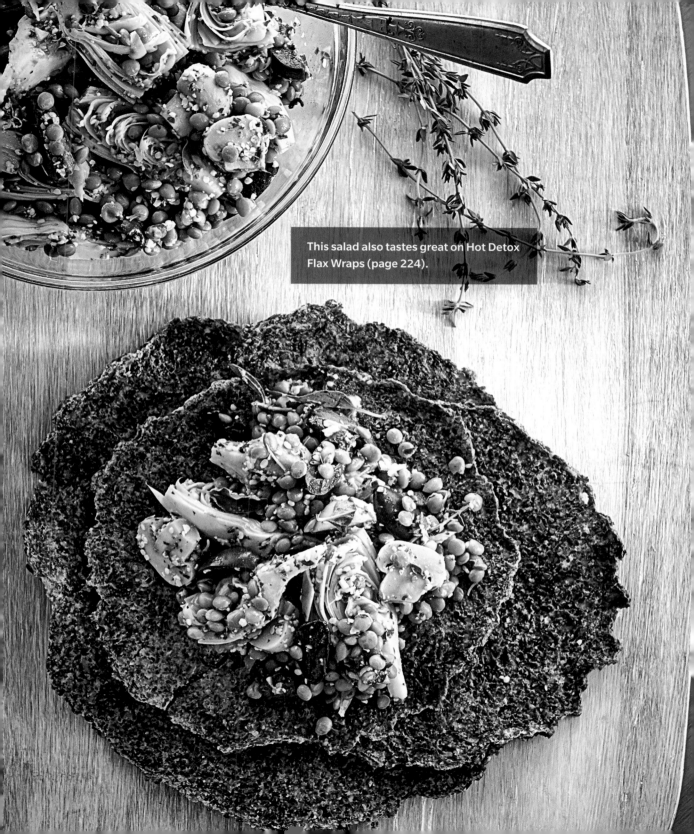

This salad also tastes great on Hot Detox Flax Wraps (page 224).

Artichoke Skordalia

Skordalia is a lemony dip from Greece that I find truly addictive. Normally made with insulin-spiking potato, this artichoke version will cleanse your liver while making accompanying food taste sweeter. Artichokes can relieve the pain and discomfort associated with indigestion, acid reflux, bloating and mild diarrhea or constipation.

3 cups	water-packed artichoke hearts (in a jar), drained well
½ cup	raw cashews
3 Tbsp	organic lemon juice
2 Tbsp	Hemp Hearts (or extra cashews)
1–2 cloves	garlic, minced
½ tsp	pink rock or gray sea salt
⅓ cup	extra virgin olive oil, more for garnish
½ cup	fresh parsley leaves
to serve	
½ tsp	dried oregano

1 In a food processor, process the artichokes, cashews, lemon juice, Hemp Hearts, garlic and salt. With the motor running, slowly add the olive oil and parsley, and process until smooth.

2 Transfer to a serving bowl. Garnish with a drizzle of olive oil and oregano.

Makes 2 cups. Will keep for up to 1 week in the fridge.

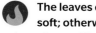 **The leaves of the artichokes should be very soft; otherwise, the dip may be slightly stringy. Save stiff artichoke leaves for stir-fries.**

Beet Cashew Dip

This dip is much easier to digest than hummus and will crush cravings quickly. The beets are incredibly energizing, so make sure to include this bright red dip for lunches and snacks when you need an extra boost.

1 cup	raw cashews
1 cup	raw sunflower seeds
2 cups	filtered water, for soaking the nuts and seeds
2 cups	cooked sliced beets
½ cup	organic lemon juice
½ cup	extra virgin olive oil
¼ cup	filtered water
2 Tbsp	organic balsamic vinegar
1 tsp	raw liquid honey
2 ½ tsp	pink rock or gray sea salt

1 Soak the cashews and sunflower seeds in 2 cups of water for 4 hours. Drain and rinse well.

2 Combine all ingredients in a food processor and process until smooth.

Makes 5 cups. Will keep for up to 1 week in the fridge.

Broccoli Wasabi Dip

Broccoli has a powerful impact on our body's detoxification system. The nutrients glucoraphanin, gluconasturtiin and glucobrassicin are a dynamic trio that neutralize and eliminate unwanted contaminants. The powerful antioxidant isothiocyanate in wasabi can increase detoxification and reduce inflammation.

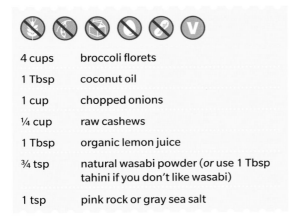

4 cups	broccoli florets
1 Tbsp	coconut oil
1 cup	chopped onions
¼ cup	raw cashews
1 Tbsp	organic lemon juice
¾ tsp	natural wasabi powder (or use 1 Tbsp tahini if you don't like wasabi)
1 tsp	pink rock or gray sea salt

1   Cook the broccoli in boiling, salted, filtered water until tender. Drain and then refresh under cold running water. Drain well.

2   In a small skillet over low heat, cook the onions in the coconut oil until soft.

3   Transfer to a food processor. Add the broccoli and cashews, and process until smooth.

4   Add the lemon juice, wasabi and salt. Process until well combined, and adjust seasoning to taste. Cover and refrigerate until ready to serve (see Tip).

Makes 2½ cups. Will keep for up to 1 week in the fridge.

 Make this dip an hour or two in advance so that the flavors have time to meld.

Onion Lentil Dip

Lentils provide protein and iron, making this dip great for vegetarians, who often struggle to get enough of these bodybuilding nutrients. Onions are packed with allicin, potassium, fiber and quercetin, which helps the liver expel toxins.

1 cup	dried lentils, rinsed well, or a 19-oz can
3 cups	filtered water
2 cups	chopped onions
2 Tbsp	coconut oil
⅓ cup	extra virgin olive oil
½ cup	raw sunflower seeds (soaked for 1 to 2 hours) or Hemp Hearts
3 Tbsp	raw apple cider vinegar
1–2 cloves	garlic (depending on how you like it)
1 ½ tsp	Julie's Curry Powder (page 269)
½ tsp	pink rock or gray sea salt

1   If starting with dried lentils, place them in a small pot with the water. Bring to a boil, then reduce the heat and simmer for 45 minutes. Drain well.

2   In a skillet over medium heat, cook the onions in the coconut oil for 5 minutes or until soft and translucent.

3   Transfer the onions and the cooked or canned lentils to a food processor, along with the rest of the ingredients. Process for 5 to 7 minutes until extra creamy.

4   Serve immediately, or transfer to a Mason jar for storing.

Makes 3 cups. Will keep for up to 4 days in the fridge.

Sunny Sunflower Pâté

Vitamin E, the fat-soluble antioxidant, is essential for the health of your cardiovascular and nervous systems, so make sure to follow the recommended intake of 15 milligrams (22 IU) each day. The sunflower seeds, hemp seeds and extra virgin olive oil in this dish will satisfy your adrenals' hunger for this vitamin.

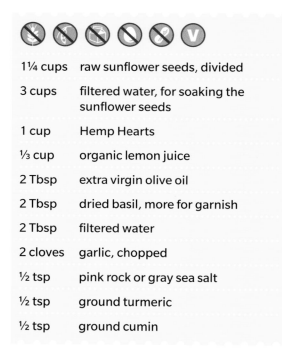

1¼ cups	raw sunflower seeds, divided
3 cups	filtered water, for soaking the sunflower seeds
1 cup	Hemp Hearts
⅓ cup	organic lemon juice
2 Tbsp	extra virgin olive oil
2 Tbsp	dried basil, more for garnish
2 Tbsp	filtered water
2 cloves	garlic, chopped
½ tsp	pink rock or gray sea salt
½ tsp	ground turmeric
½ tsp	ground cumin

1 Soak 1 cup of the sunflower seeds in 3 cups of water for 1 hour. Drain.

2 Place all the ingredients except the remaining ¼ cup of unsoaked sunflower seeds in a food processor, and process until pastelike, stopping occasionally to scrape the sides of the bowl, about 1 minute.

3 Line a small glass container with parchment paper. Spread the ¼ cup of unsoaked sunflower seeds in an even layer on the bottom.

4 Transfer the pâté to the container, pressing it down and smoothing it out with a spatula. Refrigerate for 30 minutes to set.

5 Invert onto a serving plate, and sprinkle extra dried basil on the sides if desired.

Makes 2 cups. Will keep for up to 1 week in the fridge.

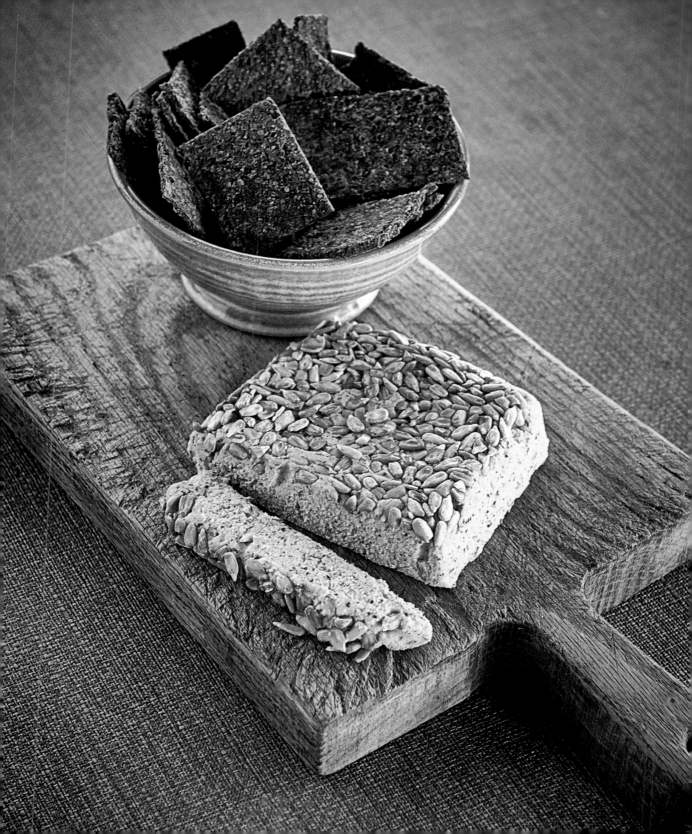

Super Guac

I've taken many trips to Cozumel, Mexico, to scuba dive in the spectacular coral reefs, and one of my favorite post-dive foods is guacamole. Avocados contain high levels of monounsaturated fats, phytosterols and antioxidants like vitamin E, vitamin C and epigallocatechin gallate (EGCG). EGCG is a polyphenol that helps with detoxification and reduces inflammation.

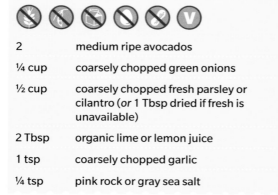

2	medium ripe avocados
¼ cup	coarsely chopped green onions
½ cup	coarsely chopped fresh parsley or cilantro (*or* 1 Tbsp dried if fresh is unavailable)
2 Tbsp	organic lime or lemon juice
1 tsp	coarsely chopped garlic
¼ tsp	pink rock or gray sea salt

Mash the avocados in a small bowl, then add the remaining ingredients and mix well.

Makes 2 cups. Will keep for up to 3 days in the fridge if well sealed.

 With just six ingredients, this recipe can be easily whipped together — perfect for a quick snack!

French White Bean Dip with Mint

Beans are a delicious source of folic acid, a key nutrient in the liver detox pathway. Rosemary and mint stimulate blood circulation and consequently the delivery of oxygen to the brain.

2 cups	white beans, cooked, *or* a 19-oz can, rinsed and drained
¼ cup	extra virgin olive oil
3 Tbsp	organic lemon juice
2 Tbsp	nut or seed butter
2 Tbsp	chopped fresh mint or basil
¼ tsp	pink rock or gray sea salt

optional boosters

½ tsp	Hawaiian spirulina powder
1 tsp	maca powder

to serve

1 Tbsp	finely chopped fresh parsley

1 In a food processor or blender, combine all the dip ingredients, including the spirulina and/or maca if using. Puree until smooth.

2 Transfer to in a serving dish, and garnish with the parsley.

3 If serving dip that's been stored in the fridge, bring to room temperature and check the seasoning before serving.

Makes 2½ cups. Will keep for up to 3 days in the fridge.

This dip is so richly flavored that you can easily slip in a dose of adrenal-boosting maca root or spirulina without affecting the taste.

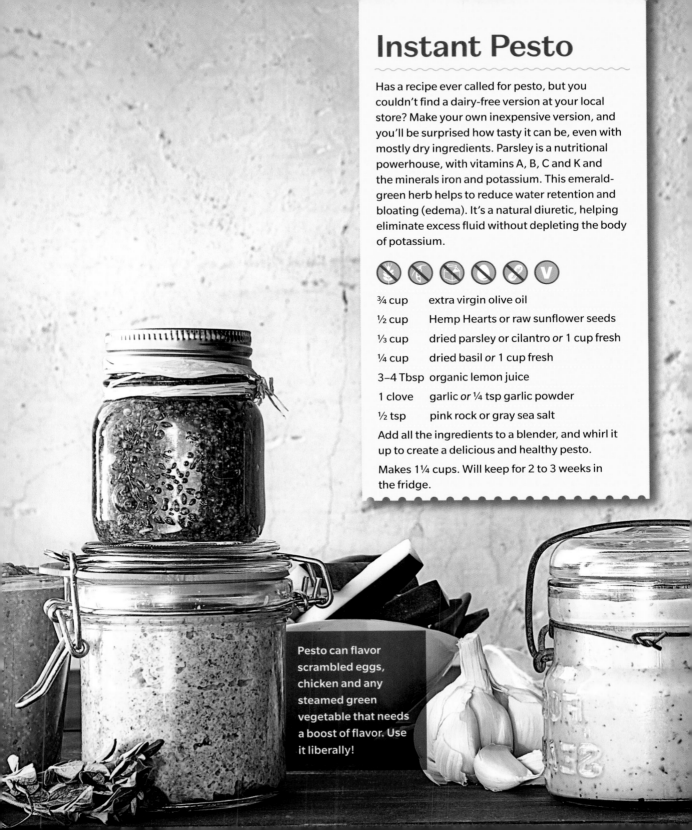

Instant Pesto

Has a recipe ever called for pesto, but you couldn't find a dairy-free version at your local store? Make your own inexpensive version, and you'll be surprised how tasty it can be, even with mostly dry ingredients. Parsley is a nutritional powerhouse, with vitamins A, B, C and K and the minerals iron and potassium. This emerald-green herb helps to reduce water retention and bloating (edema). It's a natural diuretic, helping eliminate excess fluid without depleting the body of potassium.

⊘	⊘	⊘	⊘	⊘	V

¾ cup	extra virgin olive oil
½ cup	Hemp Hearts or raw sunflower seeds
⅓ cup	dried parsley or cilantro *or* 1 cup fresh
¼ cup	dried basil *or* 1 cup fresh
3–4 Tbsp	organic lemon juice
1 clove	garlic *or* ¼ tsp garlic powder
½ tsp	pink rock or gray sea salt

Add all the ingredients to a blender, and whirl it up to create a delicious and healthy pesto.

Makes 1¼ cups. Will keep for 2 to 3 weeks in the fridge.

Pesto can flavor scrambled eggs, chicken and any steamed green vegetable that needs a boost of flavor. Use it liberally!

Chimichurri Sauce

This sauce is superversatile! It can be used as a salad dressing or veggie dip, or as a great sauce for fish or chicken. The spices are powerfully anti-inflammatory, and the high amount of sulfur in the garlic supports your liver detox enzymes, including glutathione.

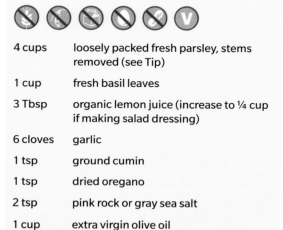

4 cups	loosely packed fresh parsley, stems removed (see Tip)
1 cup	fresh basil leaves
3 Tbsp	organic lemon juice (increase to ¼ cup if making salad dressing)
6 cloves	garlic
1 tsp	ground cumin
1 tsp	dried oregano
2 tsp	pink rock or gray sea salt
1 cup	extra virgin olive oil

1 Place all the ingredients except the olive oil in a food processor. Pulse 5 or 6 times or until roughly chopped.

2 With the motor running, slowly drizzle in the olive oil, stopping occasionally to scrape down the sides of the work bowl. Process until it reaches a saucy consistency.

3 Transfer to a Mason jar for storage.

Makes 2 cups. Will keep for up to 2 weeks in the fridge.

Wash the parsley by soaking it in a bowl of water, allowing the dirt to sink to the bottom. Just rinsing it under running water may mean some grit gets in your sauce.

Tomato-Free Ketchup or Faux Tomato Soup

I was thrilled to create this nightshade-free ketchup recipe. The alkaloids in nightshades (such as tomato, potato, peppers and eggplant) can inhibit the enzyme cholinesterase, the catalyst of the neurotransmitter acetylcholine. The enzyme is critical for relieving muscle spasms, aches and pains, and for preventing inflammation. If you suffer from chronic pain, you should definitely test your sensitivity to nightshades.

4	large unpeeled carrots
3	large unpeeled parsnips
3	medium unpeeled beets
½ cup	extra virgin olive oil
3 tsp	pink rock or gray sea salt
2 tsp	onion flakes
6 Tbsp	organic balsamic vinegar
2 Tbsp	organic lemon juice

1 Cut the carrots, parsnips and beets into cubes, and place in a large pot of water. Bring to a boil, reduce the heat and simmer for 20 to 30 minutes or until soft. Drain.

2 Place all the ingredients in a blender, and puree until smooth. Transfer to Mason jars. Let cool, cover and refrigerate.

Makes 6 cups. Keeps for 6 weeks in the fridge.

To make ketchup into **Faux Tomato Soup**, thin half of the full recipe with 2 cups of unsweetened coconut beverage (page 127 or store-bought).

Caesar Dressing

This is a dreamy dressing that you can toss on any steamed greens. The celery works as a thickener and also provides cellulose — a digestive cleanser.

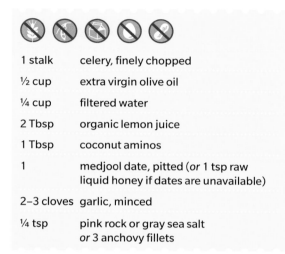

1 stalk	celery, finely chopped
½ cup	extra virgin olive oil
¼ cup	filtered water
2 Tbsp	organic lemon juice
1 Tbsp	coconut aminos
1	medjool date, pitted (*or* 1 tsp raw liquid honey if dates are unavailable)
2–3 cloves	garlic, minced
¼ tsp	pink rock or gray sea salt *or* 3 anchovy fillets

In a blender, combine all of the ingredients and blend on high speed until smooth.

Makes ¾ cup. Will keep for up to 1 week in the fridge.

 This dressing makes enough for 2 to 3 servings of steamed greens.

Detox Dressing

One of nature's perfect foods, hemp seeds contain a good balance of omega-3, -6 and -9 fats. The warming and detoxifying combo of turmeric, ginger and garlic will add a powerful kick to any meal.

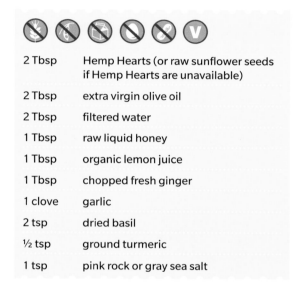

2 Tbsp	Hemp Hearts (or raw sunflower seeds if Hemp Hearts are unavailable)
2 Tbsp	extra virgin olive oil
2 Tbsp	filtered water
1 Tbsp	raw liquid honey
1 Tbsp	organic lemon juice
1 Tbsp	chopped fresh ginger
1 clove	garlic
2 tsp	dried basil
½ tsp	ground turmeric
1 tsp	pink rock or gray sea salt

In a blender, combine all of the ingredients and blend on high speed until smooth.

Makes ½ cup. Will keep for up to 1 week in the fridge.

 For more great dressing recipes, visit www.juliedaniluk.com.

Hemp Mayo

My sister, Lynn, invented this brilliant recipe to help our family avoid the sugar and processed oil found in conventional mayonnaise. I've never come across a dressing with as much protein, and it tastes just like an egg-based mayo. Hemp seeds contain more chlorophyll than any other seed, which can help purify the blood.

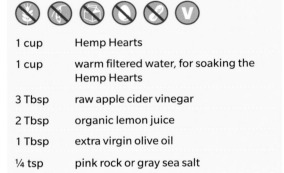

1 cup	Hemp Hearts
1 cup	warm filtered water, for soaking the Hemp Hearts
3 Tbsp	raw apple cider vinegar
2 Tbsp	organic lemon juice
1 Tbsp	extra virgin olive oil
¼ tsp	pink rock or gray sea salt

1 Soak the Hemp Hearts in the water for 1 hour.

2 Transfer the Hemp Hearts to a fine-mesh sieve, and firmly press with the back of a spoon to drain well.

3 In a blender (preferably a high-powered one; see Tip), combine the drained Hemp Hearts and the remaining ingredients. Blend on high speed until smooth and creamy. Transfer to a Mason jar and refrigerate immediately. It will thicken as it cools.

Makes 2½ cups. Will keep for 3 days in the fridge.

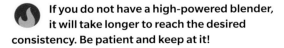

If you do not have a high-powered blender, it will take longer to reach the desired consistency. Be patient and keep at it!

If you won't use up the mayo within 3 days, cut the recipe in half.

Open Sesame Dressing

The lemon juice in this tasty dressing contains both vitamin C and flavonoids that help to reduce toxins and mucus. Carrots lower blood pressure, protect your liver and kidneys, and reduce cholesterol and your risk of cardiovascular disease and diabetes.

½ cup	organic lemon juice
1 cup	finely chopped carrots and/or radishes
½ cup	roughly chopped red onion or shallots
½ cup	raw sesame seeds
¼ cup	extra virgin olive oil
¼ cup	filtered water
2 Tbsp	coconut aminos
1–2 cloves	garlic
½ tsp	pink rock or gray sea salt

In a blender, combine all of the ingredients and blend on high speed until smooth.

Makes 2 cups. Will keep for up to 1 week in the fridge.

 Replace half of the olive oil (2 tablespoons) with sesame oil for a stronger sesame flavor.

Sunny Anti-inflammatory Dressing

I think this dressing is the bee's knees. Its creamy texture and warming spices will wrap your tummy in TLC. Tahini (aka sesame paste) contains a compound called sesamin, which prevents omega-6 fats from becoming inflammatory.

½ cup	tahini
2 Tbsp	organic lemon juice
2 Tbsp	coconut aminos (*or* ½ tsp unrefined sea salt if aminos is unavailable)
2 tsp	ground turmeric
1 tsp	freshly grated ginger *or* ½ teaspoon ground ginger
⅔ cup	filtered water

optional booster

1 tsp	raw liquid honey

In a blender, combine all of the ingredients, including the honey if using, and blend on high speed until smooth.

Makes 1½ cups. Will keep for up to 6 weeks in the fridge (it will thicken, so thin with warm water if desired).

 This dreamy dressing is perfect for any steamed green vegetable.

Very Berry Vinaigrette

This dressing is delightful over bitter greens; the combo of sweet, sour and bitter is incredibly satisfying and will boost the power of your detox by increasing bile flow.

½ cup	organic raspberries
½ cup	extra virgin olive oil
3 Tbsp	raw apple cider vinegar
1 Tbsp	chopped green onions or shallots
2 tsp	yellow mustard (look for a sugar-free mustard made with turmeric)
½ tsp	pink rock or gray sea salt

optional boosters

½ tsp	dried basil
2 tsp	raw liquid honey

In a blender, combine all of the ingredients, including the basil and/or honey if using, and blend on high speed until smooth.

Makes 1¼ cups. Will keep for up to 2 weeks in the fridge.

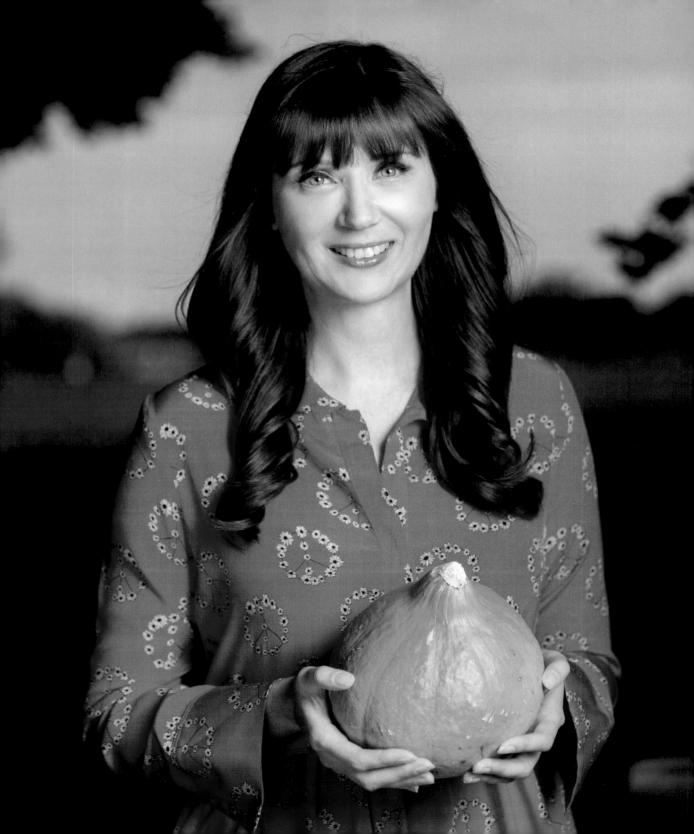

14

Main Meals

Chicken Tikka

Indian cooking can be full of flavor without lighting your mouth on fire. Try this fast and delicious recipe that is plentiful enough for leftovers on busy workdays. Coconut milk contains caprylic acid, which is known to kill the yeast candida — often overgrown due to our taking of antibiotics. The garlic and the Indian spices also help to balance the microbiome.

12	boneless, skinless organic chicken thighs
½ cup	organic coconut milk
¼ cup	finely grated fresh ginger
2 Tbsp	extra virgin olive oil
2 Tbsp	organic lemon juice
2 Tbsp	garam masala (or Julie's Curry Powder, page 269, if garam masala is unavailable)
1 clove	garlic, minced
1 tsp	pink rock or gray sea salt

optional booster

2 Tbsp	tomato paste

1 Place the chicken in a large glass baking dish.

2 In a bowl, mix together the remaining ingredients, including tomato paste if using. Pour over the chicken, and mix until evenly coated. Cover and refrigerate for several hours or up to a day to marinate.

3 Set an oven rack about 6 inches from the broiler. Broil the chicken on low for 40 to 45 minutes or until the chicken is cooked through and the juices run clear. Serve hot.

Makes 6 servings.

 Chicken thighs are cheaper and more flavorful than chicken breasts, with an added bonus: they're higher in iron! This recipe goes well with Coco Quinoa (page 210) or steamed greens.

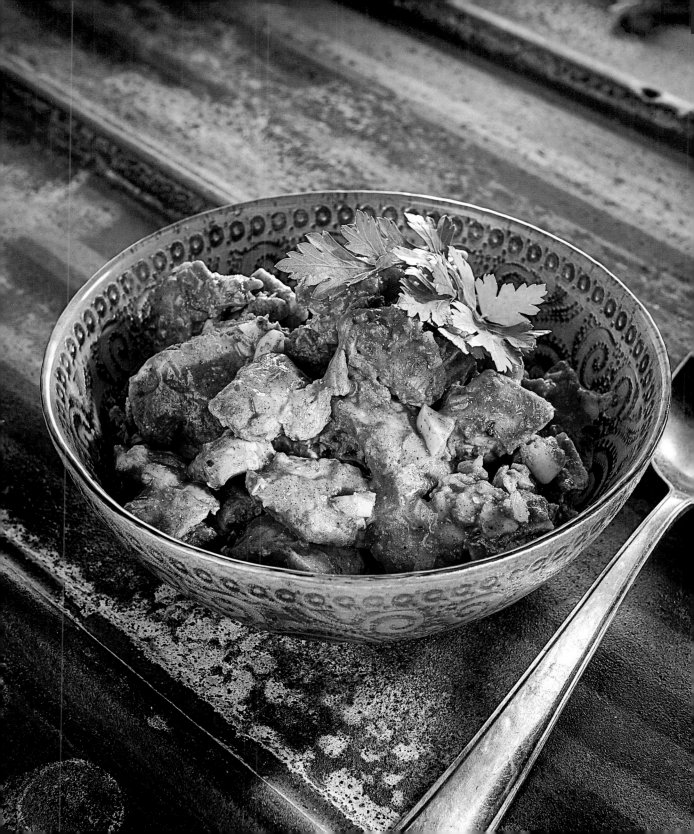

Chicken with Sugar Snap Peas and Fresh Herbs

Sugar snap peas, a staple in my home garden, are nature's candy. Because you're also eating the pods, the fiber content is higher than eating green peas alone. Snap peas are also rich in detoxifying vitamins B and C. If you want a vegetarian side dish, just skip the chicken, use vegan broth and increase the amount of seeds.

1 Tbsp	coconut oil
1 lb	boneless, skinless organic chicken breast, sliced into thin strips
1 cup	bone or vegan broth (see pages 184–187 for broth recipes)
1 tsp	Dijon mustard
½ tsp	pink rock or gray sea salt
3 cups	sugar snap peas, cut in half
14-oz jar	artichoke hearts, drained and quartered
¼ cup	finely chopped fresh herbs (such as chives, basil, tarragon or dill)
2 Tbsp	raw seeds (such as pumpkin, sunflower or sesame seeds or Hemp Hearts)
2 tsp	organic lemon juice

1 Heat the coconut oil in a large skillet over medium heat. Cook the chicken until golden, about 2 minutes per side, then set aside. Do not clean the skillet.

2 In a small bowl, whisk together the broth, mustard and salt. Return the skillet to the stove and set over high heat. Add the broth mixture, snap peas and artichoke hearts.

3 Bring to a simmer, then reduce the heat and cook, stirring constantly, for 3 minutes or until the snap peas are tender but still bright green and crisp.

4 Add the cooked chicken and heat until warmed through, 2 to 3 minutes. Add the herbs, seeds and lemon juice, toss gently and serve immediately.

Makes 4 servings.

 Splashing out on fresh herbs, like dill or basil, is worth it — they provide greater anti-inflammatory properties and ease digestion. But if you don't have fresh herbs, simply use 1 tablespoon of mixed dried herbs.

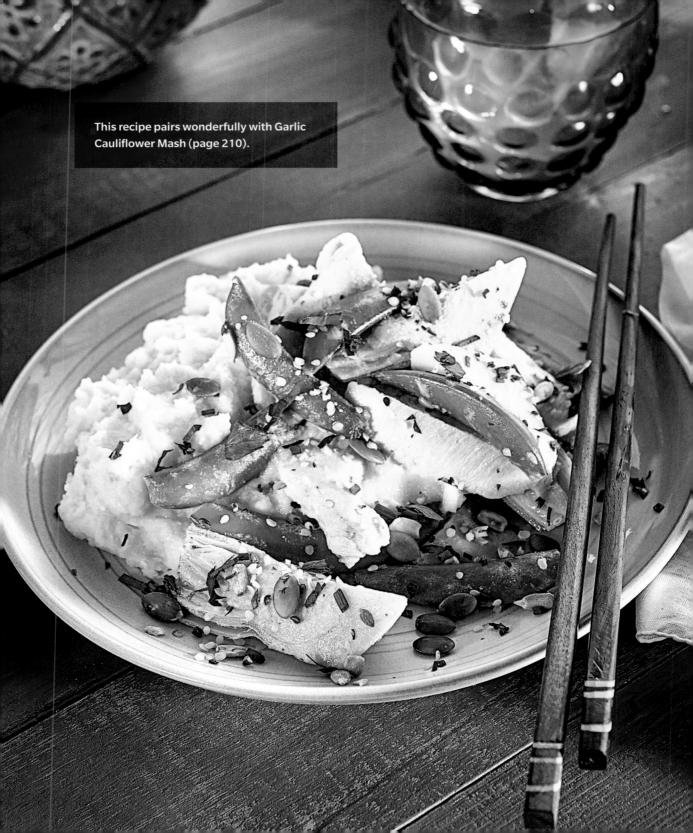

This recipe pairs wonderfully with Garlic Cauliflower Mash (page 210).

Detox Curry

Pull out the big detox guns with this recipe. Every single ingredient lends a nutrient to the detox equation: carotenoids in the squash, B vitamins in the leafy greens, vitamin C in the juice and minerals in the chicken or beans, broth and spices.

2 Tbsp	Julie's Curry Powder (opposite)
½ tsp	ground allspice
6	boneless, skinless organic chicken thighs *or* 2 cups cooked white beans
3 Tbsp	coconut oil, divided
2 cups	sliced celery
2 cups	sliced onions
3 cloves	garlic, sliced
1 Tbsp	freshly grated ginger
1 Tbsp	chopped fresh thyme *or* 1 tsp dried
1 cup	organic pomegranate juice (or any organic berry juice)
1 tsp	pink rock or gray sea salt
4 cups	cubed peeled butternut squash
5 cups	bone or vegan broth (see pages 184–187 for broth recipes)
1 cup	organic coconut milk
4 cups	chopped baby spinach or Swiss chard, including stems

optional booster

1 Tbsp	psyllium husk powder (or ground chia seeds if psyllium is unavailable)

1 In a large bowl, combine the curry powder and allspice. Add the chicken or beans, and mix until well coated. Place in the refrigerator for 1 to 2 hours.

2 In a skillet over medium-high heat, sauté the chicken pieces in 2 tablespoons of the coconut oil for 2 minutes per side. Cook in batches so that the chicken barely covers the bottom of the pan. Transfer to a plate and set aside.

3 In a large soup pot, add the remaining 1 tablespoon of coconut oil and the celery and onions, and sauté for 2 to 3 minutes. Add the garlic, ginger and thyme, and sauté for another 2 minutes.

4 Add the juice and salt, and the psyllium if using, and cook for a few minutes to blend the flavors.

5 Add the squash, broth, and cooked chicken or beans. Bring to a simmer, then cover and cook for 30 minutes.

6 Remove from the heat, add the coconut milk and spinach or Swiss chard, and stir, allowing the greens to wilt.

Makes 6 servings.

 Thyme contains high amounts of natural flavonoids and polyphenols that will help you detoxify.

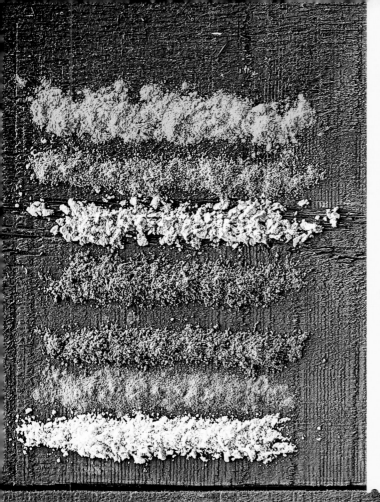

Julie's Curry Powder

If you'd like a warming spice blend that is both anti-inflammatory and free of nightshade peppers (chilies), mix this up and use it over the course of your 21-day detox. Turmeric slows down Phase 1 of the liver detox pathway while increasing Phase 2, allowing the liver to function more efficiently. Cayenne pepper is contraindicated for anyone with digestive inflammation, so it is not included in this recipe, which gets some of its heat from the mustard powder.

3 Tbsp	ground turmeric
2 Tbsp	ground cumin
2 Tbsp	ground coriander
2 Tbsp	ground cardamom
1 Tbsp	ground ginger
1 Tbsp	mustard powder
2 tsp	ground cinnamon

Mix well and store in a jar with tight-fitting lid.

Makes ¾ cup.

This spice blend can be used to spike the flavor in soups, dips, stir-fries and dressings. If you wish to grind your spices fresh, simply maintain the same ratios.

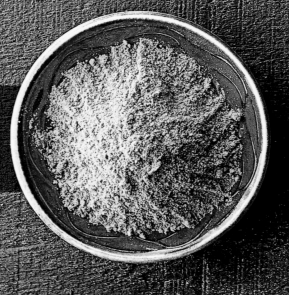

Detox Kichadi

This is a classic Ayurvedic stew with fresh ingredients. I once lived on it for 28 straight days on a yoga detox retreat, and found its balance of sweet, sour, salty, spicy and bitter flavors deeply satisfying. The spices in this dish are very healing to the digestive tract.

6 cups	bone or vegan broth (see pages 184–187 for broth recipes)
1 cup	chopped carrots
½ cup	quinoa or kasha (toasted buckwheat groats)
½ cup	dried split mung beans or split red lentils, rinsed and drained
½ cup	winter squash or pumpkin puree (see Tip on page 142)
2 Tbsp	raw apple cider vinegar
1 Tbsp	minced garlic
2 tsp	freshly grated ginger
1 tsp	ground turmeric
½ tsp	ground cumin
½ tsp	pink rock or gray sea salt (reduce to ¼ tsp if using a salted broth)
1 cup	chopped Swiss chard, kale, bok choy or broccoli, including stems

optional booster

1 cup	sliced fresh burdock root, in dime-size pieces, or 2 Tbsp dried chopped dandelion root

to serve

2 Tbsp	extra virgin olive oil or coconut oil
½ cup	fresh parsley or cilantro

1 In a medium saucepan over high heat, bring all the stew ingredients, except the 1 cup of green vegetables, to a rapid boil, stirring occasionally. Include the burdock or dandelion root if using.

2 Decrease the heat to low, cover and simmer for 20 minutes. Add the greens, and cook for 5 to 10 minutes longer.

3 Serve warm in bowls, and top with a drizzle of the olive oil or coconut oil and the fresh herbs.

Makes 6 servings.

 Keep this stew interesting by rotating the vegetables you use. Be willing to experiment for a different taste every time.

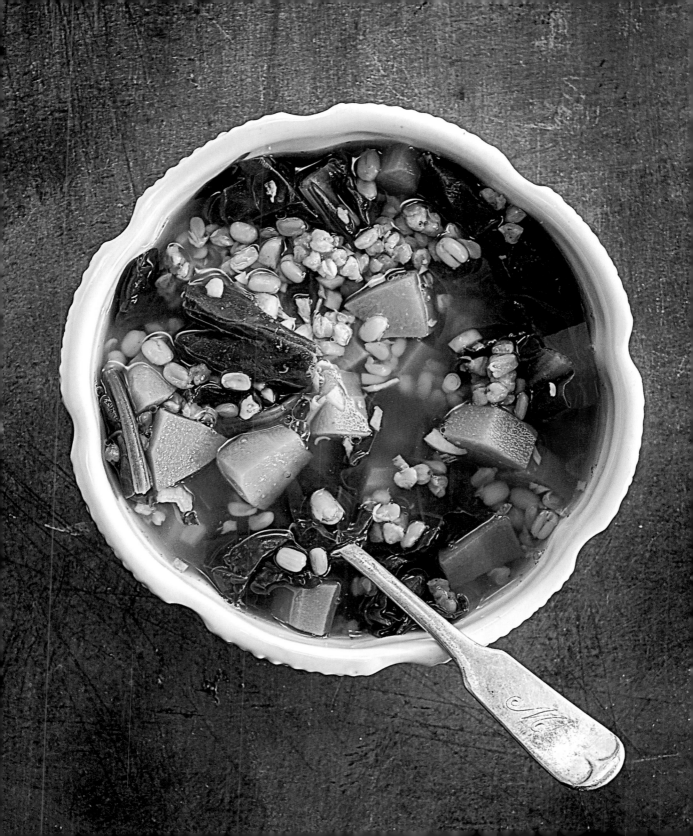

Detox Nut Butter Stew

Inspired by African cuisine, nut butter adds a richness that will keep you coming back for more. Cruciferous veggies like bok choy add an extra detox boost. Not only does bok choy contain vitamins A, B and C, it's also rich in antioxidant minerals such as zinc.

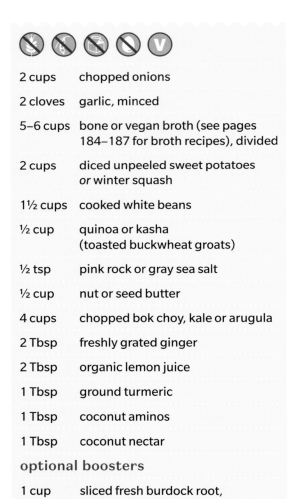

2 cups	chopped onions
2 cloves	garlic, minced
5–6 cups	bone or vegan broth (see pages 184–187 for broth recipes), divided
2 cups	diced unpeeled sweet potatoes *or* winter squash
1½ cups	cooked white beans
½ cup	quinoa or kasha (toasted buckwheat groats)
½ tsp	pink rock or gray sea salt
½ cup	nut or seed butter
4 cups	chopped bok choy, kale or arugula
2 Tbsp	freshly grated ginger
2 Tbsp	organic lemon juice
1 Tbsp	ground turmeric
1 Tbsp	coconut aminos
1 Tbsp	coconut nectar

optional boosters

1 cup	sliced fresh burdock root, in dime-size pieces

1 In a large saucepan over medium heat, cook the onion, garlic and burdock if using in ¼ cup of the broth for 3 to 5 minutes.

2 Add the remaining 4¾ cups broth (plus an extra 1 cup of broth if using burdock), sweet potatoes or squash, white beans, quinoa or kasha, and salt. Cover and simmer for 45 minutes.

3 When the quinoa or kasha is tender, scoop ½ cup liquid from the stew into a small bowl, and whisk it together with the nut or seed butter to make a paste.

4 Add this paste to the pot along with the bok choy, kale or arugula. Stir and cook for 5 minutes. Turn off the heat.

5 Add the ginger, lemon juice, turmeric, aminos and coconut nectar, and stir. Serve hot.

Makes 8 servings.

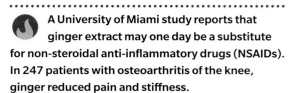

A University of Miami study reports that ginger extract may one day be a substitute for non-steroidal anti-inflammatory drugs (NSAIDs). In 247 patients with osteoarthritis of the knee, ginger reduced pain and stiffness.

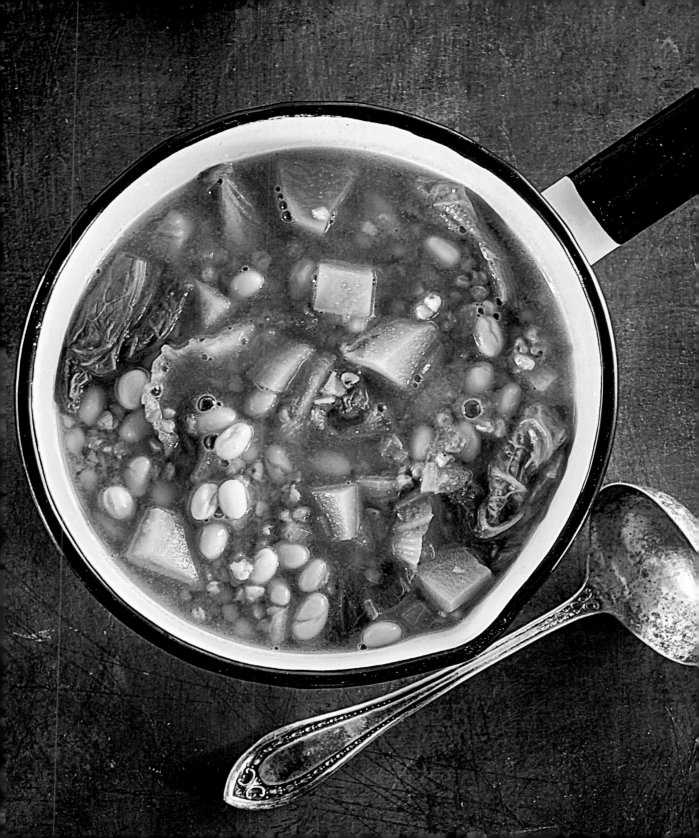

Delish Fish

This recipe works well with most medium-size fish — but choose one that's sustainable. Enjoy sablefish, Pacific cod, pollock, perch, wild salmon, local white fish or trout. You want your fillets to be half to three-quarters of an inch thick so that they cook evenly, but if you have a thinner fillet (like trout), just reduce the cooking time.

This recipe takes less than 20 minutes to cook — ideal if you have last-minute guests over for dinner. The taste is gourmet, so don't be surprised if your friends want to join you on this cleanse! If dining solo, slightly undercook the portions you keep as leftovers so they will reheat deliciously. The turmeric and garlic will help the liver detox go smoothly.

I like to serve this fish with a **Tomato Fennel Ragout. To make: Heat 1 tablespoon of olive oil in a large sauté pan over medium heat. Add 1 cup of chopped red onion and sauté until translucent, approximately 5 minutes. Add 1 chopped bulb of fennel (trimmed and cored) and 2 cloves of minced garlic and sauté for 5 minutes. Add 4 cups of chopped Roma tomatoes and season with pink rock or gray sea salt. Tie together 1 small sprig of fresh basil and 3 sprigs of fresh thyme with kitchen string and throw into pan. Cook for 15 to 20 minutes on medium-low heat until mixture has thickened. Add 1 teaspoon of apple cider vinegar and ½ cup of fish or chicken broth and cook for another 10 minutes. Remove sprigs. Check for seasoning and adjust to taste. Serves 4.**

¼ cup	chicken broth (see recipe on page 186)
2 Tbsp	yellow mustard (look for a sugar-free mustard made with turmeric)
3 Tbsp	organic lemon juice, divided
2 Tbsp	chopped fresh dill, basil, tarragon or oregano *or* 2 tsp dried if fresh is unavailable
1 tsp	coconut nectar
4 medium fillets fresh fish (about 1 lb)	
2 Tbsp	coconut oil, melted
to taste	pink rock or gray sea salt
2 cloves	garlic, minced

optional booster

¼ tsp	ground turmeric

to serve

to taste	chopped green onions

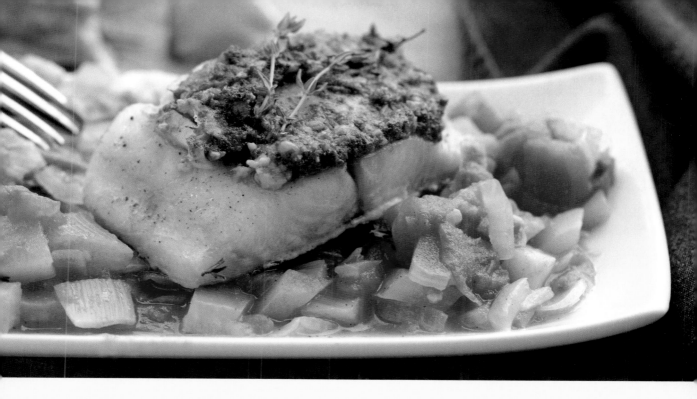

1 To make the sauce, whisk together the broth, mustard, 1 tablespoon of the lemon juice, fresh herbs and coconut nectar, and the turmeric if using, in a small bowl. Set aside.

2 Preheat the broiler to high. Place an ovenproof skillet or cast-iron pan 6 inches below the broiler for about 10 minutes to get it very hot.

3 While the pan preheats, combine the coconut oil, the remaining 2 tablespoons of lemon juice and salt in a shallow dish. Add the fish and set aside to marinate.

4 Using an oven mitt, carefully remove the pan from the oven. Transfer the fish (skin side down if the fish has skin) to the hot pan. (Reserve the marinade.) Place the pan under the broiler. The fish will cook quickly, usually in 5 to 7 minutes depending on the thickness. Test with a fork; it should flake easily. The fish tastes best when it's still rare inside. Transfer the cooked fish to a serving dish with a lid, cover and set aside in a warm spot.

5 Using the same skillet, add the reserved marinade, prepared sauce and garlic. Cook over medium heat until the mixture reduces and thickens. Pour over the fish, and serve with a garnish of green onions.

Makes 4 servings.

Hemp Burgers

These vegan burgers are perfect travel companions that pack up easily. The balance of protein, fiber and superdetox nutrients will keep you full for hours! Cashews and Hemp Hearts are excellent sources of magnesium. Every single cell in the human body needs magnesium to function. Strong bones and teeth, balanced hormones, relaxed muscles, a healthy nervous system and, most important in the Hot Detox, well-functioning detoxification pathways!

1 cup	raw cashews
2 cups	filtered water, for soaking the cashews
2 Tbsp	ground flaxseeds (freshly ground if possible)
¼ cup	filtered water, for soaking the flaxseeds
¼ cup	chopped red onion
1 cup	Hemp Hearts
½ cup	raw sunflower seeds
3 Tbsp	coconut aminos
1 Tbsp	dried basil
1 tsp	pink rock or gray sea salt
1½ cups	kasha (toasted buckwheat groats)
2 cups	grated carrots or unpeeled sweet potatoes (using a food processor)

optional booster

½ cup	dried cranberries (sweetened with apple juice)

1. In a small bowl, soak the cashews in 2 cups water for 1 hour. Drain well. In another bowl, combine the ground flax and ¼ cup water and set aside for about 5 minutes until it gels.

2. Preheat the oven to 300°F, and line 2 baking sheets with parchment paper.

3. Using a food processor, puree the soaked cashews until smooth.

4. Add the flax and the remaining ingredients, except for the kasha and carrots, and process until well combined. Then add the kasha and carrots, and the dried cranberries if using, and pulse, to avoid overmixing, until the mixture starts to form a ball.

5. Using your hands, shape the mixture into patties (about ¼ cup each). Place the patties on the baking sheet and bake for 25 minutes, flipping halfway through.

Makes 16 patties. Will keep for up to 4 days in the fridge or up to 3 months in the freezer.

 These freeze well. For an easy detox meal, just pop them into the oven or toaster oven and cook until warmed through.

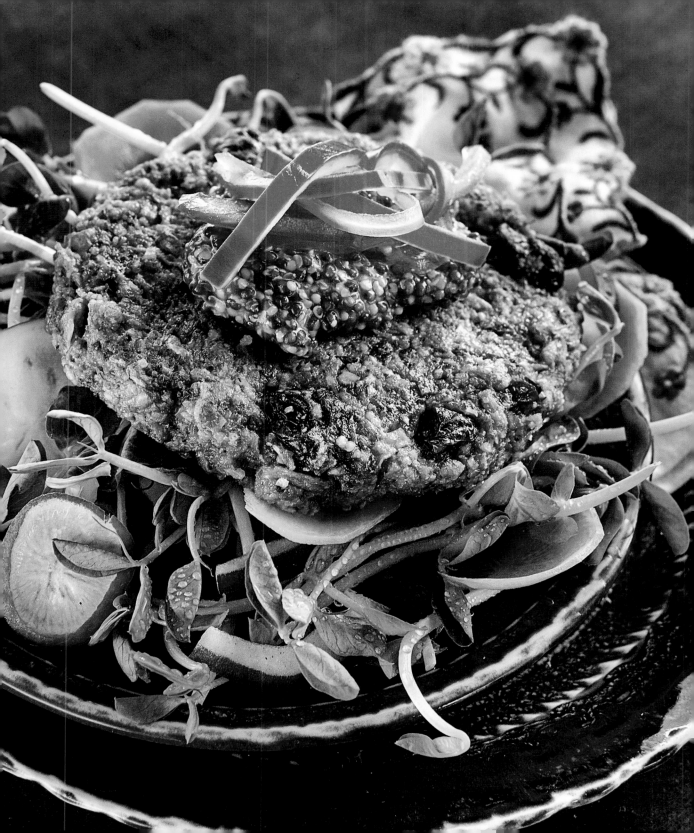

Herbed Halibut

Besides being a great source of detox nutrients, halibut has a delicately sweet flavor. It's a lean fish with snow-white flesh and is rated well for sustainability. Halibut is a very good source of magnesium, which improves the flow of blood, oxygen and nutrients throughout the body, and of omega-3 fatty acids and vitamins B6, B9 and B12, nutrients that increase detoxification and reduce inflammation.

1 lb	fresh halibut fillets
1½ cups	coarsely chopped fresh tarragon
1½ cups	coarsely chopped fresh basil
1½ cups	coarsely chopped fresh chives
2 cups	coarsely chopped fresh parsley
2 tsp	minced fresh ginger
½–1 tsp	pink rock or gray sea salt
2 Tbsp	avocado oil or extra virgin olive oil
2	organic lemons, zest and juice
2	shallots or ½ red onion, chopped

1 Preheat the oven to 400°F.

2 Cut the fillets into 4 pieces, each roughly 2-by-4 inches. Cut 4 pieces of parchment paper, each at least twice the length of a halibut piece.

3 In a large bowl, combine the fresh herbs, ginger, salt and avocado oil or olive oil, and mix thoroughly. Working with 1 piece of parchment and fish at a time, spoon one-eighth of the herb mixture evenly over the paper and lay the fish on top. Sprinkle with one-quarter of the lemon zest and juice, and then top with another one-eighth of the herb mixture and one-quarter of the shallots or red onions.

4 Wrap the paper around each piece of fish, folding over the edges to create a seal. Place the wrapped fillets in a baking dish and bake for approximately 35 minutes.

Makes 4 servings.

 Look for the premade parchment paper pockets at the grocery store to make assembly superquick and easy!

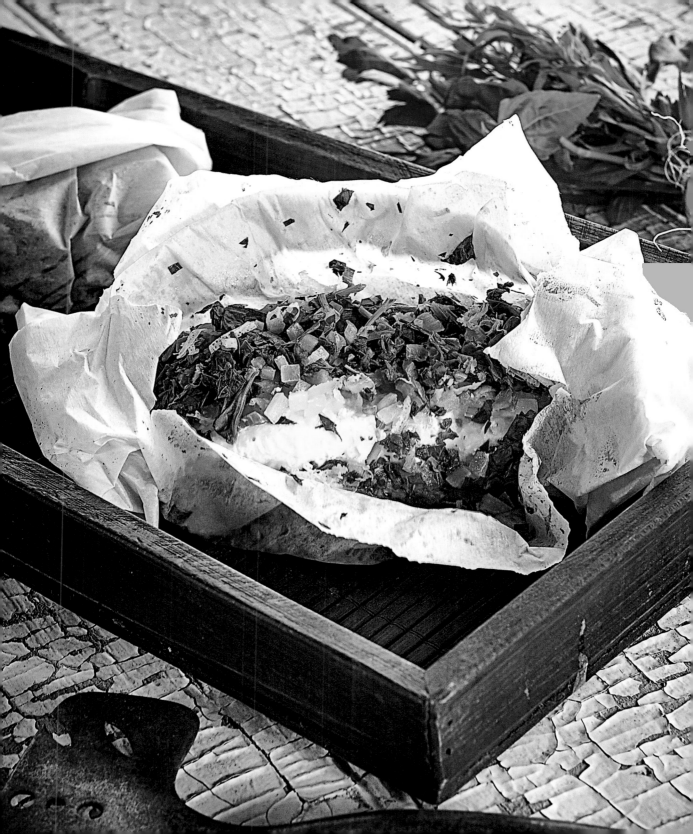

Lazy Cabbage Rolls

You'll be surprised by the sweetness of this dish, one of my sister's quick-and-easy recipes. Cabbage is filling because of its high level of fiber, which adds bulk to your stool. With only 33 calories per cup of cooked cabbage, this recipe is a natural go-to for anyone interested in controlling their weight. Cabbage is also a source of vitamin K, a nutrient essential for the upkeep of the myelin sheath, which protects nerves from damage.

2 lbs	ground organic turkey or chicken
2 Tbsp	coconut oil
1–2 tsp	pink rock or gray sea salt, divided
4 cups	sliced onions
2 cloves	garlic, chopped
12 cups	sliced cabbage, in ribbons
3 cups	sugar-free tomato sauce or diced tomatoes
2–3 Tbsp	Italian seasoning

1 Place the turkey in a large pot with the coconut oil and 1 teaspoon salt. Cook over medium heat for 5 minutes, then add the onions and garlic and cook for 2 minutes more.

2 Stir in the cabbage in batches, adding some salt each time and letting the cabbage cook down a bit before adding the next batch. Cook for at least 8 minutes or until the cabbage is soft, then add the tomato sauce or tomatoes and the Italian seasoning. Mix well and cook for 1 to 2 minutes, until the sauce is heated through.

Makes 6 servings.

Mediterranean-Style Skillet Chicken

You are going to love this easy recipe. Sour lemon, salty olives, sweet onion and currants — your palate will light up like a fireworks display. This crowd-pleasing main dish contains enough antioxidants to really keep your detox humming along.

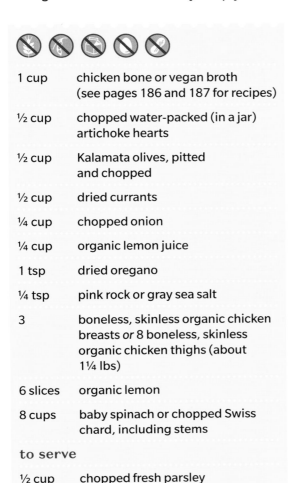

1 cup	chicken bone or vegan broth (see pages 186 and 187 for recipes)
½ cup	chopped water-packed (in a jar) artichoke hearts
½ cup	Kalamata olives, pitted and chopped
½ cup	dried currants
¼ cup	chopped onion
¼ cup	organic lemon juice
1 tsp	dried oregano
¼ tsp	pink rock or gray sea salt
3	boneless, skinless organic chicken breasts *or* 8 boneless, skinless organic chicken thighs (about 1¼ lbs)
6 slices	organic lemon
8 cups	baby spinach or chopped Swiss chard, including stems

to serve

½ cup	chopped fresh parsley

1 In a large bowl, combine the broth, artichoke hearts, olives, currants, onion, lemon, oregano and salt.

2 Slice the chicken into 3-by-1-inch strips, and add to the bowl. If time allows, cover and marinate for 30 minutes to 1 hour in the fridge.

3 In a skillet over medium heat, combine the chicken and the marinade, along with the lemon slices, and bring to a simmer. Cook for 10 minutes.

4 Add the spinach or Swiss chard, and cook for another 3 minutes or until wilted.

5 Divide the chicken between 4 serving plates. Spoon over the sauce in the skillet, and garnish with the cooked lemon slices and parsley.

Makes 4 servings.

 Olives increase blood levels of glutathione, one of the body's premier detox substances.

Power Protein Vegan Bowl

Calling all vegans! Here is a hearty bowl of tasty goodness when you need a meal that really sticks to your ribs. You may think buckwheat is a cereal grain, but it's actually the seed of a fruit that's related to rhubarb, making it suitable for people sensitive to gluten or following a grain-free detox.

¾ cup	quinoa or kasha (toasted buckwheat groats)
1½ cups	filtered water
4 cups	seasonal greens (chopped napa cabbage, baby bok choy, baby spinach)
1½ cups	cooked adzuki or black beans (*or* one 14-oz can, rinsed and drained)
¼ cup	dairy- and nut-free basil pesto (such as Instant Pesto, page 257)
3 Tbsp	raw sesame oil
3 Tbsp	organic lemon juice
¼ tsp	pink rock or gray sea salt
2 cups	grated carrots
¼ cup	chopped raw nuts or seeds of choice

1 Place the quinoa or kasha in a small saucepan with the water, and bring to a boil. Reduce the heat to low, cover and simmer for 15 minutes. Do not stir. When all the liquid is absorbed, remove from the heat and fluff with a fork.

2 Meanwhile, gently blanch the greens in a medium saucepan of salted boiling water for 5 minutes. Drain, then transfer to a medium bowl. Combine the greens with the beans and pesto.

3 In a small bowl, whisk together the sesame oil, lemon juice and salt, then toss with the cooked quinoa or kasha until well coated.

4 Divide the quinoa or kasha among 4 serving dishes. Top with the pesto-bean mixture, as well as the carrots and nuts or seeds.

Makes 4 servings.

Quinoa is the seed of a broad-leaf plant and is much easier to digest than grass grains. It also contains the antioxidant flavonoids quercetin and kaempferol in higher quantity than in some berries!

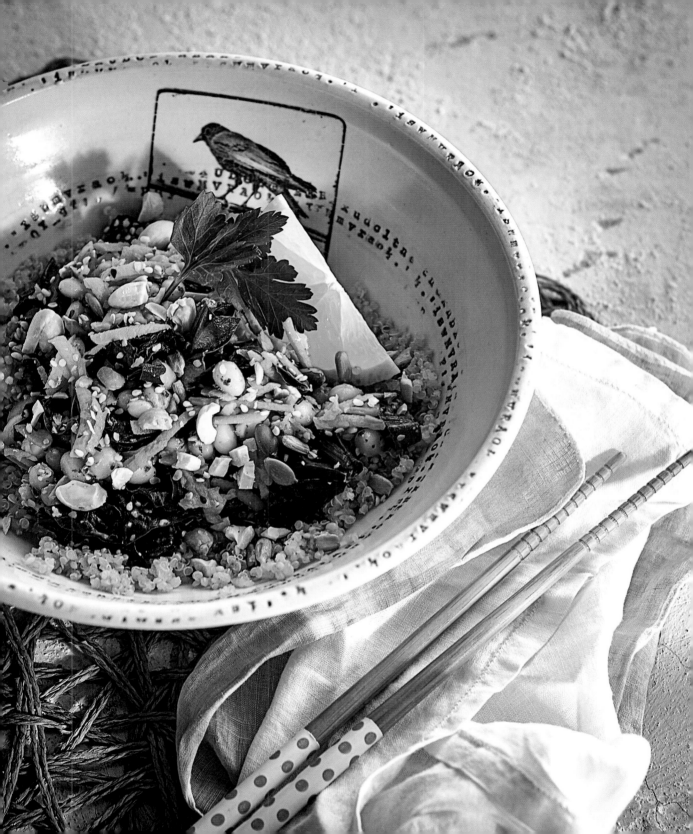

Pineapple Chai Chicken

Pineapple is a tasty tropical way to enjoy vitamin C, which defends your body against free radicals and assists in detox. Do not throw away the core. Not only is it delicious, it's full of the enzyme bromelain, which is anti-inflammatory. Thinly sliced, it has a texture similar to water chestnut. On days 1 to 5 or days 16 to 21 of the Hot Detox program, try this recipe atop Coco Quinoa (page 210).

2 cups	sliced onions
4 cloves	garlic, chopped
2 Tbsp	freshly grated ginger
1 tsp	pure vanilla extract
1 Tbsp	ground cinnamon
1 tsp	ground cardamom
¼ tsp	ground cloves
½ tsp	ground nutmeg
1 cup	organic coconut milk
2 tsp	pink rock or gray sea salt
1½ lbs	boneless, skinless organic chicken thighs (about 8 pieces), cut into strips
5 cups	cubed pineapple (and the thinly sliced core, if desired; keep separate)
6 cups	broccoli florets

optional boosters

2 cups	sliced red bell pepper

to serve

2 cups	chopped fresh cilantro

1 In a large pot over medium heat, combine the onions, garlic, ginger, vanilla, cinnamon, cardamom, cloves, nutmeg, coconut milk and salt. Bring to a simmer, and cook for 5 minutes.

2 Increase the heat to medium, then add the chicken and cubed pineapple. Cover and cook for 10 to 12 minutes. Add the broccoli, and cook for 5 more minutes. Add the red pepper and pineapple core if using, and cook for 2 more minutes.

3 Garnish with cilantro, and serve immediately.

Makes 8 servings. Will keep for up to 3 days in the fridge.

 Cardamom seeds lose their flavor and aroma quickly after being removed from their protective pods, so it's best to buy them whole. Simply crack open the pods (discard pods) and grind the seeds.

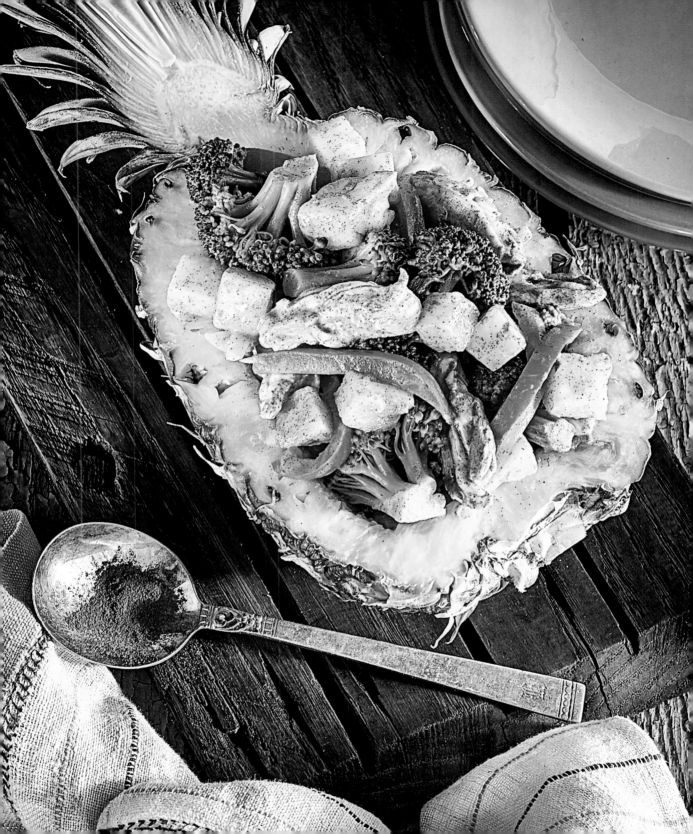

Sautéed Comfort

Sautéed leeks and squash with chicken or beans — comfort food for your cleanse. This recipe boasts a good amount of protein, which is very important on a cleanse because it provides the necessary amino acids for proper liver detoxification.

2 Tbsp	extra virgin olive oil, divided
2 Tbsp	yellow mustard (look for a sugar-free mustard made with turmeric)
2 tsp	organic lemon zest
2 tsp	chopped fresh thyme or 1 tsp dried
2 tsp	ground turmeric
8	boneless, skinless organic chicken thighs or 2 cups cooked adzuki beans
½ tsp	pink rock or gray sea salt
4 cups	chopped peeled butternut squash, in 1-inch cubes
4 cups	sliced leeks (white and green parts)
1 cup	bone or vegan broth (see pages 184–187 for broth recipes)
2 Tbsp	raw apple cider vinegar

1 Preheat the oven to 400°F.

2 In a bowl, combine 1 tablespoon of the olive oil with the mustard, lemon zest, thyme and turmeric. Reserve 1 tablespoon, and brush the rest over the chicken or drizzle over the beans. Sprinkle the chicken or beans with the sea salt.

3 Heat the remaining 1 tablespoon olive oil in a large skillet over medium heat. Add the chicken and cook for 2 minutes per side or until lightly browned.

4 Transfer the chicken to a plate. In the same skillet, sauté the squash in the pan juices for 1 minute. Add the leeks, and sauté for 2 minutes.

5 Add the broth, reserved mustard mixture and vinegar, and bring to a boil. Reduce the heat.

6 If using beans, add to the skillet, stir to combine, cover and cook for 5 minutes or until warmed through. If using chicken, place the browned chicken on the vegetables in the skillet. Cover and cook for 15 to 20 minutes or until the chicken juices run clear.

7 Remove the chicken from the skillet and slice it before serving on top of the vegetables.

Makes 4 servings.

Do you use only the white part of the leek? The dark green part tastes great and is high in nutrition. It just needs to be cooked longer to tenderize it.

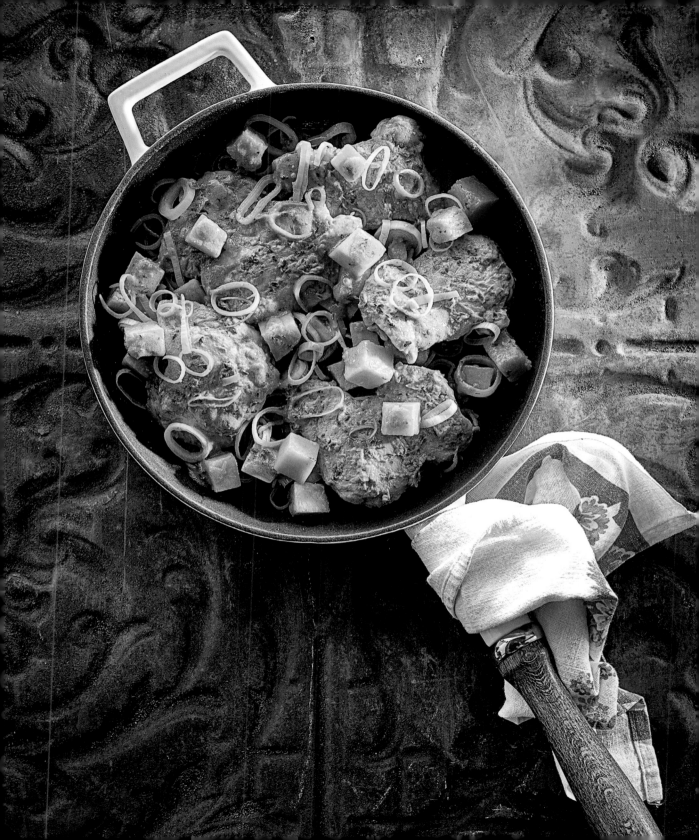

Savory Carrot Cashew Bake

This gentle and soothing casserole tastes friendly and familiar. It makes a wonderful vegan main dish that can satisfy the whole family. The psyllium husk adds a lot of fiber to clean the gastrointestinal system. The beta-carotene in the carrots converts to vitamin A, which assists in skin cell turnover and skin detox.

1 tsp	coconut oil
4¼ cups	grated carrots (use a food processor)
1 cup	chopped green onions
1 cup	chopped celery
1 cup	almond or hazelnut flour
½ cup	raw cashew pieces
⅓ cup	Hemp Hearts or raw sunflower seeds
2 Tbsp	psyllium husks
1 Tbsp	dried basil
1 tsp	dried thyme
½ tsp	dried ground sage
¼ cup	vegan broth (see page 187 for a recipe)
3 Tbsp	extra virgin olive oil
1 Tbsp	organic lemon juice
½–1 tsp	pink rock or gray sea salt

1. Preheat the oven to 350°F. Grease an 8-by-8-inch baking dish with the coconut oil.

2. In a food processor, combine all of the ingredients, and pulse until well incorporated but still chunky.

3. Press into the baking dish. Bake for 45 minutes or until the top edges begin to look dry.

Makes 10 servings. Will keep for up to 4 days in the fridge and 6 months in the freezer.

Grate the carrots in the food processer first and set aside. Then switch to the S-blade to process all the ingredients together.

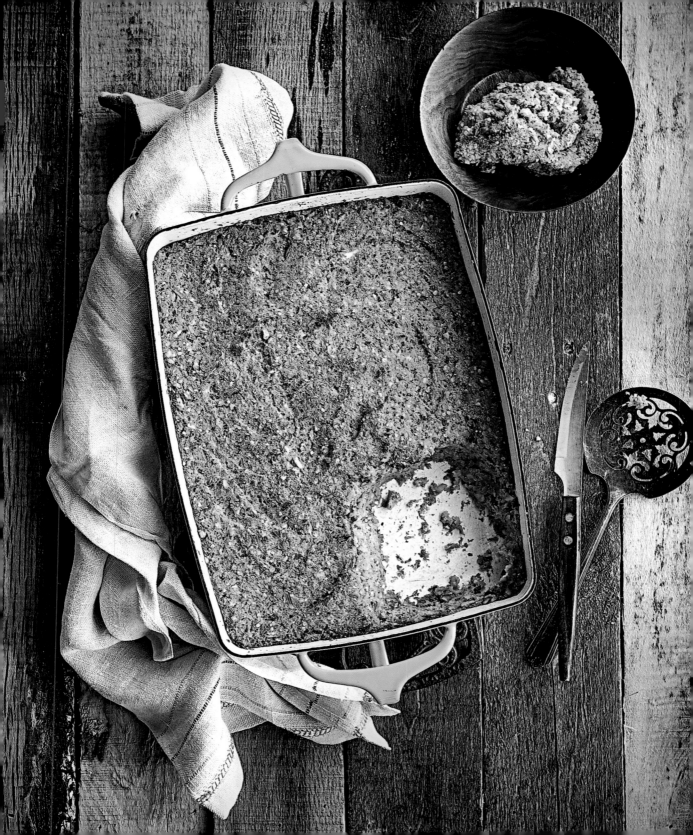

Sesame-Crusted Fish

Sesame seeds are a good source of manganese, magnesium, calcium, iron, zinc, selenium and molybdenum. Molybdenum converts the toxin acetaldehyde (created by the die-off of yeast and when you consume alcohol) into safe acetic acid; a buildup of acetaldehyde can cause joint pain, a feeling of weakness and brain fog. So sprinkle on those sesame seeds fast, and enjoy some brain-building fish today!

1 cup	fresh cilantro or basil
2 Tbsp	raw sesame oil
2 Tbsp	coconut nectar
1 Tbsp	grated fresh ginger
3 cloves	garlic
4 fillets	frozen fish (basa, pollock, perch)
⅓ cup	raw sesame seeds
½ tsp	pink rock or gray sea salt
2	organic lemons, cut into ¼-inch slices (about 16)

1 Preheat the oven to 350°F. Grease a baking dish with coconut oil.

2 In a small food processor, combine the cilantro or basil, sesame oil, coconut nectar, ginger and garlic. If your food processor is too large for this amount, chop the herbs and garlic finely by hand and mix well.

3 Arrange half the lemon slices in a single layer in the baking dish, and place the fish on top. Spread the cilantro mixture evenly over the fish. Sprinkle with sesame seeds and salt.

4 Place 2 lemon slices on top of each fillet. Bake for 35 minutes, until fish flakes easily with a fork. Serve with Chimichurri Sauce (page 258).

Makes 4 servings.

It's especially important to choose environmentally friendly and low-toxin fish while on the Hot Detox. Check out a full guide at www.seachoice.org. If you choose to use fresh fish, be sure to get 4 equal-sized fillets and reduce the cooking time by 10 minutes.

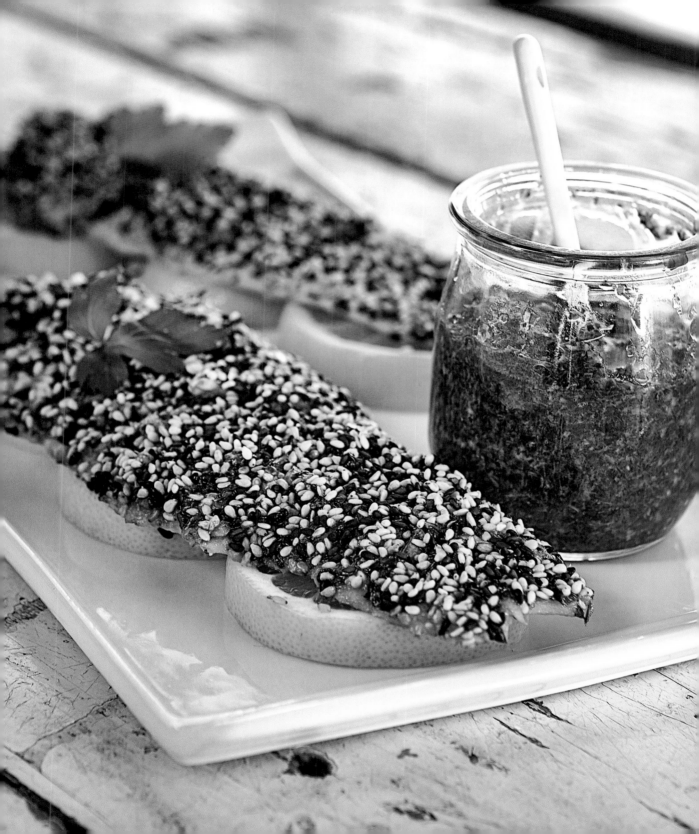

Super Shepherd's Pie

This dinner is a real crowd-pleaser. My nephews and nieces love this recipe so much, it even makes it onto their birthday meal wish list. If you use lentils, cauliflower and sweet potato, you're getting a *lot* of fiber to ensure good digestion. This recipe is tasty enough to sneak veggies into a picky eater's diet.

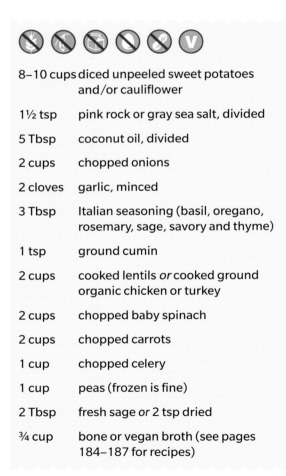

8–10 cups	diced unpeeled sweet potatoes and/or cauliflower
1½ tsp	pink rock or gray sea salt, divided
5 Tbsp	coconut oil, divided
2 cups	chopped onions
2 cloves	garlic, minced
3 Tbsp	Italian seasoning (basil, oregano, rosemary, sage, savory and thyme)
1 tsp	ground cumin
2 cups	cooked lentils *or* cooked ground organic chicken or turkey
2 cups	chopped baby spinach
2 cups	chopped carrots
1 cup	chopped celery
1 cup	peas (frozen is fine)
2 Tbsp	fresh sage *or* 2 tsp dried
¾ cup	bone or vegan broth (see pages 184–187 for recipes)

1 In a saucepan, boil the sweet potatoes and/or cauliflower in filtered water until soft; drain. Using an immersion blender or a food processor, puree the vegetables with ½ teaspoon of the salt and 3 tablespoons of the coconut oil. Set aside.

2 Preheat the oven to 350°F.

3 In a large pot over medium-low heat, melt the remaining 2 tablespoons coconut oil. Add onions, garlic, herb blend, cumin and the remaining 1 teaspoon salt. Cook for 2 minutes, and then add the lentils or chicken or turkey. Cook, stirring, for 1 minute.

4 Add the spinach, carrots, celery, peas, sage and broth, and stir to combine. Cook for 10 minutes.

5 Transfer the mixture to a 13-by-9-inch baking dish. Top with the reserved sweet potato/cauliflower. Score the top with a fork and bake for 30 minutes.

6 Move the baking dish to the top rack in the oven, and broil on low for 7 minutes or until nicely browned. Serve hot.

Makes 9 servings. Vegan version keeps up to 1 week in the fridge (the poultry variation keeps up to 3 days). Freezes well.

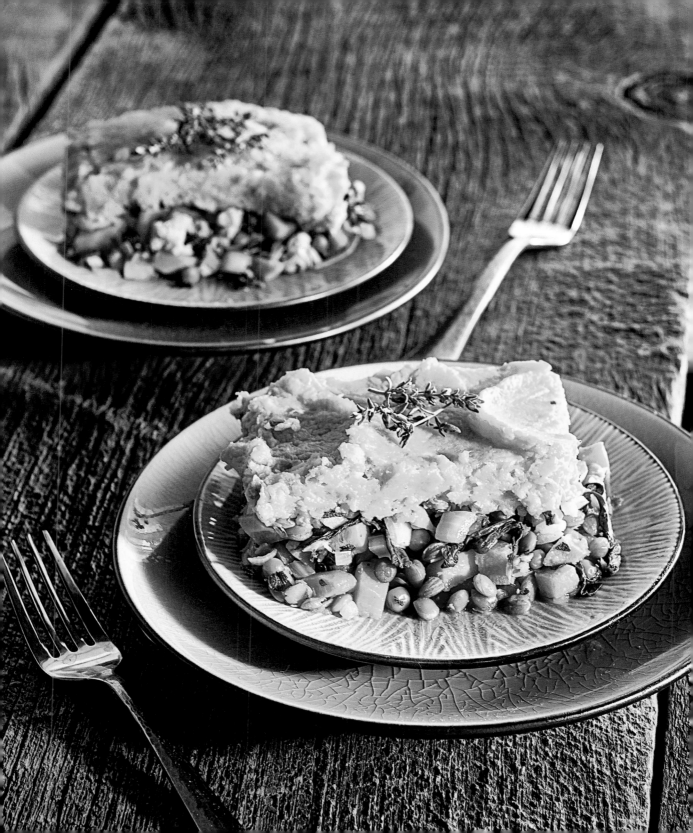

Turkey Loaf

My mother-in-law first introduced me to the idea of pickles in a meat dish. The fermented tang makes this loaf shine! Turkey is high in tryptophan, which gets converted to 5-hydroxytryptophan (5-HTP), and then to serotonin, the neurotransmitter that helps improve mood. Onions are often overlooked on the nutrition scale, but they contain some of the highest levels of an antioxidant called quercetin, which works as both an antihistamine and an anti-inflammatory.

1 tsp	coconut oil
1 lb	ground organic turkey or chicken
1 cup	chopped celery
1 cup	grated zucchini
1 cup	chopped onions
½ cup	chopped fresh dill
½ cup	chopped fresh parsley
½ cup	chopped sugar-free pickles
1 clove	garlic, minced
1 Tbsp	ground flaxseeds (freshly ground if possible)
1 Tbsp	yellow mustard (look for a sugar-free mustard made with turmeric)
1	large organic egg
¼ tsp	pink rock or gray sea salt

1 Preheat the oven to 350°F. Grease a glass loaf dish with the coconut oil.

2 In a large bowl, mix together all the ingredients (clean hands work well).

3 Press mixture evenly into the loaf dish. Bake for 45 minutes or until cooked through.

Makes 8 servings. Will keep up to 3 days in the fridge. Freezes well.

 A study published in *Clinical Gastroenterology and Hepatology* found the combination of onions and turmeric (found in the mustard) creates a synergistic effect that reduces both the size and number of precancerous lesions in the gut.

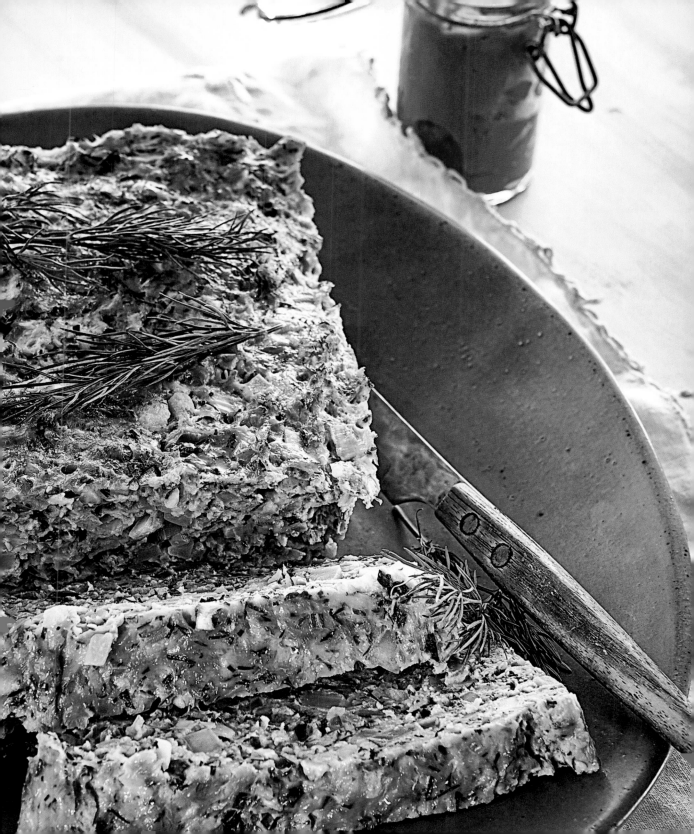

Wild Fish Cakes

I sometimes dream of roasting up fresh fish in my own backyard wood fire oven as Jamie Oliver does on his TV show *Jamie at Home*. To keep these fish cakes quick and easy, I use sustainable fish found in the frozen section of most grocery stores, such as Canadian haddock or Norwegian pollock. Fish is a wonderful source of protein and the essential fatty acids that will aid in detoxification.

1 lb	frozen haddock or pollock fillets, thawed
1 cup	almond or hazelnut flour, divided
½ cup	finely chopped green onions
1 Tbsp	dried dill *or* ¼ cup chopped fresh
1 Tbsp	mustard seeds, ground
1	large organic egg
1 tsp	pink rock or gray sea salt

optional boosters

½ cup	finely chopped celery
1 Tbsp	Julie's Curry Powder (page 269)

1 Place the thawed fish in a colander and press to remove excess liquid. Transfer the fish to a bowl and, using two forks, tear into flakes.

2 Add ¾ cup of the nut flour and the rest of the ingredients, including curry powder and celery if using, and stir well.

3 Preheat the oven to 350°F. Line a baking sheet with parchment paper.

4 Divide the mixture into eight ¼-cup portions, using your hands to shape each into a ½-inch-thick patty.

5 Place on the baking sheet, and sprinkle the remaining ¼ cup nut flour on top of the patties until well coated.

6 Bake the for 40 minutes or until lightly browned. Serve warm with the Super Guac on page 256.

Makes 10 fish cakes. Will keep up to 4 days in the fridge. Freezes well.

 You can also use canned salmon in a pinch, but be sure it's packed in BPA-free cans, as many brands coat the inside of the can in a plastic barrier that contains the toxin. Reduce the cooking time to 30 minutes.

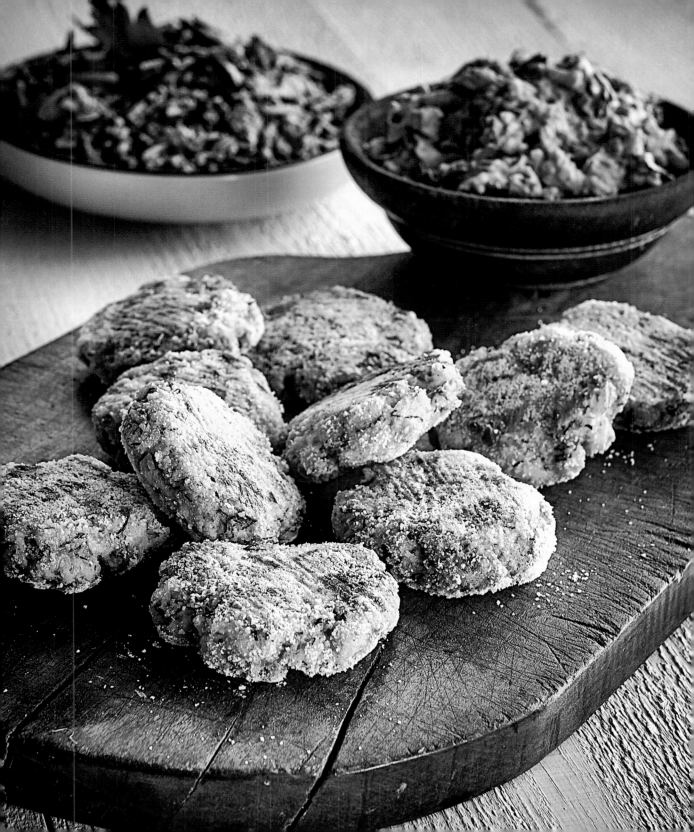

Zucchini Kasharole

This is an incredibly easy and tasty casserole that can be made ahead and enjoyed anytime (especially when prep time is in short supply). Avoid peeling zucchini because the skin contains an incredible amount of the antioxidants lutein, zeaxanthin and beta-cryptoxanthin. The onions and garlic not only complement the lovely summer squash, but also contain organosulfur compounds that aid in detoxification.

1 ½ Tbsp	coconut oil, divided
2 cups	chopped onions
½ tsp	pink rock or gray sea salt, more for the sautéed zucchini
2 cloves	garlic, minced
4 cups	sliced zucchini, in ½-inch-thick half moons
1 cup	sliced green or black olives
1 Tbsp	dried basil
1 tsp	dried thyme
1 tsp	dried rosemary
1 tsp	ground turmeric
3	large organic eggs
½ cup	organic coconut milk
1 cup	kasha (toasted buckwheat groats) or cooked quinoa

optional booster

½ cup	sliced oil-packed sun-dried tomatoes *or* ¼ cup if not packed in oil

1 Preheat the oven to 375°F. Grease a 11-by-7-inch baking dish with coconut oil.

2 Heat 1 tablespoon coconut oil over medium heat in a large, heavy skillet. Add the onions and cook, stirring, until tender, about 5 minutes.

3 Add the garlic and salt, and cook, stirring, until fragrant, 30 seconds to 1 minute.

4 Add the zucchini, olives, basil, thyme, rosemary and turmeric, and sun-dried tomatoes if using. Cook, stirring often, until the zucchini is tender but not mushy, about 10 minutes. Season to taste with salt, and remove the pan from the heat.

5 Beat the eggs and coconut milk in a large bowl. Stir in the zucchini mixture and kasha or quinoa. Mix well, and then transfer to the baking dish.

6 Bake for 30 minutes or until set. Serve hot, warm or at room temperature.

Makes 8 servings. Will keep for up to 4 days in the fridge.

 This also makes an easy stir-fry. You can serve the dish after step 4 (omitting the eggs, coconut milk and kasha/quinoa).

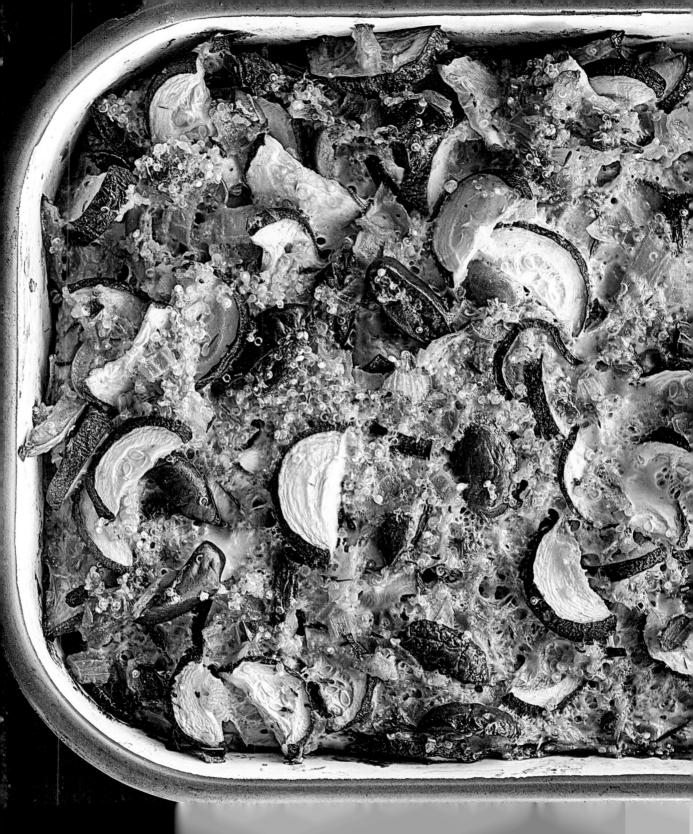

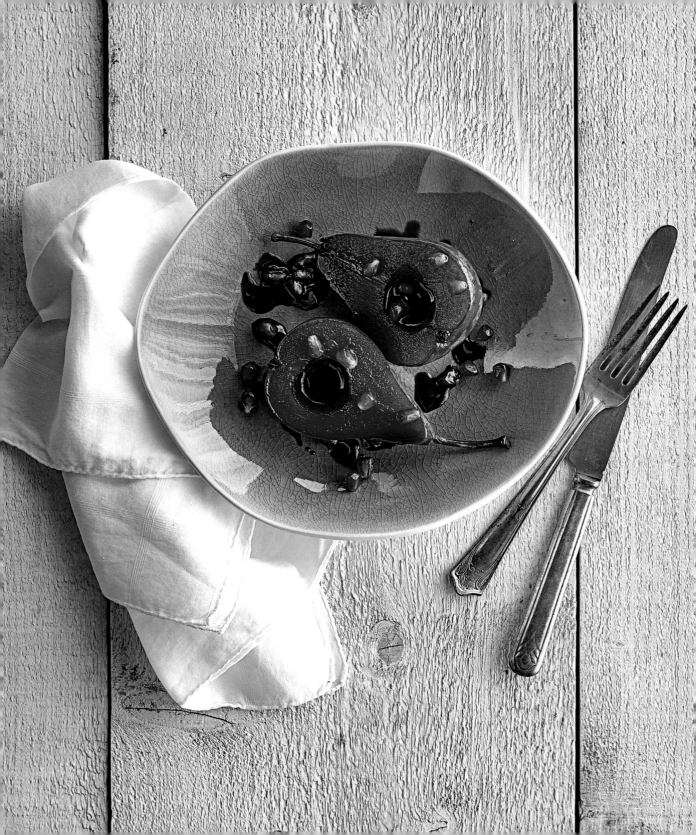

15

Special-Occasion Treats

Cherry Almond Biscotti

Cut from Scottish cloth, my husband, Alan, loves his shortbread during the holiday season. I made these biscuits for him as a healthy substitute and quickly converted him. No need for regular refined flour and butter, what with almond flour's healthy fats and rich taste! Almonds are a great source of magnesium, a mineral that is needed for both the glucuronidation and methylation liver detox pathways.

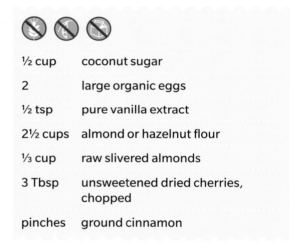

½ cup	coconut sugar
2	large organic eggs
½ tsp	pure vanilla extract
2½ cups	almond or hazelnut flour
⅓ cup	raw slivered almonds
3 Tbsp	unsweetened dried cherries, chopped
pinches	ground cinnamon

1 Preheat the oven to 350°F. Line a baking sheet with parchment paper.

2 In a medium bowl, using an electric mixer, beat together the sugar and eggs until thick and pale yellow. Beat in the vanilla. Using a wooden spoon, stir in the nut flour, then fold in the slivered almonds and dried cherries.

3 As best you can, divide the dough in half (it will be very sticky). Shape each half into a log 6 to 8 inches long and 2 inches thick. (Using wet hands will help keep the dough from sticking to them.) Transfer the loaves to the pan, spacing at least 4 inches apart. Sprinkle each loaf with a touch of cinnamon.

4 Bake for 25 minutes or until firm. Remove the pan from the oven, and lower the heat to 275°F. Let the logs cool for about 10 minutes.

5 Using a serrated knife, cut the logs into ½-inch-thick rounds, and spread out in a single layer on the same baking sheet.

6 Bake for another 20 to 25 minutes, turning over once midway through. Bake until the biscotti are firm and dry to your liking. Let cool completely on the pan before serving.

Makes 16 biscotti. Will keep for 3 to 4 weeks in an airtight container at room temperature or for several months in the freezer.

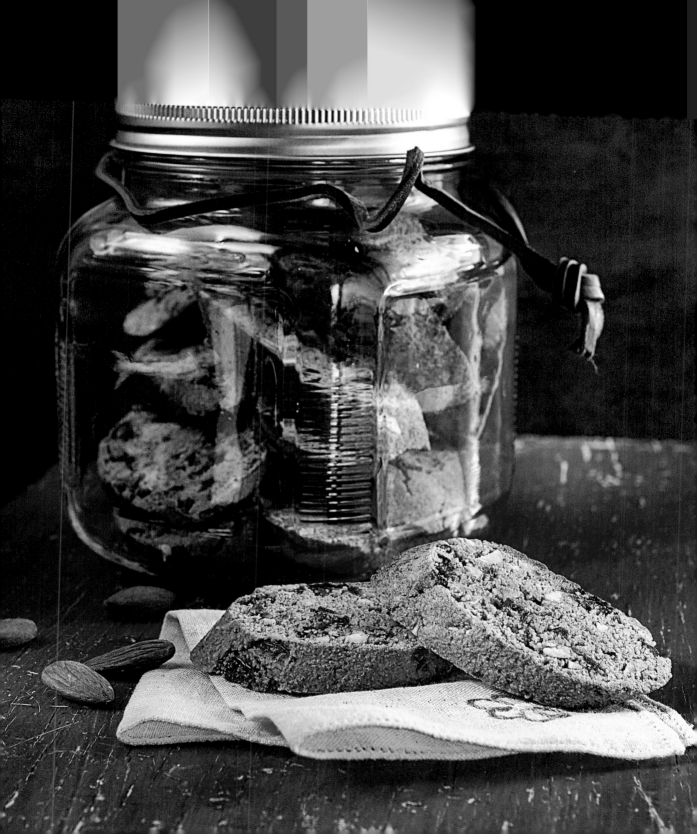

Choco-Chia Pudding

Make this pudding before you go to bed, and you will wake up to an omega-rich treat ready to go. Hemp Hearts and chia seeds both contain heart-healthy omega-3 fats, which play a crucial role in keeping inflammation under control. Two tablespoons of Hemp Hearts have 7 to 11 grams of complete protein; 2 tablespoons of chia seeds have 5 grams of fiber.

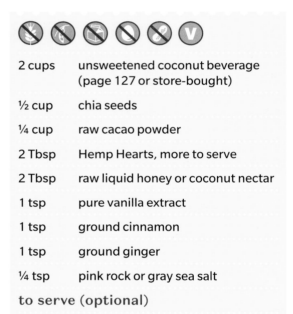

2 cups	unsweetened coconut beverage (page 127 or store-bought)
½ cup	chia seeds
¼ cup	raw cacao powder
2 Tbsp	Hemp Hearts, more to serve
2 Tbsp	raw liquid honey or coconut nectar
1 tsp	pure vanilla extract
1 tsp	ground cinnamon
1 tsp	ground ginger
¼ tsp	pink rock or gray sea salt

to serve (optional)

to taste	raw cacao nibs

1 Combine all the pudding ingredients in a 1-quart (4-cup) Mason jar. Seal with the lid and shake vigorously, or mix with a spoon until well combined.

2 For individual servings, you can transfer the pudding into four 1-cup jars, if you like. If desired, top the pudding with cacao nibs and/or more Hemp Hearts. Seal jar(s) with lids.

3 Refrigerate for a minimum of 2 hours or overnight, until thickened.

Makes 4 servings. Will keep for up to 5 days in the fridge.

It's important to include protein and fiber in your breakfast routine to keep you feeling full during the cleanse. This recipe is in the treat section because of its chocolate content; make these when you're missing caffeine!

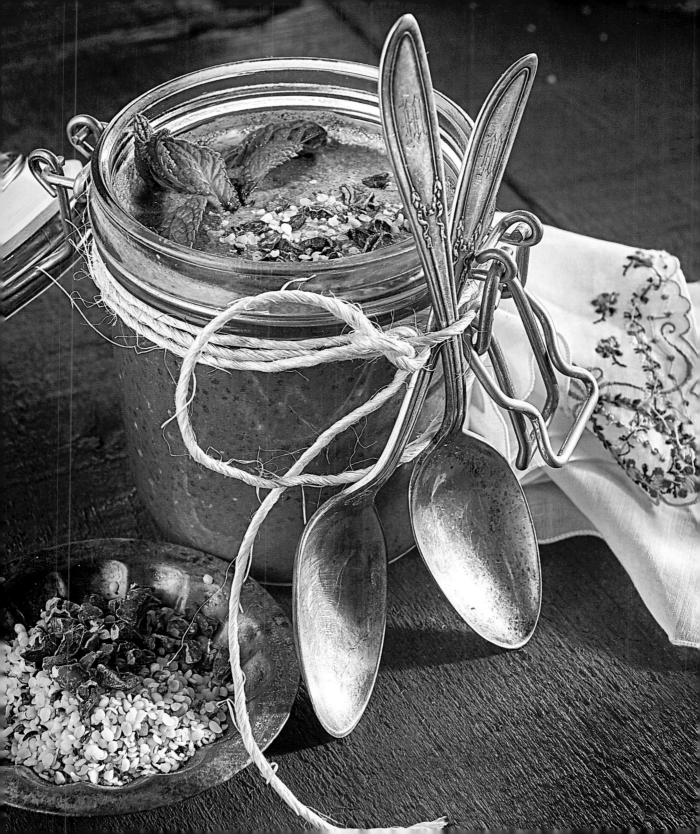

Cinnamon-Dusted Pineapple

Move over, cinnamon buns! Not only is this recipe easy to make, but it smells incredible when baking. When roasted, pineapple tastes sweeter and becomes even easier to digest. Enjoy as a special treat during Phases 1 and 3 of the Hot Detox when you are craving something sweet.

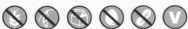

1	pineapple, peeled, cored and quartered lengthwise
1 Tbsp	coconut oil, melted
1½ tsp	ground cinnamon

1 Preheat the oven to 350°F. Line a baking sheet with parchment paper.

2 Place the pineapple wedges on the baking sheet, brush with coconut oil, then sprinkle evenly with cinnamon.

3 Bake for 30 minutes. Let cool, then slice into bite-size pieces for serving.

Makes 4 servings.

 Don't have a pineapple on hand? Try this recipe with unpeeled apples, pears or even peaches.

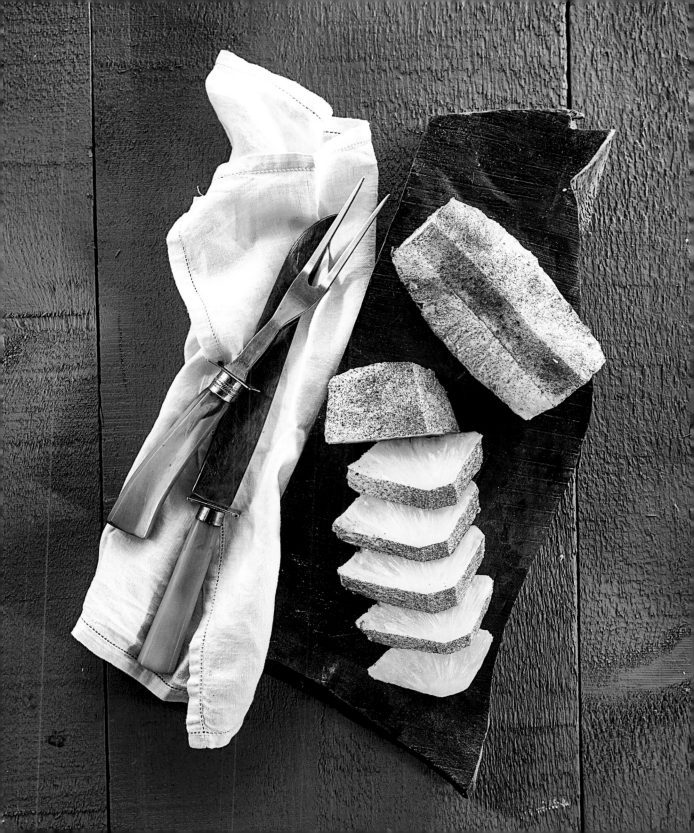

Detox Macaroons

This recipe is high in fiber, which binds to toxins to help remove them from the body. The lemon zest contains vitamin P (also known as flavonoids), which shuttles vitamin C into your cells, so I highly recommend using it here. Zest tastes like heaven, and it does heavenly work! It's important to use organic lemons to avoid the potential hormone-disrupting petrochemicals that are commonly found on conventionally grown citrus.

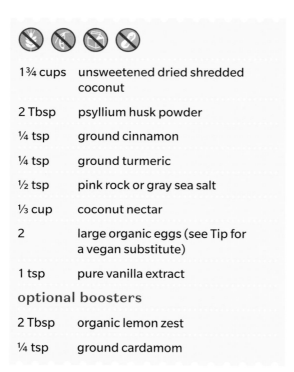

1¾ cups	unsweetened dried shredded coconut
2 Tbsp	psyllium husk powder
¼ tsp	ground cinnamon
¼ tsp	ground turmeric
½ tsp	pink rock or gray sea salt
⅓ cup	coconut nectar
2	large organic eggs (see Tip for a vegan substitute)
1 tsp	pure vanilla extract

optional boosters

2 Tbsp	organic lemon zest
¼ tsp	ground cardamom

1 Preheat the oven to 350°F. Line a baking sheet with parchment paper.

2 In a bowl, combine the coconut, psyllium, cinnamon, turmeric, salt, and the lemon zest and cardamom if using. Add the coconut nectar, eggs and vanilla, and mix well.

3 Using a tablespoon, scoop up balls of the dough and drop them onto the baking sheet. Bake for 15 minutes or until just slightly golden.

Makes 18 macaroons. Will keep for up to 7 days in an airtight container at room temperature or for 6 months in the freezer.

 Here's a vegan egg substitute: To make one "egg," stir 1 tablespoon of ground flax with 2½ tablespoons filtered water, and let sit for 5 minutes. Stir again just before adding to a recipe.

This recipe is traditionally made with honey. In Ayurvedic medicine, cooking honey is not recommended. When using coconut nectar, the cookie will be harder to shape and will appear darker.

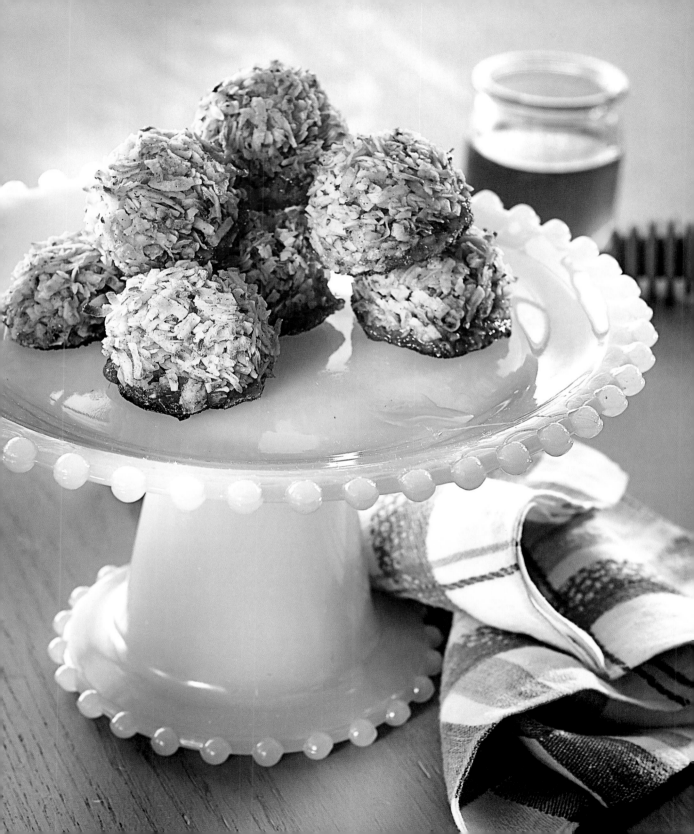

The Great Canadian Hemp Cookie

This recipe was created for my nephew one holiday season when he was following an elimination menu to figure out what he was allergic to. Now these cookies are a family favorite. Hemp Hearts add a subtle nutty flavor to this recipe.

2 ½ Tbsp	filtered water
1 Tbsp	ground flaxseeds (freshly ground if possible)
2 cups	Hemp Hearts
2 cups	unsweetened dried shredded coconut
2 tsp	ground ginger
2 tsp	ground cinnamon
¼ tsp	pink rock or gray sea salt
⅔ cup	raw liquid honey
2 Tbsp	coconut butter (or coconut oil if coconut butter is unavailable)

1 Preheat the oven to 350°F. Line 2 baking sheets with parchment paper.

2 In a medium bowl, combine the water and flax, and let sit for 10 minutes.

3 In a large mixing bowl, combine the hemp, coconut, ginger, cinnamon and salt.

4 Add the honey and coconut butter to the flax. With a hand mixer, beat until smooth, about 1 minute.

5 Fold this wet mixture into the dry ingredients, and combine well. The resulting texture should be fairly dry.

6 Scoop 1 tablespoon of the mixture, and, using your hands, roll into a ball. Place on a baking sheet. With wet fingers, flatten the top so the cookie is ½ inch thick. Repeat until all the dough is used up.

7 Bake for 10 minutes or until slightly golden.

Makes 24 cookies. Will keep for 2 weeks in an airtight container at room temperature or up to 6 months in the freezer.

This recipe was developed for people with IBS/IBD who need to use honey as a sweetener. It is not acceptable in Ayurvedic medicine to cook honey, so use at your own discretion.

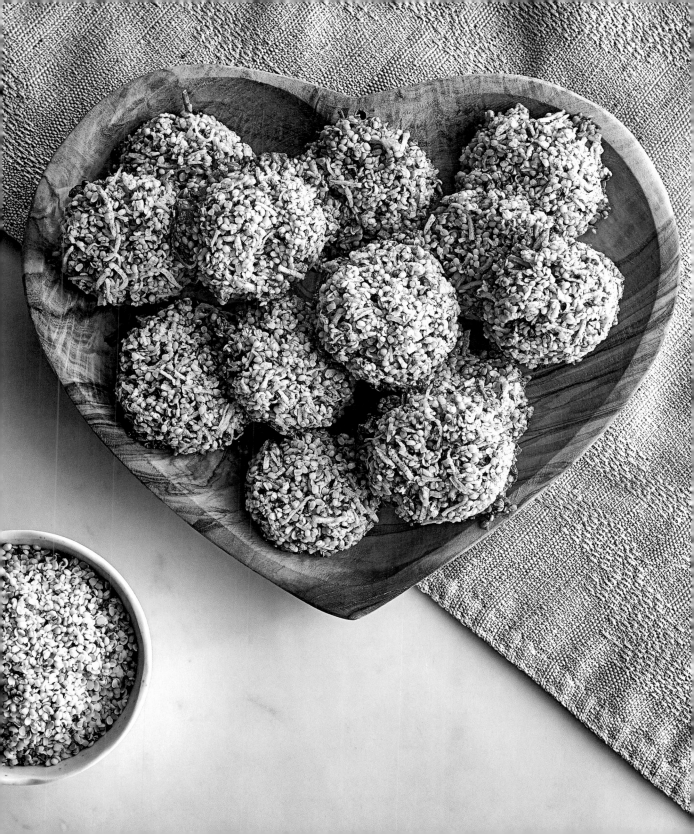

Meals-That-Heal Seed Bar

A seed bar packs a powerful nutritional punch in a small package. This recipe boasts high amounts of protein, good fats and plant sterols, which can balance both your blood sugar and immune system. By filling up on this seed bar, you are keeping your hands out of the cookie jar!

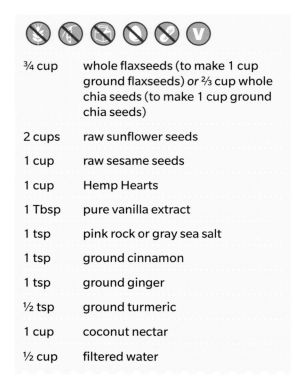

¾ cup	whole flaxseeds (to make 1 cup ground flaxseeds) *or* ⅔ cup whole chia seeds (to make 1 cup ground chia seeds)
2 cups	raw sunflower seeds
1 cup	raw sesame seeds
1 cup	Hemp Hearts
1 Tbsp	pure vanilla extract
1 tsp	pink rock or gray sea salt
1 tsp	ground cinnamon
1 tsp	ground ginger
½ tsp	ground turmeric
1 cup	coconut nectar
½ cup	filtered water

1 Using a clean spice or coffee grinder, roughly grind the whole flax- or chia seeds. (If you don't have a grinder, use preground seeds.) Roughly grind the sunflower seeds. (If you don't have a grinder, use a small food processor.)

2 Preheat the oven to 300°F. Line a 18-by-12-inch baking pan with parchment paper, leaving several inches of overhang on all sides.

3 In a large bowl, combine all the ingredients except the coconut nectar and water, and stir until well combined.

4 Add the coconut nectar and water and mix with a fork until everything is well incorporated.

5 Spread the mixture evenly into the baking pan, firmly pressing it into the sides and corners. Bake for 35 minutes.

6 Remove from the oven and place the pan on a wire rack to cool slightly. Using the parchment overhang to protect your hands, press down to firmly compact the bars before leaving them to cool for about 30 minutes.

7 Once the bars have cooled, invert them onto another piece of parchment laid on the wire rack.

8 Let cool completely, then cut into 2- to 3-inch bars. Wrap individually for quick snack-size packages.

Makes 16 bars. Will keep for up to a week in an airtight container at room temperature.

Pineapple Coconut Upside-Down Cake

My sister, Lynn, wanted to create a new birthday cake so you could celebrate even when on a cleanse. It has a whole pineapple in it, so get ready to smile!

6	pineapple rings, cut ½ inch thick
4 tsp	ground cinnamon, divided
20	frozen cherries
½ cup	pecan pieces
⅔ cup	whole white chia seeds
½ cup	full-fat organic coconut milk
2 cups	mashed banana
¼–⅓ cup	coconut nectar
2 Tbsp	lemon juice
1 Tbsp	pure vanilla extract
1 cup	coconut flour
2 tsp	baking soda
½ tsp	pink rock or gray sea salt

1 Preheat oven to 350°F. Line a 13-by-9-inch baking pan with parchment paper.

2 Sprinkle pineapple rings with 1 teaspoon of the cinnamon and arrange evenly on the bottom of the pan. Arrange cherries around the pineapple rings. Sprinkle pecans evenly over top. Set aside.

3 Using a clean spice or coffee grinder, grind the chia seeds finely to make a flour. (If you don't have a grinder, use 1 cup preground seeds.) In a large bowl, combine the chia and coconut milk and mix well.

4 Add the mashed banana, coconut nectar, lemon juice and vanilla. Mix well.

5 In a bowl, whisk together the coconut flour, baking soda, salt and remaining 3 teaspoons of cinnamon. Add to the wet ingredients and mix until it forms a dough.

6 Press the dough evenly over the top of the fruit and nut mixture in the pan. Bake for 45 minutes.

7 Let cool completely. Before serving, lift the cake from the pan by the parchment paper and place on a baking sheet or tray. Place a serving tray on top, then carefully invert the baking sheet onto the tray. Peel away the parchment paper to reveal the pineapple.

Makes 12 servings. Serve warm or at room temperature. Will keep for up to 1 week in an airtight container in the fridge.

Pomegranate Poached Pears

Sometimes the most delicious treats are also the simplest to make. This dessert is super-easy to prepare while you cook your main meal. Pears are one of the highest of the high-fiber fruits, offering 5 to 6 grams per medium-size pear, well on the way to meeting the daily requirement of 25 to 35 grams. Filling up on fiber keeps your digestion regular and prevents a belly bloated by constipation. Pears also contain the detox vitamins C, B2, B3, B6 and B9 (folate), as well as magnesium, potassium and manganese.

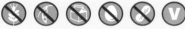

4	unpeeled Bosc or Bartlett pears, halved and cored
2 cups	organic pomegranate juice

to serve (optional)

½ cup	fresh pomegranate seeds
3 Tbsp	raw sliced almonds or Hemp Hearts

1 Place the pears in a 3- to 4-quart saucepan, then add the pomegranate juice. Bring to a low boil over medium-high heat.

2 Cover and reduce the heat to low. Let the pears simmer, gently turning occasionally so they color evenly, for 30 to 45 minutes, until tender.

3 Using a slotted spoon, divide the pears evenly among 4 serving plates, and set aside.

4 Reduce the remaining poaching liquid to ½ cup by boiling for 15 to 20 minutes.

5 Drizzle the reduced sauce over the pears, and if desired sprinkle with pomegranate seeds and the almonds or Hemp Hearts.

Makes 4 servings.

Save any leftover poaching liquid in a Mason jar in the fridge. Just add hot filtered water for a tasty warm drink.

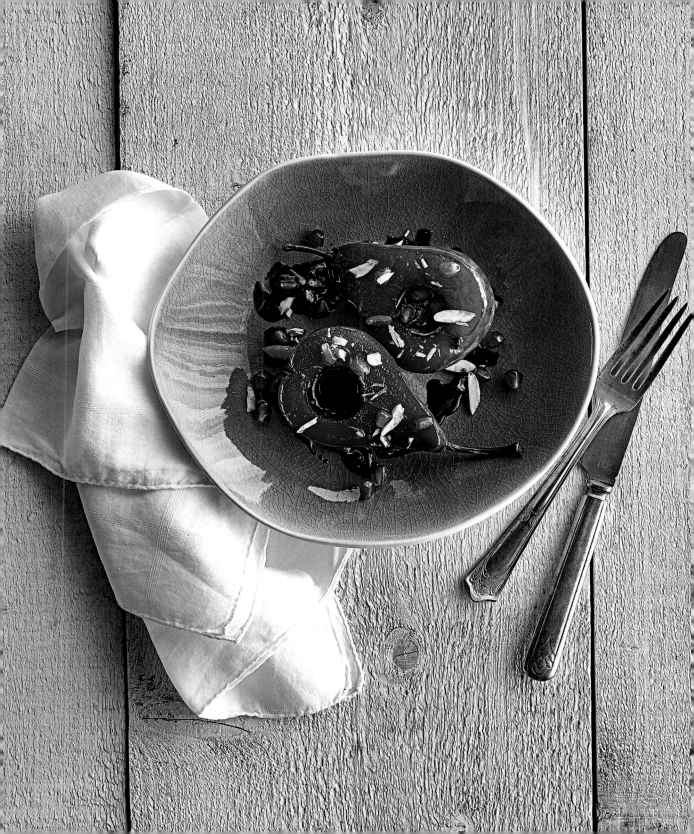

Resources

For appliance suggestions, check out www.JulieDaniluk.com.

Nature's Way
NutraSea Omega-3, herbs, and probiotics
825 Challenger Drive
Green Bay, WI 54311
www.naturesway.com

Fresh Hemp Foods Ltd.
Top-quality hemp seed products
69 Eagle Drive
Winnipeg, MB R2R 1V4
Canada
Tel: 204-953-0233
www.manitobaharvest.com

Bioforce USA
A.Vogel/BioSnacky
Sprouting supplies, herbal seasonings, Biotta Juice
6 Grandinetti Drive
Ghent, New York 12075
Tel: 1-800-641-7555
www.bioforceusa.com

Eden Foods, Inc.
Beans, sauces, seeds, dried fruit
701 Tecumseh Road
Clinton, MI 49236
Tel: 517-456-7854
www.edenfoods.com

ILIADA Olive Oil
6th klm National Highway Kalamata-Messini
24100 Kalamata
Greece
Tel: +30 2721069269

SaunaRay
Far-infrared saunas
620 Sixth Street
Collingwood, ON L9Y 3Y9
Canada
Tel: 877-992-1100
www.saunaray.com

Lemon Lily Tea
Certified Organic Teas
184 Davenport Road
Toronto, ON M5R 1J2
Canada
Tel: 416-846-1057
www.lemonlily.ca

The Hot Detox Tea (page 141)
is available at www.JulieDaniluk.com

Traditional Medicinals Tea
Certified Organic Teas
4515 Ross Road
Sebastopol, CA 95472
Tel: 1-800-543-4372
www.traditionalmedicinals.com

Shambu Yoga
Hatha yoga techniques
Box 123
Lynden, ON L0R 1T0
Canada
Tel: 613-265-5847
www.shambuyoga.com

The Institute for Functional Medicine
505 S. 336th Street
Suite 600
Federal Way, WA 98003
Tel: 1-800-228-0622
www.functionalmedicine.org

New York College of Traditional Chinese Medicine
200 Old Country Road
Suite 500
Mineola, NY 11501
Tel: 516-739-1545
www.nyctcm.edu

American College of Traditional Chinese Medicine (ACTCM)
450 Connecticut Street
San Francisco, CA 94107
Tel: 415-282-9603
www.actcm.edu

Wrap It Up ~ Raw Inc.
Grain-free flax wraps
Fenwick, ON L0S 1C0
Canada
Tel: 905-691-6551
www.wrapitupraw.com

Paleo Wraps
Coconut wraps
624 Garrison Street
Suite 101
Oceanside, CA 92054
Tel: 1-800-982-7323
http://paleowrap.com

Take Your Hot Detox to the Next Level with Julie's 21-Day Online Program!

Are you needing a helping hand to commit to the Hot Detox? Let me share more great techniques that will ensure your success.

People who have taken the Hot Detox Online Program report more energy, weight loss, clear skin, positive moods, less bloating, improved digestion and reduced pain!

This online program allows you to activate the Hot Detox with:

- Daily emails to support and motivate you during your detox
- Special coaching on how to mentally prepare yourself for success

> "Thank you, Julie, and all your team members who put this extraordinary 21-Day Hot Detox Online Program together. I really looked forward to the videos. It felt like I was doing it with a friend and really kept me motivated to stay the course. I feel great with more energy and more mental clarity. I feel more at peace and have a sense of calm. Teaching kindergarten ... I need all the calm I can get!"
> — Martha M.

PLUS...

Extensive guides and how-to videos to show you just how easy a detox can be, including:

- Powerful detox yoga videos
- Clearing your cupboards guide
- Tips on how to prepare and store food
- Cooking methods and demonstration videos
- Bonus activities and techniques to deepen your cleanse

Even more satisfying, delicious, nutritionally balanced recipes:

- Powerful elixirs
- Tasty teas
- Crave-busting, fast and easy snacks
- Superfood shakes that leave you happy and satisfied

Weekly menu plans and shopping list:

- Suggested weekly menu plans
- Daily menu planners and journals
- Printable weekly shopping lists
- Vegan menu plan for my plant-loving posse

Available at www.JulieDaniluk.com

Be sure to claim your bonuses for purchasing this book by visiting www.hotdetox.com.

References

Note: Throughout the book, I used the U.S. Department of Agriculture's "National Nutrient Database for Standard Reference," Release 28, September 2015 (ndb.nal.usda.gov) as a reference for nutrient content of foods. Please refer back to it for nutrition information.

For a detailed glossary, online resources and a complete list of references (with active links), visit www.JulieDaniluk.com.

Chapter 1: Creating Fire: The Benefits of the Hot Detox Program

Albright J.F., and Goldstein R.A. 1996. *Otolaryngoly–Head and Neck Surgery*. 114(2): 232–238.

Allen J., et al. 2011. *Journal of Alternative and Complementary Medicine*. 17(12): 1175–80.

Arnett T. 2008. *Journal of Nutrition*. 138: 4155–4185.

Baillie-Hamilton P.F. 2002. *Journal of Alternative and Complementary Medicine*. 8(2): 185–192.

Beasley J.D., and Swift J.J. 1989. The Kellogg Report. Annandale-on-Hudson, NY: Institute of Health Policy and Practice, Bard College Center. 4: 171.

Beinfield H., and Korngold E. 1991. *Between Heaven and Earth*. New York: Ballantine Books.

Bland J., et al. 1995. *Altern Ther Health Med*. 1: 62–71.

Butler L., et al. 2003. *American Journal of Epidemiology*. 157: 434–445.

Centers for Disease Control and Prevention. 1998. "*Helicobacter pylori*: Fact Sheet for Health Care Providers." Atlanta: CDC. http://www.cdc.gov/ulcer/files/hpfacts.pdf.

Chan D. n.d. "Chinese Nutrition by Food Group." *Acupuncture.com*. http://www.acupuncture.com/nutrition/chinut1.htm.

Cohen M. 1996. *The Chinese Way to Healing: Many Paths to Wholeness*. New York: Berkley Publishing Group.

Colbin A. 1986. *Food and Healing*. New York: Ballantine Books.

Conaway C., et al. 2000. *Nutrition and Cancer*. 38: 168–178.

Coronado-González J.A., et al. 2007. *Environmental Research*. 104(3): 383–389.

Gao D. 2013. *Traditional Chinese Medicine: The Complete Guide to Acupressure, Acupuncture, Chinese Herbal Medicine, Food Cures, and Qi Gong*. London: Carlton Books.

Hedren E., et al. 2002. *European Journal of Clinical Nutrition*. 56: 425–430.

Huang C.F., et al. 2011. *Kaohsiung Journal of Medical Sciences*. 27(9): 402–410.

Jarvis M., et al. 2003. *Plant, Cell, and Environment*. 26: 977–989.

Kastner J. 2009. *Chinese Nutrition Therapy: Dietetics in Traditional Chinese Medicine*. Stuttgart, NY: Thieme.

Kilburn K.H., et al. 1989. *Archives of Environmental Health*. 44(6): 345–250.

Klein A., and Kiat H. 2014. *Journal of Human Nutrition and Dietetics*. 28(6): 1–12.

Lamb J.J., et al. 2011. *Alternative Therapies in Health and Medicine*. 17(2): 36–44.

Lane R. 2011. "Day 13: Why Consider a Spring Detox?" http://www.turningpointnutrition.ca/tag/exotoxins.

Lim S., et al. 2010. *Annals of the New York Academy of Sciences*. 1201: 166–176.

Liska D.J. 1998. *Alternative Medicine Review*. 3(3): 187–198.

Mishra V. 2013. "Xenoestrogens: The Curse of Civilization." Chapter 185 in *Medicine Update 2013*. Mumbai: Association of Physicians of India. 815–820.

Mlynek V., and Skoczyńska A. 2005. *Advances in Hygiene and Experimental Medicine*. 59: 1–8.

Murphy R. 2006. "Homeopathic Toxicology." http://lotushealthinstitute.com/index.php/homeopathic-medicine-mainmenu-33/19-homeopathic-toxicology.

Navas-Acien A., et al. 2008. *Journal of the American Medical Association*. 300(7): 814–822.

Obtułowicz K. 2001. *Przegl Lek*. 58(4): 204–207.

Page L. 2008. *Healthy Healing's Detoxification: Programs to Cleanse, Purify & Renew*. Eden Prairie, MN: Healthy Healing Enterprises, LLC.

Pappas A. 2009. *Dermatoendocrinology*. 1: 262–267.

Percival M. 1997. "Nutritional Support for Detoxification." *Applied Nutritional Science Reports*. http://acudoc.com/Detoxification.PDF.

Pitchford P. 2002. *Healing with Whole Foods: Asian Traditions and Modern Nutrition*. Berkeley, CA: North Atlantic Books.

Schnare D.W., et al. 1982. *Medical Hypotheses*. 9(3): 265–282.

Schook L.B., and Laskin D.L., eds. 1994. *Xenobiotics and Inflammation: Roles of Cytokines and Growth Factors*. San Diego, CA: Academic Press.

Schwalfenberg G. 2012. *Journal of Environmental and Public Health*. 6: 1–12.

"Sulforaphane Glucosinolate Monograph." 2010. *Journal of Alt Med Review* 15: 352–360.

Tierra M., and Tierra L. 1998. *Chinese Traditional Herbal Medicine, Volume 1: Diagnosis and Treatment.* Twin Lakes, WI: Lotus Press.

Unlu N., et al. 2005. *American Society for Nutritional Sciences.* 135(3): 431–436.

Van het Hof K., et al. 2000. *Journal of Nutrition.* 130: 503–506.

Vereczkey L., et al. 1998. *Acta Pharmaceutica Hungarica.* 68(5): 284–288.

Verhagen M., et al. 1998. *Neurogastroenterol Mot.* 10: 175–181.

Vormann J., and Remer T. 2008. *Journal of Nutrition.* 138: 4135–4145.

Zinn A., and Palmer B. 2010. *American Journal of Medical Sciences.* 340: 481–491.

Zmrzljak U.P., and Rozman D. 2012. *Chemical Research in Toxicology.* 25(4): 811–824.

Chapter 2:
Start with the Gut

Abd Malek R., et al. 2010. *Current Research Technology and Education Topics in Applied Microbiology and Microbial Biotechnology.* 2: 1196–1204.

Aroutcheva A., et al. 2001. *Infect Dis Obstet Gynecol.* 9: 33–39.

Asai T., et al. 2000. *British Journal of Anaesthesia.* 85: 861–864.

Badet M., et al. 2001. *Journal of Applied Microbiology.* 90: 1015–1018.

Bassioni G., et al. 2015. *Int J Electrochem Sci.* 10: 3792–3802.

Bergqvist S., et al. 2005. *Food Microbiology.* 22: 53–61.

Chang J., et al. 2012 *Journal of Medical Microbiology.* 61: 361–368.

Chilton S., et al. 2015. *Nutrients.* 7: 390–404.

Coconnier M., et al. 1997. *Antimicrobial Agents and Chemotherapy.* 41: 1046–1052.

Craig C., and Stitzel R. 2004. *Modern Pharmacology with Clinical Applications.* Philadelphia: Lippincott Williams & Wilkins.

Crinnion W. 2010. *Alt Med Rev.* 15: 190–196.

Cross M., et al. 2001. *International Immunopharmacology.* 1: 891–901.

Dhingra D., et al. 2012. *J Food Sci Technol.* 49: 255–266.

Donato K., et al. 2010. *Microbiology.* 156: 3288–3297.

Drouault S., et al. 2002. *Appl Environ Microbiol.* 68: 938–941.

Giovannini M., et al. 2007. *Pediatric Research.* 62: 215–220.

Gomes A., and Malcata F. 1999. *Trends in Food Science and Technology.* 10: 139–157.

Groeger D., et al. 2013. *Gut Microbes.* 404: 325–339.

Guglielmetti S., et al. 2011. *Alimentary Pharmacology and Therapeutics.* 33: 1123–1132.

Hamada E., et al. 1997. *Biochimica et Biophysica Acta.* 1356: 198–206.

Heidelbaugh J. 2013. *Therapeutic Advances in Drug Safety.* 4: 125–133.

Hong S., et al. 2014. *Environmental Health and Toxicology.* 29: 1–6.

Ito T., and Jensen R. 2010. *Curr Gastroenterol Rep.* 12: 448–457.

Iwamoto T., et al. 2010. *Mosby.* 110: 201–208.

Jolliffe D. 2009. *Contin Educ Anaesth Crit Care Pain.* 9: 173–177.

Jungersen M., et al. 2014. *Microorganisms.* 2: 92–110.

Kabeerdoss J., et al. 2011. *Nutr J.* 10: 138.

Kelesidis T. 2012. *Therap Adv Gastroenterol.* 5: 111–125.

"Lactobacillus rhamnosus LGG." 2008. *Metagenics.* 2: 1–8.

Leiper J. 2015. *Nutrition Reviews.* 73: 57–72.

Lim B., et al. 2005. *Japanese J Can Res.* 93: 36–41.

Linsalata M. et al. 2010. *Current Pharmaceutical Design.* 16: 847–853.

Madara B., and Pomarico-Denino V. 2008. *Quick Look Nursing: Pathophysiology.* Mississauga, ON: Jones and Bartlett Publishers Canada.

Martinsen T., et al. 2005. *Basic and Clinical Pharmacology and Toxicology.* 96: 94–102.

Munoz J., et al. 2011. *Applied and Environmental Microbiology.* 77: 8775–8783.

National Research Council. 2005. *Dietary Reference Intakes for Energy, Carbohydrate, Fiber, Fat, Fatty Acids, Cholesterol, Protein, and Amino Acids (Macronutrients).* Washington, DC: National Academies Press.

Niku-Paavola M., et al. 1999. *Journal of Applied Microbiology.* 86: 29–36.

Nunamaker E., et al. 2013. *Journal of the American Association for Laboratory Animal Science.* 52: 22–27.

Ogata T., et al. 1999. *Microbial Ecology in Health and Disease.* 11: 41–46.

Okada H., et al. 2010. *Clinical and Experimental Immunology.* 160: 1–9.

Ouwehand A., et al. 2002. *Anton Leeuw Int J G.* 82: 279–289.

Parvez S., et al. 2006. *Journal of Applied Microbiology.* 100: 1171–1185.

Petrova P., et al. 2013. *Starch.* 65: 34–47.

Picard C., et al. 2005. *Ailment Pharmacol Ther.* 22: 495–512.

Reddy B., and Rivenson A. 1993. *Cancer Research.* 53: 3914–3918.

Sardesai V. 2012. *Introduction to Clinical Nutrition.* Boca Raton, FL: CRC Press.

Selhub E., et al. 2014. *Journal of Physiological Anthropology.* 33: 1–12.

Sharma R., et al. 2014. *Journal of Pharmacy and Biological Sciences.* 9: 52–58.

Shockey K., and Shockey C. 2014. *Fermented Vegetables: Creative Recipes for Fermenting 64 Vegetables and Herbs*. North Adams, MA: Storey Publishing.

Sonnenburg E., and Sonnenburg J. 2014. *Cell Metabolism*. 20: 779– 786.

Taipale T., et al. 2011. *British Journal of Nutrition*. 105: 409–416.

Tennant S., et al. 2008. *Infection and Immunity*. 76: 639–645.

Turroni F., et al. 2014. *Microbiology*. 5: 1–8.

Vani M., et al. 2012. *Indian Journal of Clinical Practice*. 23: 224–230.

Vargas S., et al. 1993. *Infection and Immunity*. 61: 619–626.

Vighi G., et al. 2008. *Clinical and Experimental Immunology*. 153: 3–6.

Weiss S. 2002. *New England Journal of Medicine*. 347: 930–931.

Yildirim Z., et al. 1999. *Journal of Applied Microbiology*. 86: 45–54.

Chapter 3: Give Back to Your Liver

Ahmad M., et al. 2000. *South Med J*. 93: 261–264.

Albright J.F., and Goldstein R.A. 1996. *Otolaryngoly – Head and Neck Surgery*. 114(2): 232–238.

Allen J., et al. 2011. *Journal of Alternative and Complementary Medicine*. 17(12): 1175–80.

Al-Malki A., et al. 2013. *Journal of Medicinal Plants Research*. 7: 1494–1505.

Alnouti Y. 2009. *Toxicol Sci*. 108: 225–46.

Anderson J., et al. 2009. *Nutrition Reviews*. 67: 188–205.

Anzenbacher P., and Zanger U. 2012. *Metabolism of Drugs and Other Xenobiotics*. Weinheim, Germany: Wiley-VCH.

Arterburn L. et al. 2006. *Am J Clin Nut*. 83: 1467–1476.

Atkuri K., et al. 2007. *Current Opinion in Pharmacology*. 7: 355–359.

Baillie-Hamilton P.F. 2002. *Journal of Alternative and Complementary Medicine*. 8(2): 185–192.

Baranski M., et al. 2014. *British Journal of Nutrition*. 112: 794–811.

Beasley J.D., and Swift J.J. 1989. The Kellogg Report. Annandale-on-Hudson, NY: Institute of Health Policy and Practice, Bard College Center. 4: 171.

Behara Y. 2011. *Journal of Pharmaceutical and Biomedical Sciences*. 11: 1–6.

Beinfield H., and Korngold E. 1991. *Between Heaven and Earth*. New York: Ballantine Books.

Bellows C., et al. 2005. *AAFP*. 72: 637–642.

Bottiglieri T. 2002. *American J of Clin Nutr*. 76: 1151–1157.

Brown A., et al. 1987. *Gut*. 28: 1426–1432.

"Calcium-D-glucarate." 2002. *Altern Med Rev*. 7: 336–339.

Capdevila J., et al. 2000. *Lipid Research*. 41: 163–181.

Chen M., et al. 2007. *Can J Gastroenterol*. 21: 155–158.

Cheng N., et al. 2013. *Food and Chemical Toxicology*. 55: 234–240.

Craig S. 2004. *Am J Clin Nutr*. 80: 539–549.

Coronado-González, J.A., et al. 2007. *Environmental Research*. 104(3): 383–389.

Das S., and Vasudevan D. 2006. *Indian J Biochem Biophys*. 43: 306–311.

Farahmandfar M., et al. 2012. *Surgical Science*. 3: 332–338.

Fife B. 2010. *The Healing Crisis*. Colorado Springs, CO: Empire Publishing Service.

Frahm D. 2000. *A Cancer Battle Plan Sourcebook*. Los Angeles: Tarcher.

Gaby A. 2009. *Alt Med Rev*. 14: 258–267.

Gamage N., et al. 2006. *Toxicological Sciences*. 90: 5–22.

Gebhard R., et al. 1996. *Hepatology*. 24: 544–548.

Gordon F. 2006. *100 Questions and Answers about Liver Transplantation: A Lahey Clinic Guide*. Burlington, MA: Jones & Bartlett Learning.

Griffin G. 1992. *Journal of Antimicrobial Chemotherapy*. 29(6): 613–616.

Higdon J., et al. 2007. *Pharmacol Res*. 55: 224–236.

Hinson J., et al. 2010. *Handb Exp Pharmacol*. 196: 369–405.

Houghton P., et al. 1984. *Br Med J*. 289: 1350.

Hsu C., et al. 2015. *Food and Nutrition Research*. 9: 1–7.

Huang C.F., et al. 2011. *Kaohsiung Journal of Medical Sciences*. 27(9): 402–410.

Jancova P., et al. 2010. *Biomed Pap Med Fac Univ*. 154: 103–116.

Johnston C., et al. 1993. *Am J Clin Nutr*. 58: 103–105.

Joseph M., et al. 2004. *Nutrition and Cancer*. 50: 206–213.

Keck A., and Finley J. 2004. *Integrative Cancer Therapies*. 3: 5–12.

Kelly G. 2011. *AltMed Review*. 16: 263–274.

Kilburn K.H., et al. 1989. *Archives of Environmental Health*. 44(6): 345–250.

King R., et al. 2006. *Curr Drug Metab*. 7: 745–753.

Kisker C., et al. 1997. *Annu. Rev. Biochem*. 66: 233–267.

Kopf R. 2015. *Schuessler Salts Cell Salts: Biochemistry Simply Explained*. Munich, Germany: BookRix.

Lamb J.J., et al. 2011. *Alternative Therapies in Health and Medicine*. 17(2): 36–44.

Lampe J., et al. 2000. *Carcinogenesis*. 21: 1157–1162.

Lampe J., et al. 2002. *Journal of Nutrition*. 132(6): 1341–1344.

Lane, R. 2011. "Day 13: Why Consider a Spring Detox?" http://www.turningpointnutrition.ca/tag/exotoxins.

Langmead L., et al. 2002. *Aliment Pharmacol Ther*. 16: 197–205.

Lattanzio V., et al. 2009 *Journal of Functional Foods*. 1: 131–144.

Lieber C. 2002. *Am R Clin Nutr*. 76: 1183–1187.

Lim S., et al. 2010. *Annals of the New York Academy of Sciences*. 1201: 166–176.

Lin S., et al. 2002. *J Biomed Sci*. 9: 401–409.

Liska, D.J. 1998. *Alternative Medicine Review*. 3(3): 187–198.

Maruti S., et al. 2008. *Cancer Epidemiol Biomarkers Prev*. 17: 1808–1812.

Maurer N., et al. 2012. *Food Chemistry*. 134: 1173–1180.

Mizutani T. 2009. *Journal of Environmental and Public Health*. 2009: 1–9.

Mlynek V., and Skoczyńska A. 2005. *Advances in Hygiene and Experimental Medicine*. 59: 1–8.

Mohamed M., and Frye R. 2011. *Drug Metab Dispos*. 39: 1522–1528.

Murphy R. 2006. "Homeopathic Toxicology." http://lotushealthinstitute.com/index.php/homeopathic-medicine-mainmenu-33/19-homeopathic-toxicology.

Murray M., and Pizzorno J. 2012. *The Encyclopedia of Natural Medicine*. 3rd edition. New York: Atria.

Navas-Acien A., et al. 2008. *Journal of the American Medical Association*. 300(7): 814–822.

Nimni M., et al. 2007. *Nutrition and Metabolism*. 4: 1–12.

Obeid R. 2013. *Nutrients*. 5: 3481–3495.

Obtułowicz, K. 2001. *Przegl Lek*. 58(4): 204–207.

Ogu C., and Maxa J. 2000. *BUMC Proceedings*. 13: 421–423.

Okwu D., and Emenike I. 2006. *International Journal of Molecular Medicine and Advance Sciences*. 2: 1–6.

Ozturk N., et al. 1998. *Phytomedicine*. 5: 283–288.

Page, L. 2008. *Healthy Healing's Detoxification: Programs to Cleanse, Purify & Renew*. Eden Prairie, MN: Healthy Healing Enterprises.

Palipoch S., et al. 2014. *Complementary and Alternative Medicine*. 14: 1–8.

Papaioannou R., and Pfeifer C. 1984. *Journal of Orthomolecular Psychiatry*. 13: 107–110.

Pearson J., et al. 1989. *Cancer*. 64: 911–915.

Percival, M. 1997. *Nutritional support for detoxification*. Applied Nutritional Science Reports. http://acudoc.com/Detoxification.PDF.

Perreault M., et al. 2013. *PLOS One*. 8: 1–9.

Platel K., et al. 2004. *Indian J Med Res*. 119: 167–179.

Powers H., and Thurnham D. 1981. *Br J Nut*. 46: 257–266.

Pu H., et al. 2012. *Evidence-Based Complementary and Alternative Medicine*. 2012: 1–7.

Radu D., et al. 2012. *Journal of Agroalimentary Processes and Technologies*. 18: 219–222.

Raftogianis R., et al. 2000. *J Natl Cancer Inst Monogr*. 27: 113–124.

Rakel D. 2012. *Integrative Medicine*. Philadelphia: Elsevier.

Rhoades R., and Bell D. 2013. *Medical Physiology: Principles for Clinical Medicine*. Philadelphia: Lippincott Williams & Wilkins.

Rideout T., et al. 2008. *Vascular Health and Risk Management*. 4: 1023–1033.

Rodriguez-Fragoso L., and Reyes-Esparza, J. 2013. "Fruit/Vegetable-Drug Interactions: Effects on Drug Metabolizing Enzymes and Drug Transporters." Chapter 1 in *Drug Discovery*, ed. H.A. El-Shemy. Rijeka, Croatia: In Tech.

Schnare D.W., et al. 1982. *Medical Hypotheses*. 9(3): 265–282.

Shay K., et al. 2009. *Biochem Biophys Acta*. 10: 1149–1160.

Shenfield G. 2004. *Clin Biochem Rev*. 25: 203–206.

Shimada T., et al. 2012. *Chem Res Toxicol*. 21: 2313–2323.

Stinton L., and Shaffer E. 2012. *Gut and Liver*. 6: 172–187.

Strasberg S. 2008. *NEMJ*. 358: 2804–2811.

Sun J. 2007. *Alt Med Rev*. 12: 259–264.

Surai P. 2015. *Antioxidants*. 4: 204–247.

Sweeney B., et al. 2006. *Anaesthesia*. 61: 159–177.

Tchounwou P., et al. 2012. *EXS*. 101: 133–164.

Timby B., and Smith N. 2014. *Introductory Medical-Surgical Nursing*. Philadelphia: Lippincott Williams and Wilkins.

Ueng T., et al. 1998. *Journal of Toxicology and Environmental Health*. 54: 509–527.

Val, S., et al. 2009. *Inhalation Toxicology*. 21 Suppl 1: 115–122.

Velpen G., et al. 1993. *Gut*. 34: 1448–1451.

Vereczkey, L., et al. 1998. *Acta Pharmaceutica Hungarica*. 68(5): 284–288.

Volak L., et al. 2008. *Drug Metab Dispos*. 36: 1594–1605.

Wallwork J., et al. 1985. *Journal of Nutrition*. 115: 252–262.

Wauthier V., et al. 2007. *Current Medicinal Chemistry*. 14: 745–757.

Wu B., et al. 2011. *Curr Drug Metab*. 12: 900–916.

Wu G., et al. 2004. *J. Nut*. 134: 489–492.

Wu J., et al. 2008. *Drug Metabolism and Disposition*. 36: 589–596.

Yang C., et al. 1992. *FASEB Journal*. 6: 737–744.

Zanger U., et al. 2013. *Pharmacology and Therapeutics*. 138: 103–141.

Zhang D., and Surapaneni, S. 2012. Appendix: Drug Metabolizing Enzymes and Biotransformation Reactions. *ADME-Enabling Technologies in Drug Design and Development*. Hoboken, NJ: Wiley.

Zmrzljak U.P., and Rozman D. 2012. *Chem Res Toxicol*. 25(4): 811–824.

Chapter 4: Love Your Lymph

Angeli V., and Randolph G. 2006. *Lymphat Res Biol*. 4(4): 217–228.

Beuth J., and Moss R. 2006. *Complementary Oncology: Adjunctive Methods in the Treatment of Cancer*. New York: Thieme.

Canadian Cancer Society's Advisory Committee on Cancer Statistics. 2015. *Canadian Cancer Statistics 2015*. Toronto: Canadian Cancer Society.

Chaitow L. 2008. *Naturopathic Physical Medicine: Theory and Practice for Manual Therapists and Naturopaths*. Toronto: Elsevier.

"Echinacea Monograph." 2001. *Alt Med Rev*. 6: 411–414.

Feldman E., et al. 1983. *J of Lipid Res*. 24(8): 967–976.

Ferracane R., et al. 2010. *Journal of Pharm Biomed Anal*. 51(2): 399–404.

Goats G. 1994. *British Journal of Sports Medicine*. 28(3): 153–156.

Hoffmann D. 2003. "Materia Medica." Chapter 26 in *Medical Herbalism: The Science and Practice of Herbal Medicine*. Rochester: VT: Healing Arts Press. 528–600.

Jones J., et al. 1997. *Journal of Experimental Biology*. 200: 1695–1702.

Kastner J. 2004. *Chinese Nutrition Therapy: Dietetics in Traditional Chinese Medicine*. New York: Thieme.

Lachance P., et al. 2013. *PlosOne*. 8(9): 1–12.

Lane K., et al. 2005. *Sports Med*. 35(6): 461–471.

Ligor M., et al. 2013. *Food Anal Methods*. 6: 630–636.

Miller S. 2005. *Evid Based Complement Alternat Med*. 2: 309–314.

Rayman M. 2005. *Proceedings of the Nutrition Society*. 64: 527–542.

Rutto L., et al. 2013. *International Journal of Food Science*. 2013: 1–9.

Vairo G., et al. 2009. *Journal of Manual and Manipulative Therapy*. 17(3): 80–89.

Williams A., et al. 2002. *European Journal of Cancer Care*. 11: 254–261.

Yadav R., et al. 2013. *International Journal of Agriculture and Food Science Technology*. 4(7): 707–712.

Chapter 5: Be Kind to Your Kidneys

Bolignano D., et al. 2007. *Journal of Renal Nutrition*. 17: 225–234.

Brasnyó P., et al. 2011. *British Journal of Nutrition*. 106(3): 383–389.

Breslau N., et al. 1988. *Journal of Clinical Endocrinology & Metabolism*. 66(1): 140–146.

Crandall, J., et al. 2012. *Journals of Gerontology Series A: Biological Sciences and Medical Sciences*. 67(12): 1307–1312.

Drezner M. 2015. "Patient Education: Vitamin D Deficiency." UpToDate: Wolters Kluwer. http://www.uptodate.com/contents/vitamin-d-deficiency-beyond-the-basics.

Garland C., et al. 2006. *Am J Public Health*. 96: 252–261.

Hall J., and Guyton A. 2011. *Textbook of Medical Physiology*. Philadelphia: Elsevier.

Health Canada. 2012. "Vitamin D and Calcium: Updated Dietary Reference Intakes." http://www.hc-sc.gc.ca/fn-an/nutrition/vitamin/vita-d-eng.php.

Hosseini F., et al. 2009. *Pakistan Journal of Biological Sciences*. 12: 1140–1145.

Johnson R., et al. 2007. *Am J Clin Nut*. 86: 899–906.

Kim C., and Kim S. 2014. *Korean J Intern Med*. 29: 416–427.

Kitada M., et al. 2013. *Oxidative Medicine and Cellular Longevity*. 2013: 1–7.

Lee J., et al. 2009. *Cancer Epidemiol Biomarkers Prev*. 18: 1730–1739.

Massey L., et al. 2004. *Journal of Urology*. 172(2): 555–558.

Orth S., and Hallan S. 2008. *Clin J Am Soc of Neph*. 3(1): 226–236.

Real Salt Elemental Analysis. Heber City, UT: Redmond Trading Company, LC. http://redmond.life/pdfs/IsYourSaltRealBooklet.pdf.

Ross A.C., et al. 2011. *Dietary Reference Intakes for Calcium and Vitamin D*. Washington, DC: National Academies Press.

Saldana T., et al. 2007. *Epidemiology*. 18: 501–506.

Tofovic S., et al. 2002. *Kidney International*. 61: 1433–1444.

Trujillo J., et al. 2013. *Redox Biology*. 1: 448–456.

United States Department of Agriculture. 2003. *Agriculture Fact Book 2001–2002*. Washington, DC: USDA. http://www.usda.gov/factbook/2002factbook.pdf.

Williams S., et al. 2009. *Ethn Dis*. 19: 1–7.

Wood R. 2010. *The New Whole Foods Encyclopedia*. New York: Penguin.

Yang, W., et al. 2014. *American Journal of Kidney Diseases*. 63(2): 236–243.

Chapter 6: Exercise the Breath with Lung Detoxification

Amra B., et al. 2006. *Respiratory Medicine*. 100: 110–114.

Asokan S., et al. 2008. *J Indian Soc Pedod Prev Dent*. 26(1): 12–7.

Asokan S., et al. 2009. *Indian J Dent Res*. 20(1): 47–51.

Asokan S., et al. 2011. *Indian J Dent Res*. 22(1): 34–7.

Asokan S., et al. 2011. *J Indian Soc Pedod Prev Dent*. 29(2): 90–4.

Button B., and Button B. 2013. *Cold Spring Harb Perspect Med*. 3(8): 1–16.

Carbone J., and Marini J. 1984. *Western Journal of Medicine*. 140: 398–402.

Claudio L. 2011. *Environ Health Perspect*. 119: a426–a427.

Consolazio C., et al. 1963. *Journal of Applied Physiology*. 18(1): 65–68.

Dean W. 1981. *JAMA*. 246: 623.

Dodd S., et al. 2008. *Expert Opin Biol Ther.* 8: 1955–1962.

Field T. 2011. *Complementary Therapies in Clinical Practice.* 17: 1–8.

Guo Y., et al. 2014. *Int J Clin Exp Med.* 7: 5842–5846.

Hermelingmeier K., et al. 2012. *American Journal of Rhinology and Allergy.* 26: 119–125.

Kobayashi K., et al. 2007. *Using Houseplants to Clean Indoor Air.* Honolulu, HI: College of Tropical Agriculture and Human Resources.

Kukkonen-Harjula K., et al. 2006. *International Journal of Circumpolar Health.* 65: 195–205.

Lansley K., et al. 2011. *J Appl Physiol.* 110: 591–600.

Masuda A., et al. 2005. *J Psychosom Res.* 58(4): 383–7.

Masuda A., et al. 2005. *Psychosomatic Medicine.* 67(4): 643–7.

Masuda A., et al. 2007. *Nippon Rinsho* [in Japanese]. 65(6): 1093–8.

Matveïkov G.P., et al. 1993. Ter. Arkh. [in Russian]. 65(12): 48–51.

McDonald E., et al. 2002. *Chest Journal.* 122: 1535–1542.

McEwen B.S. 1998. *Annals of the New York Academy of Sciences.* 840: 33–44.

Mero A., et al. 2015. *SpringerPlus.* 4: 1–7.

Natural Resources Defense Council. n.d. "How to Buy a Safer Sofa." https://www.nrdc.org/stories/how-buy-safer-sofa.

Nurmikko T., et al. 1992. *Pain.* 49(1): 43–51.

Oliver N., and Sharp R. 2015. "Five Couches without Fire Retardants You Can Buy Right Now." Environment Working Group. http://www.ewg.org/enviroblog/2015/03/five-couches-without-flame-retardants-you-can-buy-right-now.

Price S., and Price L. 1999. *Aromatherapy for Health Professionals.* 2nd edition. Toronto: Churchill Livingston.

Riedl M., et al. 2009. *Clinical Immunology.* 130: 244–251.

Schmidt K.L. 1991. *Zeitschrift für die gesamte innere Medizin und ihre Grenzgebiete* [in German]. 46(10–11): 370–4.

Schnaubelt K. 2011. *The Healing Intelligence of Essential Oils: The Science of Advanced Aromatherapy.* Toronto: Healing Arts Press.

Scoon G.S., et al. 2007. *Journal of Science and Medicine in Sport / Sports Medicine Australia.* 10(4): 259–62.

Singh S., et al. 2012. *Indian J Physiol Pharmacol.* 56: 63–68.

Tsatsoulis A., et al. 2006. *Annals of the New York Academy of Sciences.* 1083: 196–213.

United States Environmental Protection Agency. 2000. "Vinyl Chloride." https://www3.epa.gov/airtoxics/hlthef/vinylchl.html.

Valderramas S., and Nagib A. 2009. *Respiratory Care.* 54: 327–333.

Wilson R. 1995. *A Complete Guide to Understanding and Using Aromatherapy for Vibrant Health.* New York: Avery Publishing Group.

Wolverton B.C., et al. 1989. *Interior Landscape Plants for Indoor Air Pollution Abatement.* NASA Final Report.

Young G. 2003. *Essential Oils: Integrative Medical Guide.* Lehi, UT: Essential Science Publishing.

Zinchuk V., and Zhadzko D. 2012. *Medicina Sportiva.* 8: 1883–1889.

Chapter 7: Love the Skin You're In

Baker B.S. 2006. *Clin Exp Immunol.* 144 (1): 1–9.

Baronzio G., et al. 2006. *In Vivo.* 20: 689–696.

Bieuzen F., et al. 2013. *PLOS One.* 8: 1–15.

Bowe W., and Logan A. 2011. *Gut Pathogens.* 3: 1–11.

Chaitow L. 2008. *Naturopathic Physical Medicine: Theory and Practice for Manual Therapists and Naturopaths.* Toronto: Elsevier.

Chen Y., and Lyga J. 2014. *Inflammation and Allergy: Drug Targets.* 13: 177–190.

Chia K., and Tey H. 2013. *JEADV.* 27: 799–804.

Crinnion W. 2007. *Altern Ther Health Med.* 13: 154–156.

Dahl M.V. 1993. *J Am Acad Dermatol.* 28(5): S19–S23.

Dierendonck D., and Nijenhuis J. 2005. *Psychology and Health.* 20: 405–412.

Fiscus K., et al. 2005. *Arch Phys Med Rehabil.* 86: 1404–1410.

Flora S., and Pachauri V. 2010. *Int J Environ Res Public Health.* 7: 2745–2788.

Forton F. 2012. *J Eur A Derm Vener.* 26: 19–28.

Frey B., et al. 2012. *Int J. Hyperthermia.* 28(6): 528–542.

Genuis S., et al. 2003. *ISRN Toxicology.* 2003: 1–7.

Genuis S., et al. 2010. *Arch Environ Contam Toxicol.* 2: 1–15.

Genuis S., et al. 2012. *Journal of Environmental Medicine and Public Health.* https:www.hindawi.com/journals/jeph/2012/185731.

Genuis S. et al. 2013. *The Scientific World Journal.* 4: 1–3.

Guo Y., et al. 2014. *Int J Clin Exp Med.* 7: 5842–5846.

Jarmuda, S., et al. 2012. *J Med Microbiol.* 61(11): 1504–10.

Jonsson K., et al. 2014. *E J Int Med.* 6: 601–609.

Juliff L., et al. 2014. *J of Streng Cond Res.* 28: 2353–2358.

Kjellgren A., et al. 2008. *Qualitative Report.* 13: 636–656.

Kjellgren A., and Westman J. 2014. *Complementary and Alternative Medicine.* 14: 417–425.

Kober M., and Bowe W. 2015. *Int J Women's Derm*. 1: 85–89.

Kudesia R., and Bianchi M. 2012. *ISRN Neurology*. 2012: 1–7.

Laake D., and Compart P. 2013. *The ADHD and Autism Nutritional Supplement Handbook*. Beverley, MA: Fair Winds Press.

Lambers H., et al. 2006. *Int J Cosmet Sci*. 28(5): 359–70.

Liu Y., et al. 2014. *PLOS One*. 9: 1–9.

Morgan P., et al. 2013. *J of Stren Cond Res*. 27: 3467–3474.

Muizzudin N., et al. 2012. *Journal of Cosmetic Science*. 63(6): 385–395.

Neal, A., and Guilarte T. 2013. *Toxic Res*. 2(20): 99–114.

Olszowski T., et al. 2012. *Acta Biochimica*. 59: 475–482.

Parodi A., et al. 2008. *Clin Gastro Hep*. 6: 759–764.

Paulino L.C., et al. 2006. *J Clin Microbiol*. 44(8): 2933–41.

Rae W. 1997. *Chemical Sensitivity, Volume 4: Tools of Diagnosis and Methods of Treatment*. Boca Raton, FL: Lewis Publishers.

Sears M., and Genuis S. 2012. *J Env Pub Health*. 2012: 1–15.

Sears M., et al. 2012. *Journal of Environmental and Public Health*. 2012: 1–10.

Turner J., and Fine T. 1983. *Applied Psychophysiology and Biofeedback*. 8(1): 115–126.

Warburton D., et al. 2006. *CMAJ*. 176: 801–809.

Waring R. 2006. "Report on Absorption of Magnesium Sulfate across the Skin." http://www.epsomsaltcouncil.org/wp-content/uploads/2015/10/report_on_absorption_of_magnesium_sulfate.pdf.

Chapter 9: The Hot Detox

Ahima R.S., et al. 2000. *Front Neuroendocrinolgy*. 21(3): 263–307.

Arguin H.I. 2012. *Menopause*. 19(8): 870–876.

Bland J.E. 1995. *Alternative Therapies in Health and Medicine*. 1(5): 62–71.

Breuss R. 1995. *Breuss Cancer Cure*. Burnaby, BC: Alive Books

Cunningham M. 1986. *AAOHN Journal*. 34(6): 277–279.

Dannecker E.Y. 2012. *Experimental Gerontology*. 48(10): 1101–1106

de Rosa G., et al. 1983. *Experimental and Clinical Endocrinology*. 82(5): 173–177.

Dulloo A.G., and Jacquet J. 1998. *American Journal of Clinical Nutrition*. 68(3): 599–606.

Dulloo A.G., and Samec S. 2001. *British Journal of Nutrition*. 86(2): 123–139.

Duncan B.B. 2000. *Obesity*. 8(4): 279–286.

Faris M.S.-K. 2012. *Nutrition Research*. 32(12): 947–955.

Friedl K.E., et al. 2000. *Journal of Applied Physiology*. 88(5): 1820–1830.

Gerson M. 1958. *A Cancer Therapy: Results of Fifty Cases and the Cure of Advanced Cancer by Diet Therapy: A Summary of 30 Years of Clinical Experimentation*. San Diego, CA: Gerson Institute.

Goff J.L. 2000. *Advanced Nutrition and Human Metabolism*. Belmont, CA: Wadsworth/Thomson Learning.

Grant E.C. 1988. *British Medical Journal*. 296(6622): 607–609.

Heilbronn L.K., et al. 2005. *American Journal of Clinical Nutrition*. 81(1): 69–73.

Horne B.D., et al. 2008. *American Journal of Cardiology*. 102(7): 814–819.

Immamura M.T. 1984. *American Journal of Industrial Medicine*. 5(1): 147–153.

Kilburn K.R. 1989. *Archives of Environmental Health*. 44(6): 345–250.

Klein S., et al. 2000. *American Journal of Physiology Endocrinology and Metabolism*. 278(2): E280–E284.

Kozusko F. 2001. *Bulletin of Mathematical Biology*. 63(2): 393–403.

Lamb J.V. 2011. *Alternative Therapies in Health and Medicine*. 17(2): 36–44.

Mansell P., and MacDonald M.P. 1988. *British Journal of Nutrition*. 60(1): 39–48.

MacIntosh A., and Ball K. 2000. *Alternative Therapies in Health and Medicine*. 6(4): 70–76.

Meyer W.C., et al. 2001. *International Journal of Obesity and Related Metabolic Disorders*. 25(5): 593–600.

Müller H. 2001. *Scandinavian Journal of Rheumatology*. 30(1): 1–10.

National Research Council/Committee on the Toxicological Effects of Methylmercury. 2000. *Toxicological Effects of Methylmercury*. Washington, DC: National Academy Press.

Schnare D.G. 1982. *Medical Hypotheses*. 9(3): 265–282.

Schteingart D.L. 2002. *Endocrinology and Metablolism Clinics of North America*. 31(1): 173–189.

Stohs S.J. 2011. *Journal of Basic Clinical Physiology and Pharmacology*. 6(3): 205–228.

Thune I.T. 1997. *New England Journal of Medicine*. 336(18): 1269–1275.

Wan R.I. 2009. *Journal of Nutritional Biochemistry*. 21(5): 413–417.

Watson B. 2008. *The Detox Strategy: Vibrant Health in 5 Easy Steps*. New York, NY: Free Press.

Williams K.M. 1998. *Diabetes Care*. 21(1): 2–

Acknowledgments

My gratitude overflows toward the team that created this book with me:

Brad Wilson was my editor at HarperCollins. His loveable and gentle soul believed in this book when it was just a phantom of an idea. He made sure that this book is as beautiful as it is useful. Also kudos to managing editor Noelle Zitzer, my publisher Iris Tupholme and my publicist Melissa Nowakowski for their support.

My publisher at Hay House, Reid Tracy, has stuck with me through my early growth. Being part of Louise L. Hay's special family of authors means the world to me. Hay House editor Sally Mason is so diligent and appreciates my healthy gourmet recipes.

My naturopathic adviser, Dr. Lynne Racette, ND, helped to clarify and fact check information and contributed to the lymph and liver sections. She also did a great job of making sense of the hundreds of references. Thank you for your diligence!

Medical illustrator Leanne Chan brought my analogies to life. Video producer Katie Stewart created the lovely infographics and captured the Hot Detox Online Program. Their artistic spirit is delightful.

Katie Mitton captured some of my thoughts by dictation while I recovered from a back injury. Her joyful work ethic made sure we could hit our deadline.

Photographer Shannon Ross was so insightful and generous. Along with fab food stylist Chantel Payette and her husband, Sean, Shannon made my Hot Detox recipes prettier than in my wildest daydreams. Other great styling help came from Kirstin Johns, Julia Hrivnak and Tanya Scata. Thanks also to Christine Buijs for the fun cover photo!

Thanks to my book designer, Gareth Lind.

Lead recipe testers Angela Gagnon, Kaydn Gangnier and Laura James have been such a loving presence in my test kitchen. Thanks also to Beverley Szandtner, Erica Liebenberg, Andre Stringari and Marilyn Denis.

My literary agent and friend Rick Broadhead will stop at nothing to ensure I am taken care of.

Fellow nutritionists Sarah Britton and Marni Wasserman contributed tasty recipes. Freelance editors Grace Yaginuma and Tracy Bordian helped with precision.

Thanks to fellow healers Dr. Zoltan Rona, Kate Kent, Dr. Susan Sun, Bryce Wylde, Sarah Dobec, Taevan Gangnier, Melissa Ramos, Kris Carr, Gabrielle Bernstein, Dr. Ted Chung, Dr. Kate Wharton, Penny Hopp, Sarah Walton and Dr. Patricia McCord. Their therapeutic talents opened my eyes to new concepts that influenced this book.

My book tour supporters, Geoff Wills of Nature's Way, Mackie I. Vadacchino and Manon Bibeau of Bioforce Canada Inc., and Mike Fata and Kelly Sanderson of Manitoba Harvest Hemp Foods, provided assistance to ensure that we can reach the readers with live workshops that motivate true vitality.

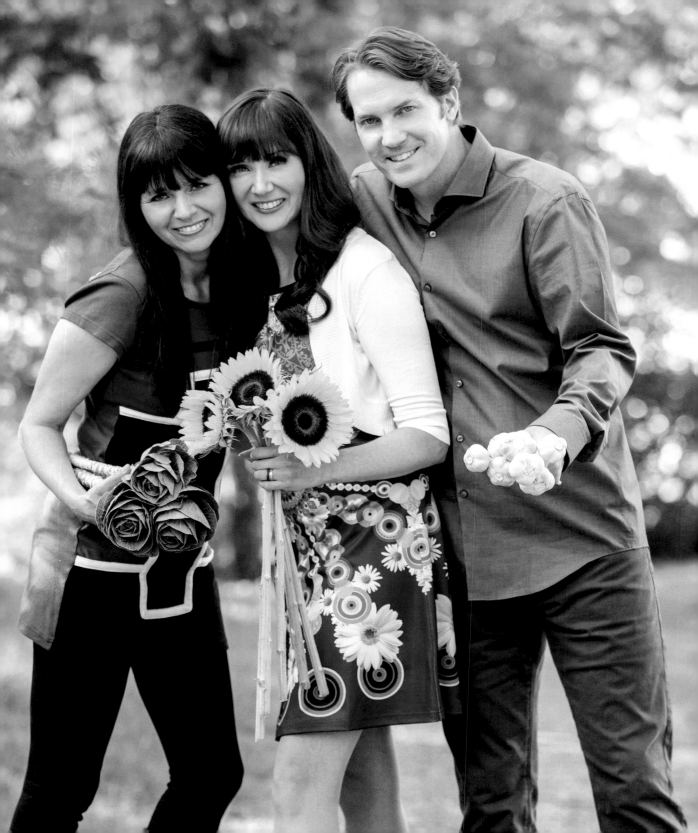

Index

Chinese traditional medicine (*cont.*)
  on dampness and mucus, 52, 62, 68, 194
  energetics of food, 17–18t
  on kidneys and adrenal glands, 60
  on sweet cravings, 193
  yin and yang states, 15, 18, 60
cleavers, 52
cold or cooling foods
  in Ayurvedic and Chinese traditions,
    14–19, 105, 144, 205
  food energetics, 16–17t
  fruits, 94
  raw foods, 12, 15, 86
  vegetables, 92
cold weather, 2, 9–20, 18, 58
colitis, 12, 128
colon, 28–9, 31
constipation. See stools and bowel
    movements
contractive foods, 18
contrast hydrotherapy, 75–6
cooking
  advance preparation, 86–7, 99
  ingredients and shopping lists, 85–6
  tools and equipment for, 84–5
cortisol, 60, 79, 105
cortisone creams, 79
Crohn's disease (inflammatory gastroin-
    testinal disease), 12, 128
curcumin, 195
cutting boards, 84
cytokines, 12, 20t, 34

dehydration
  constipation with, 29
  headaches with, 99
  vs hunger, 103
dehydrators, 85
diabetes
  benefits of cinnamon for, 194
  benefits of exercise for, 72
  benefits of fiber for, 30, 150
  toxins linked to, 20
diarrhea. See stools and bowel
    movements
digestive fire (*agni*), 9, 14
doshas, 14

eggs
  selection and guidelines for, 89, 93
energetics of food, 16–17t
Epsom salt
  for flotation bath, 76
  for salt scrub, 79

essential oils
  actions and indications, 70t
  for respiratory system, 68
  for salt scrubs, 79
exercise
  cardiovascular, 64
  for kidney function, 60
  for lungs and respiration, 63–4, 103–4
  sweating with, 72
expansive foods, 18

fatigue (during detoxification), 100
fiber
  with juicing or blending, 86, 128–9
  role in detoxification, 30, 32, 45
  soluble vs insoluble, 30–1, 32t, 45
  sources of, 31, 32t
fibromyalgia, 12, 21–2, 69
flavonoids
  in asparagus, 248
  in citrus fruits, 45, 133, 162, 260, 308
  in fennel and anise, 136
  in kudzu, 174
  in quinoa, 282
  in thyme, 268
food allergies. See under allergies
food dyes, 96
food preservatives, 97
food processors, 84, 85
food rainbow, 44, 45, 128
food reintroduction (after cleanse),
    116–19
food shopping, 85, 90
frozen foods
  impact of, 9, 15, 130
  for storage, 86–7, 200, 223

gallbladder and gallstones, 25, 27, 36,
    46–9, 195
gastrointestinal tract, 23–36
gastrointestinal transit times, 28
glass canning jars (Mason jars), 30, 84
glucuronic acid and glucuronidation, 41,
    42t, 302
glutathione (enzyme), 31, 41, 42t, 52, 57, 64
glycine, 41, 42t, 172
grapefruit essential oil, 70t
graters, 84
green foods, 45t, 86, 128
green-light food guidelines, 92–5

H. pylori, 13, 35, 131, 210
headaches, 99–100

heartburn, 14, 24, 136
heat therapies, 22, 69, 72–5
heavy metals. See metal toxins
HEPA filters, 65
Hot Detox Plan, 83–119
  3-day version, 83, 87, 114–15
  10-day version, 83, 87, 110–11, 112–13
  21-day version, 83, 87, 106–9
  benefits, 4, 9–22
  Busy Person's Plan, 112–13
  commitment to, 83, 86, 88
  cravings during, 103–5
  dining out during, 103
  focus of, 1–4, 83
  guidelines for, 92–7
  phases of (see Phase 1; Phase 2; Phase 3)
  preparation for, 83–90
  reintroducing foods after, 102–3, 116
  rules for, 99
  scheduling of, 87–8
  scientific perspectives on, 21–2
  social support during, 90, 103
  spices for, 194–5
Hot Detox Solutions, 29–36, 44–6, 58–60
Hot Detox yoga flow, 54, 60, 73
house plants, 65
humidifiers, 68
hydration, 29–30, 58–9, 95, 99
hydrochloric acid, 10, 26, 27
hydrotherapy, 54, 75–6

immune system
  benefits of broth for, 182
  reactions of, 12
  role of digestive tract, 34
  role of lymphatic system, 51
inflammation
  with cooling foods, 17, 18
  with food allergies, 17, 29
  with food particles in blood, 12, 13
  with grilling or frying, 18
  with hot spices, 14
  impact of, 9, 10, 62
  with intestinal hyperpermeability,
    12–13
  in lungs, 62–3
  with nightshades, 96
  in sinuses, 67
  with sugars, 96, 97
  with toxins, 20t
  yellow- and red-light guidelines for,
    92, 95–7
inflammatory bowel disease (IBD), 31, 89,
    92, 240
insulin, 27

intestinal hyperpermeability (leaky gut syndrome), 12, 13, 29
intestines, 27–8
irritable bowel syndrome (IBS), 28, 63, 89, 92, 240

juicing
    compared to blending, 128–9
    health benefits, 44, 59
    juice extractors or presses, 129

kapha dosha, 14–15
kidneys, 55–60
    and blood pressure, 57–8
    and energy production, 60
    function of, 55–6
    hormones produced by, 56
    toxins affecting, 19, 57
kitchen tools and equipment, 84–5, 87
knives, 84

leaky gut. See intestinal hyperpermeability
Lee, Bruce, 139
lemon essential oil, 70
light-headedness, 100
lipase (enzyme), 10
liver, 37–49
    detoxification phases, 38–43
    nutrients for, 40, 42–3, 45–6, 195
    rainbow of foods for, 44, 45
    toxins processed by, 19, 39
lobelia, 62
lungs, 61–70
    foods and herbal remedies for, 62
    function of, 61
    and gastrointestinal conditions, 63
    and pet allergies, 66
    respiration exercises, 63–4, 103–4
    salt air for, 68
    sinus cleansing, 67
    toxins affecting, 19, 64–8
lutein, 45t, 298
lymph drainage massage, 54
lymphatic system, 51–4

magnesium
    for headaches, 100
    sources of, 76, 79, 93, 222, 276, 278, 302
mechanical digestion, 10
meditation, 60, 105
menu plans (for Hot Detox)

for 3-day version, 114–15
for 10-day version, 110–11
for 21-day version, 106–9
adaptation of, 91
for busy people, 112–13
mercury, 20t, 22, 73, 74, 212
metal toxins (heavy metals), 20t, 73, 75, 223
methylation, 41, 42t, 43, 230, 302
milk thistle, 46
mouthcare
    oil pulling, 66, 78
    tongue cleaning, 68, 78
    tooth brushing, 105
mucus
    excess of, 14–15, 62, 63
    in gastrointestinal tract, 26, 32, 52, 63
    in respiratory tract, 62–3, 69
mullein, 62

N-acetylcysteine (NAC), 41, 64
nature therapy (*shinrin-yoku*), 64
neti pot (*jala neti*), 67
neutral foods, 16–17t, 94
nightshades, 96, 195, 258, 269
Nordic spa techniques, 66

oils and fats
    for bowel lubrication, 36
    for cooking, 94
    during detoxification, 44–5, 94, 104–5
    omega-3 oils, 36, 45, 94
    for salt scrubs, 79
omnivore cleansing, 88, 89–90
orange foods, 18, 45t, 48, 128, 193
oregano, oil of, 68

packaged or processed food, 97
pancreas, 24, 26, 27
peristalsis, 10, 24, 27, 29
pets, 66
pH balance, 10–12
Phase 1 (of Hot Detox Plan)
    10-day menu plan, 110–11
    21-day menu plan, 106–7
    description and focus of, 98
    joy and clarity during, 101
    omnivore option for, 88
    repetition or extension of, 101
    vegan option for, 88
    vegetarian option for, 88
Phase 2 (of Hot Detox Plan)
    10-day menu plan, 110–11
    21-day menu plan, 106–7

description and focus of, 99–101
    symptoms and solutions during, 99–100
    vegan liquid meal plan for, 99
    weight loss during, 99
Phase 3 (of Hot Detox Plan)
    10-day menu plan, 110–11
    21-day menu plan, 108–9
    description and focus of, 102
    omnivore option for, 88
    vegan option for, 88
    vegetarian option for, 88
pitta dosha, 14, 144, 195
potassium, 58, 59, 222, 229
pranayama, 63–4, 104
prebiotics, 29, 31–2
preparation phase (of Hot Detox), 84–90
probiotic mask, 78
probiotics, 32–6
    and intestinal transit times, 28
    soil-based organisms, 36
    sources of, 29, 33t, 34–5, 208
probiotics: types of
    Bifidobacterium bifidum, 35, 78
    Lactobacillus acidophilus, 34, 35
    Saccharomyces boulardii, 35
    Streptococcus thermophilus, 78
protein
    balance with calories, 103
    for food cravings, 103
    green-light guidelines, 93
    omnivore options, 93
    vegan options, 93, 103
purple coneflower, 53
purple foods, 45t, 128

qigong, 60
quercetin, 52, 66, 133, 136, 253, 282

raw foods, 12, 15, 86
red foods, 18, 45t, 128
red-light food guidelines, 92, 96–7
relaxation
    with breathing exercises, 63–4
    with hot ginger baths, 196
    for kidney energy, 60
    with salt scrubs, 79
    with salt-water flotation, 76
    with spa techniques and treatments, 66, 69
resveratrol, 45t, 57
Rona, Zoltan, 99

Recipe Index

Squeaky Clean Granola, 175
star anise
    Asian Onion Soup, 188
stinging nettle
    nutritional benefits, 53
    The Hot Detox Tea, 141
strawberries
    Berry Chia Jam, 153
    Detox Rocket, 136
    Heart Blush, 140
    Joint-Healing Gell-O, 172
    Vegan Lemon Gell-O, 174
sunflower lecithin powder. *See* lecithin
sunflower seeds
    to make milk from, 124–5
    Asian Salad Bowl, 234
    Beet Cashew Dip, 252
    Blueberry Seed Soak, 153
    Carrot Cake Bars, 154
    Detox Olive Crackers, 227
    Extreme Ginger Bake, 163
    Hemp Burgers, 276
    Hot Detox Bread, 168
    Instant Pesto, 257
    JFC Coleslaw (or Stir-Fry), 240
    Meals-That-Heal Seed Bar, 312
    Onion Lentil Dip, 253
    Savory Carrot Cashew Bake, 288
    Squeaky Clean Granola, 175
    Sunny Sunflower Pâté, 254
    Sweet Seed Milk, 126
Sunny Anti-inflammatory Dressing, 261
Sunny Sunflower Pâté, 254
Super Shepherd's Pie, 292
sweet potatoes
    nutritional benefits, 226, 229
    Comforting Chicken Soup, 198
    Detox Nut Butter Stew, 272
    Dijon Chicken or Lentil Soup, 200
    The Early Riser, 164
    Hemp Burgers, 276
    Messy Gingered Sweet Potatoes, 226
    Probiotic Cashew Cheese, 229
    Spiced Sweet Potato Mash, 229
    Super Shepherd's Pie, 292
    Sweet Potato and Asparagus Salad, 248
Sweet Seed Milk, 126
sweeteners, 95
Swiss chard. *See* chard (Swiss chard)

tahini (sesame paste)
    nutritional benefits, 261
    Broccoli Wasabi Dip, 253
    Extreme Ginger Bake, 163

Sunny Anti-inflammatory Dressing, 261
    See also sesame seeds
tangerines. *See* oranges, mandarins, and tangerines
tarragon, fresh
    Chicken with Sugar Snap Peas and Fresh Herbs, 266
    Delish Fish, 274–5
    Herbed Halibut, 278
Tea-Time Eggs, 212
thyme
    nutritional benefits, 268
    Comforting Chicken Soup, 198
    Detox Curry, 268
    Detox Olive Crackers, 227
    Sautéed Comfort, 286
Tiger Spice Smoothie, 144
Tomato Fennel Ragout, 274
Tomato-Free Ketchup, 258
Tomato Soup, Faux, 258
tomatoes, fresh
    Lazy Man's Cabbage Rolls, 280
    Tomato Fennel Ragout, 274
tomatoes, sun-dried
    The Early Riser, 164
    Zucchini Kasharole, 298
    Zucchini Stir-Fry, 298
triticale, 97
turkey
    nutritional benefits, 294
    Asian Salad Bowl, 234
    Lazy Man's Cabbage Rolls, 280
    Super Shepherd's Pie, 292
    Turkey Loaf, 294
turmeric
    health benefits, 56, 143, 194–5
    Detox Dressing, 259
    Detox Nut Butter Stew, 272
    Detox Olive Crackers, 227
    Gentle Healing Dal, 201
    Golden Chicken Bone Broth, 186
    The Green Goddess, 222
    Julie's Curry Powder, 269
    Oh-So-Hardcore Detox Drink, 143
    Paleo Pumpkin Bagels, 178
    Sautéed Comfort, 286
    Spiced Sweet Potato Mash, 229
    Sunny Anti-inflammatory Dressing, 261
    Turmeric Spice Latte, 145
turnips
    Dijon Chicken or Lentil Soup, 200

umeboshi paste
    The Green Goddess, 222

Vanilla Cinnamon Pecan Milk, 126
Vegan Broth, 187
Vegan Detox Macaroons, 308
Vegan Lemon Gell-O, 174
vegetable side dishes
    Baba's Sautéed Cabbage, 212
    Beet Kvass, 206
    Butternut Squash Puree or Soup, 193
    Cauliflower Crust Pizza, 211
    Coco Quinoa, 210
    Fasolakia Lemonata (Lemon Green Beans), 214
    Garlic Cauliflower Mash, 210
    Garlic Dandelion Greens, 216
    Garlic Roasted Asparagus, 218
    Garlic Steamed Artichokes, 220
    Ginger Kimchi, 206
    The Green Goddess, 222
    Messy Gingered Sweet Potatoes, 226
    Pretty Purple Sauerkraut, 208–9
    Probiotic Cashew Cheese, 229
    Roasted Garlic, 223
    Roasted Leeks with Olives and Garlic, 230
    Tomato Fennel Ragout, 274
vegetables
    to blanch and freeze, 87
    to cook, 91
    cruciferous, 44, 62
    green-light guidelines for, 92
    raw vs cooked, 12, 15, 86
    reintroduction of, 118
    vegetable juice, 104
    See also specific varieties
venison bones
    Rich Bone Broth, 184
Very Berry Vinaigrette, 261
vinegar, 95, 105

walnuts
    omega-3 fats in, 94
    rancidity of, 124
    Faux-tmeal Breakfast, 166
Warm ACV and Honey Drink, 145
wasabi powder
    health benefits, 253
    Broccoli Wasabi Dip, 253
water chestnuts
    pineapple core substituted for, 205, 284
    Salad Soup, 205

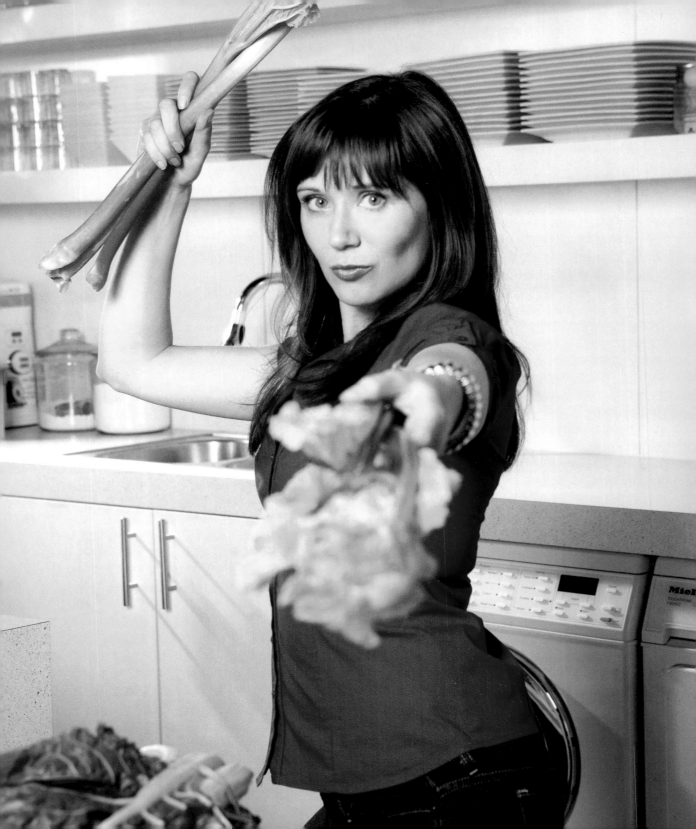